CREATIVITY AND ILLNESS: HOW SUFFERING AFFECTS LITERATURE, ART, AND MUSIC

LUND UNIVERSITY

LUND UNIVERSITY PRESS

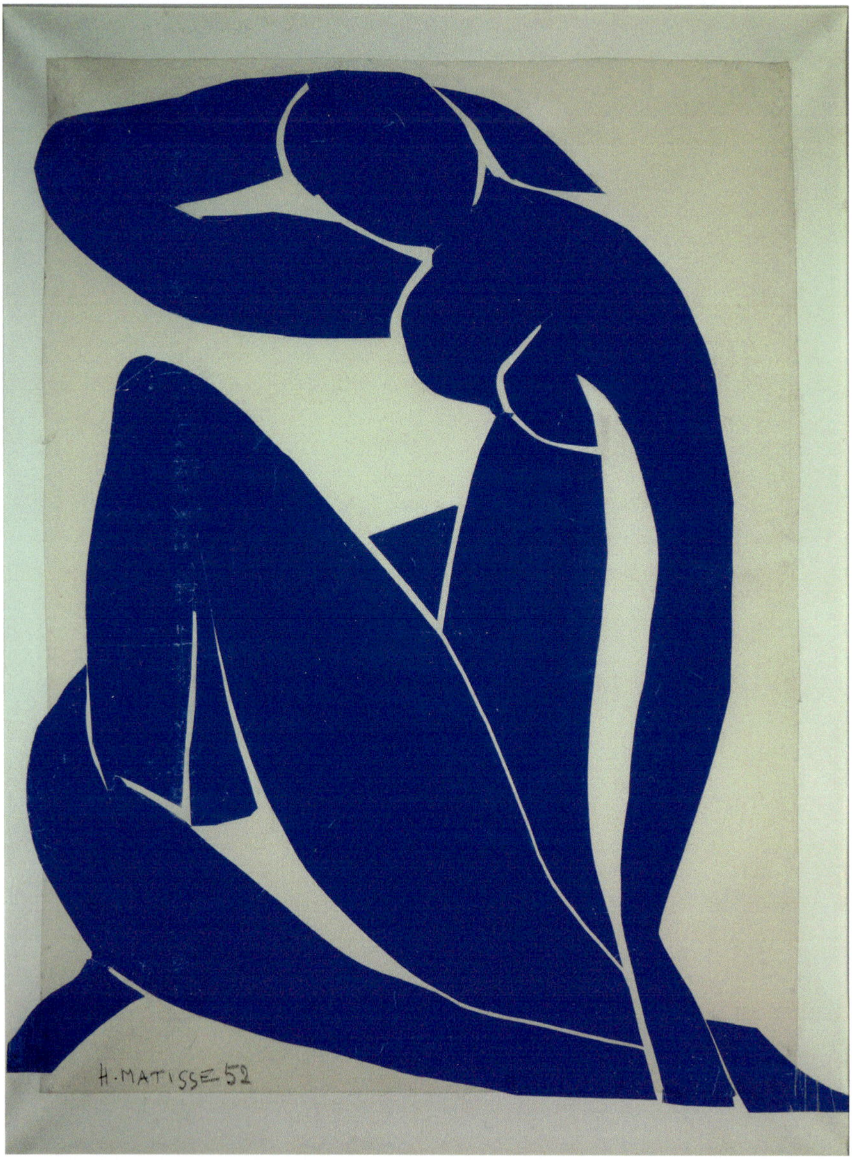
H. MATISSE 52

Creativity and illness

How suffering affects literature, art, and music

PHILIP SANDBLOM

Lund University Press

Lund University Press
The Joint Faculties of Humanities and Theology

LUND UNIVERSITY

LUND UNIVERSITY PRESS

P.O. Box 192
SE-221 00 LUND
Sweden
https://lunduniversitypress.lu.se

Lund University Press books are published in collaboration with Manchester University Press.

British Library Cataloguing-in-Publication Data
A catalogue record for this book is available from the British Library

ISBN 978 91 987405 2 3 hardback

First published 2025

The translation, copyright permissions, and production costs of this book were funded by the Einar Hansen Allhem Foundation. Lund University Press also gratefully acknowledges publication assistance from the Grace S. Sandblom Fund and the Thora Ohlsson Foundation.

EU authorised representative for GPSR:
Easy Access System Europe, Mustamäe tee 50, 10621 Tallinn, Estonia
gpsr.requests@easproject.com

MIX
Paper | Supporting responsible forestry
FSC® C013056
FSC
www.fsc.org

Typeset
by Cheshire Typesetting Ltd, Cuddington, Cheshire
Printed in Great Britain
by TJ Books, Padstow

To Grace
My well-beloved
since 1932 in the Nationalmuseum in Stockholm

… A countenance in which did meet
Sweet records, promises as sweet;
A Creature not too bright or good
For human nature's daily food;
For transient sorrows, simple wiles,
Praise, blame, love, kisses, tears, and smiles.

And now I see with eye serene
The very pulse of the machine;
A Being breathing thoughtful breath,
A Traveller between life and death;
The reason firm, the temperate will,
Endurance, foresight, strength, and skill;
A perfect Woman, nobly planned,
To warn, to comfort, and command;
And yet a Spirit still, and bright
With something of angelic light.

William Wordsworth, from 'She was a
Phantom of delight', 1804/1807

Contents

Illustrations

Publisher's note

This English-language edition of Philip Sandblom's celebrated work *Skapande och sjukdom: Hur lidande påverkar litteratur, konst och musik* is a professional translation of what the author himself regarded as the final version of his book. There had been editions in English before, most recently from Marion Boyars Publishers, and these editions – all called *Creativity and Disease* – relied on English texts supplied by Sandblom himself (see the Foreword below). However, although a fair proportion of Sandblom's English texts could be incorporated in the present version, they diverge from the final Swedish version in so many ways that an adaptation of one of them was not felt to do justice to the work.

For all his profound knowledge of the arts, Philip Sandblom was a medical man, not a Humanities scholar, and the ultimate Swedish version of his book is full of quotations for which no sources are supplied. It does contain some references, but they fall far short of what would normally be expected from a scholarly book; and where references are provided, they hardly ever offer information on publishers and pages, nor are all of them entirely accurate. For the present edition, a qualified researcher, Dr Lena Olsson, has spent two months tracking down sources to the extent that this was at all possible (where it was not, the quotation has, regrettably, been left without an adequate reference), as well as checking and correcting the quotations in the running text. In my capacity as publisher and editor/translator of the present volume, I would like to express my gratitude and admiration for Dr Olsson's sterling contribution.

Quotations from classic literary texts such as Shakespeare's plays and Keats's Odes have not been deemed to require references to particular editions.

A number of Sandblom's quotations derive from Swedish sources and have been directly translated for the present edition. Others come from sources in other languages than Swedish and English. Consistently reproducing original quotations in French and German was found to result in too comprehensive annotation, though some short quotations in these languages are provided. A number of quoted works originally in other languages than English exist in English translations, and where possible such translations have been consulted and reproduced.

Lund, October 2024
Marianne Thormählen
Publishing Director, Lund University Press, 2015–2024

Foreword

'My husband devoted much of his life to the writing of this book. The present edition was finished just before an accident suddenly ended his life.' Those were the words with which Grace Sandblom signed her husband's last Swedish version of *Skapande och sjukdom* (2002), previously published in English as *Creativity and Disease*. For 70 years of marriage she had accompanied her Philip along his life's path as a young doctor, as a professor, and in due course as Vice-Chancellor of Lund University. The author of this book, soon after his 97th birthday, had declared that the 2002 volume was 'the final version', cautiously adding, 'at least for the present'. His reservation was to prove justified. After Sandblom's death in 2001, two posthumous Swedish versions appeared. The most recent one was published in 2022 by the Faculty of Medicine at Lund University, an edition with an entirely new design which did Sandblom's brilliant narrative art the greatest possible justice in its interplay between his text and an increased and refined selection of illustrations.

It is this most recent edition – in all likelihood the 'final' one in Swedish – that is now published in a new English translation which is, like all Lund University Press books, the product of collaboration between Lund University Press and Manchester University Press. The publication of this book constitutes the completion of an extraordinary publishing history. *Creativity and Disease* was originally written in English and first published in 1982. As the years went by, it was revised and expanded up to its twelfth edition in 1999. The book, Sandblom's life's work, has continually been in demand in research and education, a classic in its treatment of the connection between artistic creativity and the experience of serious illness. Hence the label 'A Lund Classic'.

In Philip Sandblom (1903–2001), medicine and love of the arts came together in one person. Having begun at the Karolinska Institute in Stockholm, his scientific career led to a doctoral dissertation on wound healing in 1944, a work that came in for a good deal of attention. He had established the basis for his international reputation as a scientist as early as ten years before his doctorate, by means of a study of the function of the gall bladder; it was especially concerned with the pathological condition that Sandblom named *haemobilia*, subsequently an internationally accepted term for the presence of blood in bile. As a clinician, he first specialised in pediatric surgery. Following studies and practice in the United States, he evolved advanced operating techniques for, among other things, surgery on infants with congenital heart defects, so-called 'blue babies'. His demonstrations of experimental surgery were soon in demand all over Europe, and he came to be regarded as one of the pioneers in the field.

As an internationally established researcher and clinician, Philip Sandblom was appointed to the Chair of General Surgery at Lund University in 1950. The one-time specialist now became a generalist, with an abundant repertoire both as a research leader and as an instructor. As the head of a clinic, he occupied a role which afforded him limited scope for devoting time and effort to his research on the connection between suffering from illness and artistic creativity. But the fellowship of medicine and the Humanities, between scientific rigour and human compassion, remained the ethical foundation of his professional identity, an identity in which a focus on caring for the individual patient was a crucial factor. There are numerous witnesses to his patient, gentle approach during operations, where his aesthetic vision became a natural component in his technical skill. To Sandblom, surgery was literally an *ars medicinae*, an artistic medical craft and one of *les beaux arts*. His self-description remains memorable: 'I am one of those to whom surgery is one of the fine arts' – with his typical addition, 'maybe the finest'.

In the middle of his life, at the apex of his professional career as a surgeon, Sandblom was elected Vice-Chancellor of Lund University, his official honorary title being *Rector Magnificus*. His ten years of office became legendary. With his wide-ranging vision, his intellectual mobility, and his diplomatic skills, he represented the university in all its variety. Surrounded by the trust and admiration of his staff, he gained the affection as well as the confidence of the students. Nationally and internationally, he displayed unfailing commitment to the freedom of research and the autonomy of universities. The appointment of Sandblom as Sweden's delegate at the European Rectors' Conference (the CRE), formed in 1964, was a matter of course. At the same time, he developed his long-standing contacts with several leading universities in the United States, evolving new forms of collaboration.

In every situation, official and informal alike, Philip Sandblom evinced an elegance which commanded universal respect as well as an idiosyncratic combination of academic dignity and mischievous detachment. He would frequently temper the scientist's awe-inspiring objectivity with gently humorous scepticism. Sandblom's eloquence was widely admired, not least in his home city of Lund where it was regarded as a true expression of 'the spirit of the place'. His distinctive persona, a grand seigneur with a whiff of student-like irreverence, made the epithet *magnificus* seem peculiarly apt.

In 1968, the Philip Sandblom era at Lund University reached a pinnacle as he was made an Honorary Doctor at the Faculty of Arts and Humanities. After retiring as Vice-Chancellor, and with double doctorates in medicine and the arts, he left Lund in 1970 and established himself as one of the great dignitaries of international surgery, based in Lausanne. For more than two decades, into his eighties, he was summoned to various visiting professorships at universities all over the world, from Taipei in the east to San Diego in the west. His honorary doctorates became increasingly numerous, as did his memberships of the most prestigious societies of surgery worldwide.

Alongside his international career as a star surgeon, Sandblom developed his scientific interest in the effects of ill health on artistic creation in its various manifestations. Even as a medical student, with newly awakened fascination, he had begun to study and – cautiously – collect modern art. His marriage to the young American Grace Schaefer became life-defining in every sense of the word, not least in respect of their shared life in the arts. Having known each other for just under 24 hours, Philip proposed to Grace, on the Skeppsbron quay in Stockholm. A quarter of an hour later, at the adjacent Nationalmuseum, Grace accepted him. For the remainder of their lives they were united in art, as art lovers and collectors. Their personal tastes harmonising, they built the extraordinary collection of masterpieces they named 'Samling ['Collection'] S' as a joint effort – a collection in which, among many other rarities, French jewels shone, by Delacroix, Courbet, Cézanne, Braque, and Picasso. When the couple left Sweden, a large proportion of the most exquisite works in 'Samling S' was donated to Nationalmuseum and the Moderna museet in Stockholm as well as to Lund University.

In his dual role as a medical expert and a connoisseur of the arts, it was natural for Sandblom to draw attention to the ways in which pictorial artists have experienced ill health. After all, it was obvious that varying pathological conditions affected their zest for creation and their power to create, as well as their choice of themes and their aesthetics. During the last thirty years of his long life, Sandblom was increasingly absorbed in what was to be his lasting scholarly-scientific legacy, his *pièce de résistance* for posterity. Each successive revision of *Creativity and Disease* saw its field of vision expand. As time went by, literature and music came to capture his interest as much as the pictorial arts. The index at the back of the final edition of the book bears witness to its magnificent panorama of eminent artists, authors, and composers. The range of pathological conditions covered by the book is equally impressive. With his close scrutiny of the artistic dimensions of painting, writing, and musical composition as performed by about 150 geniuses afflicted by illness, Sandblom examines the ways in which the particular variant of ill health that each of them suffered from left traces in his or her work. Taken altogether, he looks at over a hundred diagnoses which are seen – applying the split vision of the scientist and the student of the arts – to influence the inspiration of the creator and the emergence of the individual work of art.

When the first edition of *Creativity and Disease* appeared in 1982, a new field of research had recently been launched at a small number of medical schools in the United States. It was called 'the Medical Humanities', an overarching designation for the application of Humanities-related perspectives to medical research and training. In the course of the ensuing decades up to the turn of the millennium, the field expanded swiftly, becoming established in Great Britain as well as at a number of American universities. Today, it exists all over the world. The respective orientation of the richly various interdisciplinary activities covered by the term differs from one university to the next. But all are united in the desire to maintain and justify medicine as an intrinsically 'human science', in the service of humanity and humaneness. The very basis of the Medical Humanities was splendidly articulated by the legendary Medical Ethics scholar Edmund Pellegrino: 'Medicine is the most humane of the sciences, the most empiric of arts, and the most scientific of humanities.'

As time went by, the aesthetic disciplines – literature, art, music – came to play an increasingly prominent role in the international development of the Medical Humanities. Sandblom soon perceived that he, with his book project which grew organically during successive decades, was moving in step with the times. He had a colleague and friend at Lund University, Professor of Physiology Håkan Westling, his junior by just over 25 years. The two men went to the United States on joint quests for inspiration, journeys which – in the spirit of Sandblom – stimulated Westling to undertake a number of projects aimed at bringing medicine closer to the Humanities. In addition, Westling became one of Sandblom's successors as Vice-Chancellor, as brilliant in office and as well-loved as his predecessor, a man who belonged to the Humanities as well as to medicine. After Sandblom's death, Westling became his unchallenged biographer.

Among Sandblom's immediate heirs in his self-imposed endeavour to promote the establishing of the Medical Humanities at Lund University, the art-and-literature historian Birgit Rausing was prominent from the outset. During their many encounters in Lund and Lausanne she became one of his closest associates in the field, brought together by the aesthetic and historical interests they shared. Thanks to her commitment, the Birgit Rausing Centre of Medical Humanities could be established in 2021, at the Faculty of Medicine in Lund. She was deservedly presented with the accolade of *doctor honoris causa*, both at the Faculty of Medicine and at the Faculty of Humanities.

This final version of *Creativity and Disease* – now renamed *Creativity and Illness* – was made possible by the Grace S. Sandblom Fund, created by Grace in memory of her husband and dedicated to the co-operation of the Humanities and medicine. In the name of the Fund, the Sandblom Day is arranged in Lund each year, in connection with Philip's birthday, 29 October. The translation, copyright permissions for the abundant illustrations, and production costs were funded by a munificent grant from the Allhem (Einar Hansen) Foundation, administered by Lund University Press.

All editions of Philip's book are dedicated to Grace. This one, published in memory of both husband and wife, is no exception.

Anders Palm
Professor Emeritus of Comparative Literature,
Lund University
M.D.h.c. (Lund)

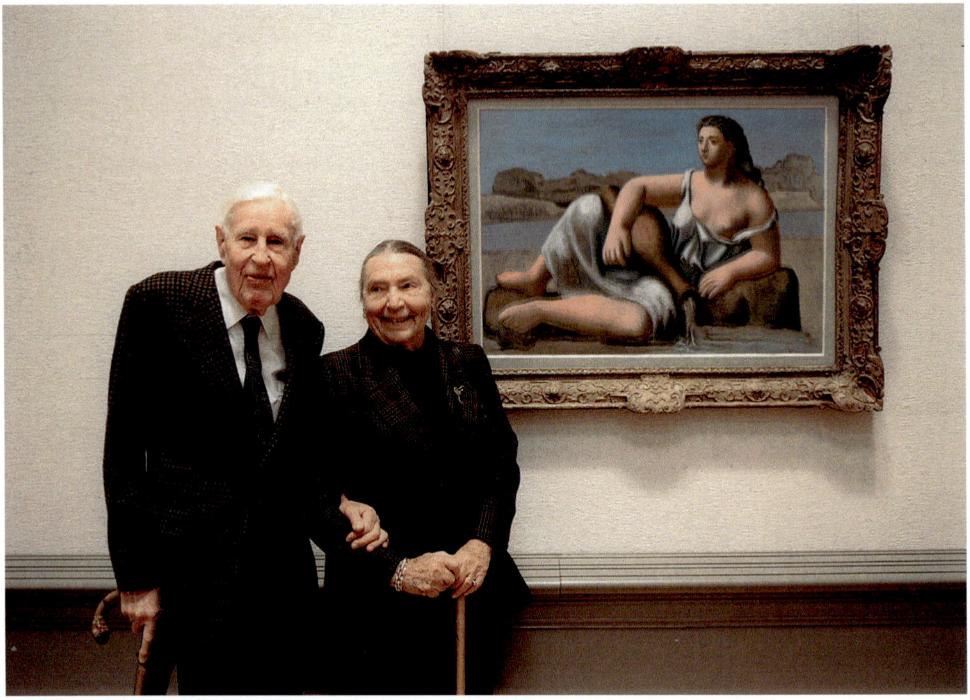

Grace and Philip Sandblom in front of Pablo Picasso's 'La source', one of the masterpieces in 'Samling S'.

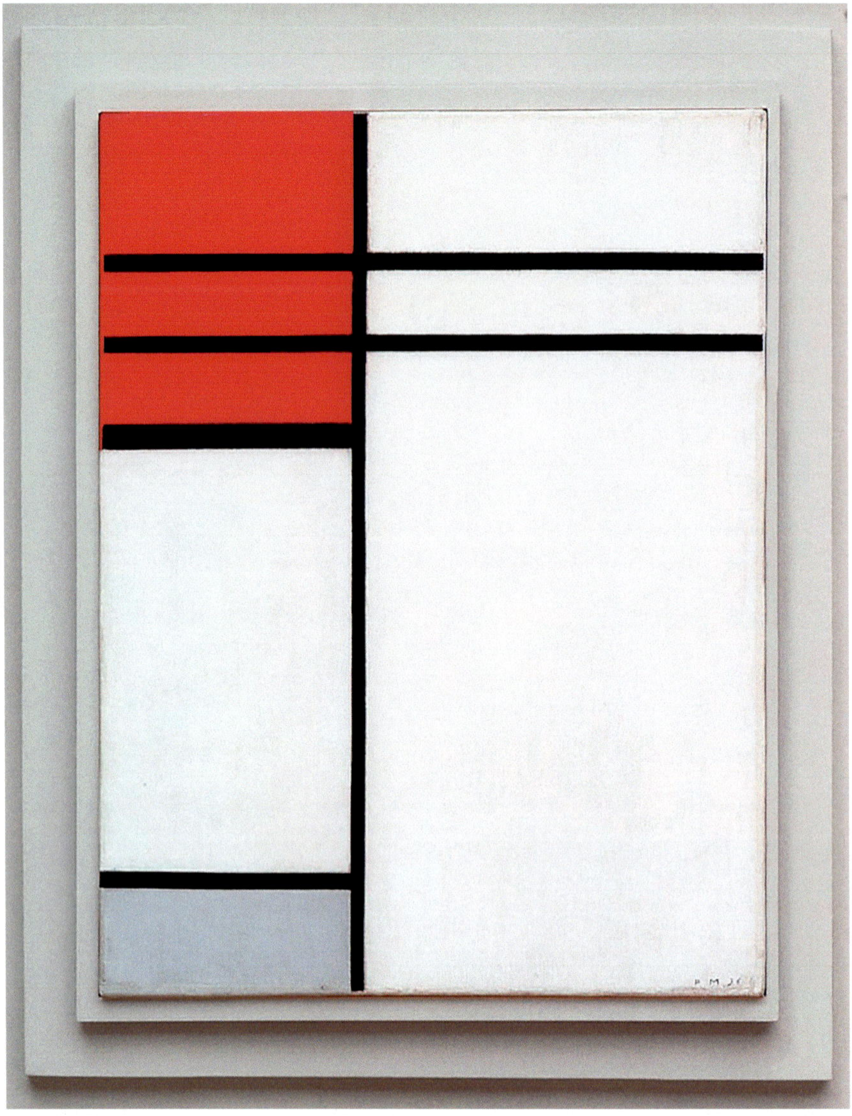

Figure 1 Piet Mondrian, 'Composition with red', 1936. Mondrian maintains that '[i]t is the line, the color and their relations which must "bring into play the whole sensual and intellectual register of the inner life"'; Piet Mondrian, *Plastic Art and Pure Plastic Art, 1937, and Other Essays, 1941–1943* (New York: Wittenborn, 1945), p. 59 (the source of Mondrian's quotation could not be identified). Michel Butor assures us that 'Mondrian is clearly aware of the tragic significance of a cross in his composition', asserting that 'the red spot represents the fatal twilight with the sun tragically setting'; Michel Butor, 'Le Carré et son habitant', originally in *Nouvelle Revue Française* 97 (1961); there is a reprint in Michel Butor, *Repertoire III* (Paris: Les Editions de Minuit, 1968), pp. 307–324 (pp. 319 and 320).

Introduction

Per varios usus artem experientia fecit.
Art is created out of experience in a variety of ways.

Manilius

'To most poets, poetry is merely a running commentary on their personal lives, a translation into verse of the prose of their own fates.'[1] Expressing this thought, the Swedish poet Esaias Tegnér might well have extended it to artists in general, for art is always based on experience – nobody can create out of nothing. Although self-evident, this still appears to be a point worth making, since it is so often repeated and pondered.

Anton Chekhov observed that he was not one of those 'literary men who take up a sceptical attitude towards science; and to the class of those who rush into everything with only their imagination to go upon, I should not like to belong'. As it was, he was able to draw on both medical training and his own tuberculosis.[2]

Henri Matisse explains how 'the artist works by observing and in due course assimilating external reality until that which he wishes to depict has finally become as it were a part of himself, so that he is able to reproduce it on the canvas as his own creation'.[3]

Gustav Mahler joins the same line of thought, arguing that creative art and the person's own experience are one and the same; '*only when I experience something* do I compose, and only when composing do I experience!' At the same time, he indicates a modification, intensely experienced in his sensual music flowing from hidden sources, '[a] residue of mystery always remains – even for the creator!'[4] Even so, he does make an attempt to

1 *Esaias Tegnérs brev, vol. II: 1818–1823*, letter to C. P. Hagberg of 6 December 1818. The volume was edited by Nils Palmborg (Malmö: Allhems, 1954), p. 77.

2 Letter to Grigory Ivanovich Rossolimo, 11 October 1899, in *Letters of Anton Chekhov to His Family and Friends*, trans. Constance Garnett (New York: Macmillan, 1920), p. 370.

3 'Propos recueillis par Régine Pernoud', *Le Courier de l'UNESCO* 1953, p. 6.

4 The first quotation comes from a letter from Gustav Mahler to Arthur Seidl of 17 February 1897, an English translation of which is found in *Selected Letters of Gustav Mahler*, ed. by Alma Mahler and Knud Martner, trans. Eithne Wilkins, Ernst Kaiser, and Bill Hopkins (New York: Farrar, Straus, Giroux, 1979). The second quotation comes from an undated letter from Mahler to Max Kalbeck; see p. 262 in the *Selected Letters*.

explain the mystery in words by describing it as the steady intensification of feeling, from the dark and hard elemental state (of the forces of nature) to the sweetest conceptions of the human heart, which in turn point towards and finally reach the divine – a subtle reminder that experience is merely the raw material out of which art is made; a diamond glitters only after it has been cut.

Scrutinising the thesis from a variety of perspectives in order to test its validity, one cannot but stop before abstract art and music with their specific, non-verbal language: can they be anything but the outcome of sheer speculation? A poetic connoisseur of art comes to our aid (see Michel Butor's comment on Mondrian, Figure 1 caption); but it is still a relief to find that Piet Mondrian himself, a leading representative of abstract art, was eager to offer his own contention, though it may not persuade everybody, explicitly stating that 'all that the non-figurative artist receives from the outside is not only useful but indispensable, because it arouses in him the desire to create that which he only vaguely feels and which he could *never represent in a true manner without the contact with visible reality and with the life which surrounds him*'.[5]

The connection between art and experience is easier to perceive in realistic painting and may be movingly evident, as in the case of Frida Kahlo, the Mexican Surrealist painter, married to Diego Rivera. She claimed that she painted her own reality, and a distressing subject it was, her reality being full of tears, blood, and pain.

Kahlo did not exaggerate when counting the causes of her suffering, claiming to hold a record in the number of operations – she underwent no fewer than 32 of them. Some were ill-advised; she is said to have insisted on them in order to secure the attention of her unfaithful husband when threatened by a new love in his life. A famous American surgeon, Leo Eloesser, who became her doctor and soon also her friend, discovered that she had a congenital malformation of the spine, a failed closure of its lower part.[6] The thus unprotected nerves degenerated, causing progressive ulcerations of the legs and feet.

As is often the case with disabled people, Kahlo preferred to blame her condition on an external cause. She had good reason to do so: not only had she had polio as a child, which left her with a permanent weakness in one leg; she had also been badly injured in a traffic accident aged 18. Her spine, her pelvis, and one foot were crushed, but not her forceful spirit. At first she was given up as a hopeless case, and then she endured years of inadequate medical care. Her severe physical injuries ultimately healed, but she never recovered her health. Declaring that she painted because she had to, she transmuted her pain into art with remarkable candour, tempered by humour and imagination.

---

5 Piet Mondrian, 'Plastic and Pure Plastic Art', in Piet Mondrian, *The New Art – The New Life: The Collected Writings of Piet Mondrian* (London: Thames and Hudson, 1987), p. 299 (italics in the original).

6 Harris Shumacker, *Leo Eloesser, M.D.: Eulogy for a Free Spirit* (New York: Philosophical Library, 1982). Unfortunately, it was not possible to locate the page.

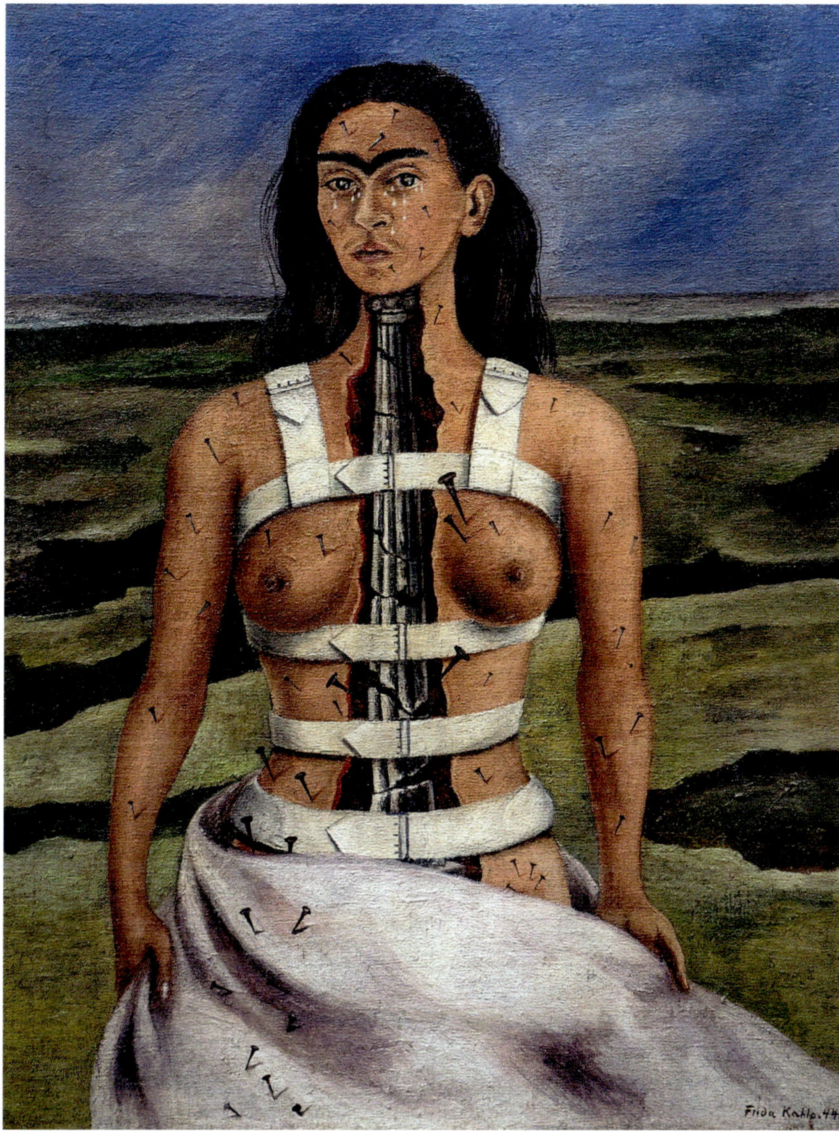

Figure 2 Frida Kahlo, 'The broken column', 1944. Self-portrait of the suffering artist, her spine shattered, encased in orthopaedic bandaging.

Kahlo expressed her suffering in a number of moving self-portraits which form a veritable 'Song of songs' of pain. In one of them (Figure 2), she is weeping with pain rendered visible as wounding nails. The crushed spine to which she attributes her condition is portrayed as a broken column. In this way, she misled both the people around her and her biographers, but her doctor was not deceived; Eloesser recorded in his reminiscences: 'I doubt whether the accident was responsible. Subsequent X-rays showed

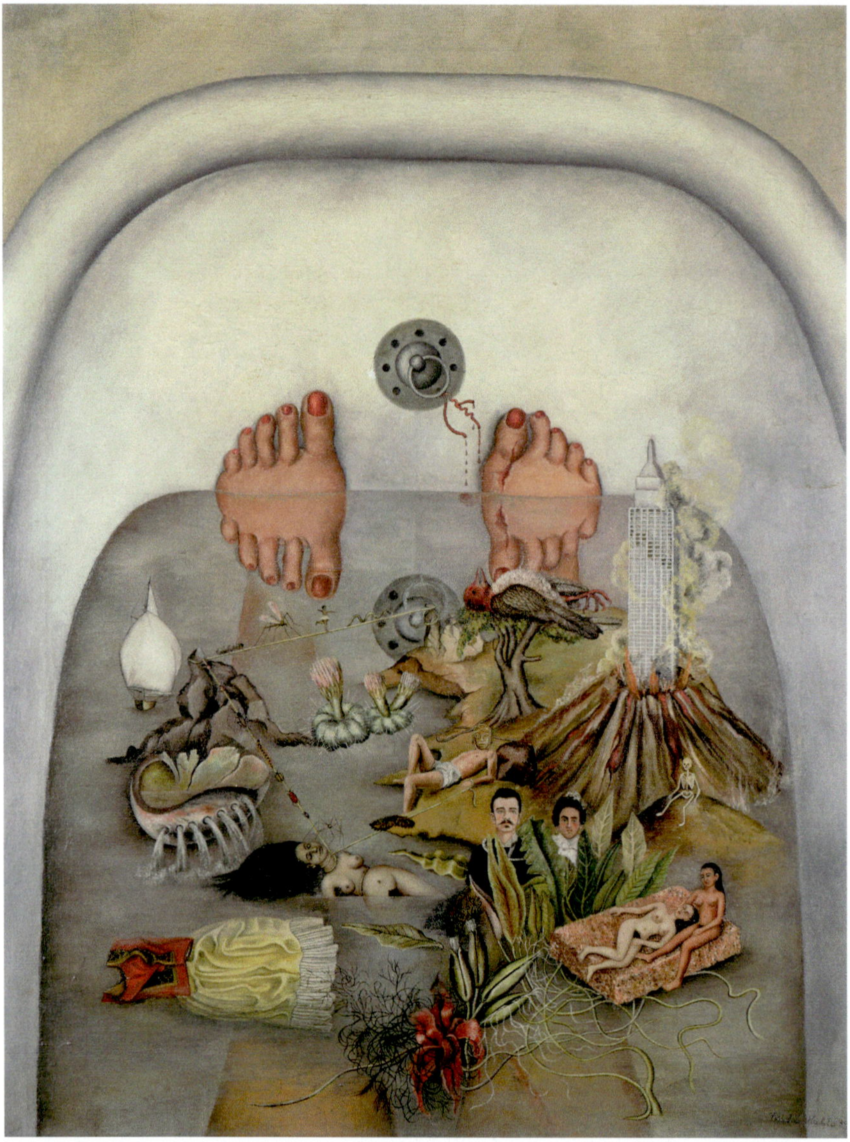

Figure 3 Frida Kahlo, 'What the water gave me', 1938. The artist represents herself in her bath. Between her toes are the sores that are typical lesions attending the congenital defect called *spina bifida*; she said that her foot was still sick. Even the broken stopper-chain bleeds in sympathy.

a *spina bifida*. The decreased sensitivity in the lower part of her body was characteristically compatible with this disorder.'[7] In words as well as in her images, Kahlo herself reveals the true state of things. She appears to have been informed, remarking 'I don't remember which doctor diagnosed it as

7 Ibid.

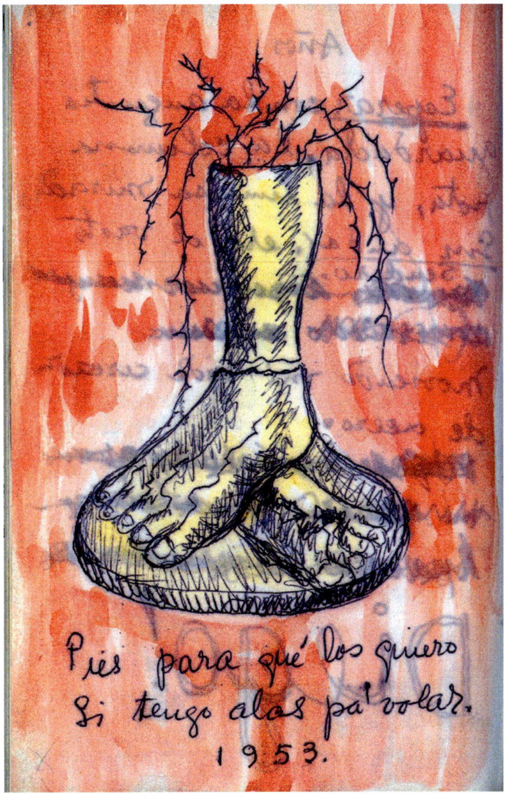

Figure 4 Frida Kahlo, 1953. This drawing in the artist's diary, with an emotional accompanying note, represents her diseased amputated leg.

a trophic ulcer. What is that[?]'[8] She was in fact well acquainted with their nature and reproduced them in another painting (Figure 3), which shows her in her bath with her feet visible above the water; the sores we see between her toes have the typical appearance of the lesions that accompany this congenital defect. Her condition gradually deteriorated, and a number of operations on her left leg and foot only made matters worse.

Kahlo could no longer count on being able to control her pain by means of the distraction afforded by painting, and she became increasingly dependent on strong painkillers. Under their influence, not only did her personality suffer but also her art, colours growing cloudy and brushwork uncertain. In the end, her left leg had to be amputated, a grievous blow, 'footless through the vast / Path', as she puts it along with a picture of the severed leg. Beneath the image, she wrote, 'Feet what do I need them for / If I have wings to fly'.[9] She was

8 Letter by Frida Kahlo to Dr Leo Eloesser, of 26 May 1932, in *The Letters of Frida Kahlo: Cartas Apasionadas*, ed. by Martha Zamora, trans. Jorge Gonzalez Casanova (San Francisco: Chronicle Books, 1995), pp. 44–45.

9 From Kahlo's diary: *The Diary of Frida Kahlo: A New Perspective*, trans. Louise Mereles Gras (n.p.: La Vaca Independiente, 2017), p. 217; pp. 163 and 164 in the diary.

referring to her ability to escape from the horrors of reality, metaphorically as well as physically. Kahlo met an inexplicable death, probably self-inflicted, registered as 'pneumonia'. She was said to have been comparatively well in the morning, but was found dead in the afternoon.

Frida Kahlo is a striking example of the fact that severe illness is an experience which may have a decisive influence on our lives as well as on our work. We can accustom ourselves to a great deal, but never to pain, always with us. The effects of pain on artistic creativity ought to be particularly apparent to physicians, given their special knowledge of the nature of illnesses. No two people look on the surrounding world with the same eyes, and our attention is drawn to those things with which we are especially closely acquainted. For example, I would think that only a medical colleague could wholly identify with poor Dr Bovary's horror (in Flaubert's novel), when he had been persuaded to try a new method of treating clubfoot by enclosing the reset foot in a home-made traction device and soon discovered that the foot had become dark blue and swollen – a terrifying foreboding of incipient gangrene. It made the good doctor himself sick, and he visited his patient day and night to see what was happening. We, his colleagues, recognise the physician's self-reproaches. Suppose the patient died, would it be his fault? The more scrupulous among us would be inclined to replace the question mark with an exclamation mark. Our perception of a work of art – and for that matter of everything that goes on around us – is hence dependent on our experience, to which the ill health we have suffered makes a significant contribution.

Chapter 1

The relationship between illness and creativity

In view of my medical background and my many years spent studying the arts in their various manifestations, it was natural for me to pay attention to the illnesses of creative artists. I would often observe that their artistic creations were affected by those illnesses. Hence, I do not share the view of one physician who reduces the significance of ill health to a matter of speculation, feeling that everyday incidents and trivialities are equally or more important.[1]

On the contrary, there are very good reasons for assuming a close relationship between illness and the arts. When a number of patients in a sanatorium were encouraged to paint pictures as a form of occupational therapy, it was observable that the course of their illness was reflected in their paintings with surprising clarity: 'The apprehension and despondency prior to haemoptysis or surgery, the sadness and apathy which follow such an event, the freshness and gaiety during convalescence – all are registered on the patient's pictures like entries in a diary.'[2]

Studying the relationship between suffering and professional activity in artists who had suffered serious illness may enhance our understanding of their works; we saw this in the case of Frida Kahlo, where knowledge of the diagnosis – frequently overlooked – helps us comprehend why the misery caused by the pain she suffered reached such a level of despair. She knew that the cause, which she wished to keep secret, was an incurable malformation of her spine accompanied by progressive lesions on her legs, and not, as she wished everyone else to believe, her traumatic physical injuries which were in fact curable. I cannot share the notion that the only thing of interest is the finished work, whereas the personal circumstances of its creator are irrelevant and uninteresting.

Few people have tried to follow, and even fewer have succeeded in following, Flaubert's exhortation to the effect that the author must, like God in the universe, be omnipresent but invisible, making posterity doubt that he

1 F. H. Franken, *Krankheit und Tod grosser Komponisten* (Baden-Baden: Witzstrock, 1979). (Reference supplied by the author; it was not possible to locate a page.)

2 Joyce H. Laing, 'Tuberculous Paintings', *Ciba Symposium* 12 (1964), 135–143 (p. 135).

ever existed. His declaration 'Madame Bovary, that is me' only increases our curiosity about his personality.[3]

***

There is a close connection between the arts with regard to form as well as content, and their development often takes place in parallel. That is understandable, since each of the arts forms an expression of cultural developments in a general sense. But the element of agreement is never complete. At times, pictorial art moves close to literature (occasionally even resembling the political pamphlet); at other times it can be seen to be associated to music with its abstract form. The latter resides at a deeper level in the life of the human soul, and has a fainter connection to external circumstances, than the other arts. Many people place music at the top of the hierarchy of the arts, owing to its power of expression and its ability to make our souls tremble with emotion.

While thoughts expressed in words or images speak directly to our reason, the path that music takes towards our inmost self is less obvious. For what reason does a certain combination of rhythm and tone engender and transmit a particular feeling, shared by most listeners? A vibrating string cannot account for the endless miracle that resides in music, in tones; 'there is no unilateral equivalent between the tonal event and a particular verbal meaning or emotion'.[4]

By descending from the height of bliss to which Beethoven raises us through his 'Hymn of Thanksgiving' (see p. 42) down to the depth of despair expressed by Shostakovich in 'Agony of Death' (see p. 185), we appreciate the full range of emotional expressions commanded by music.

These qualities enable the composer to describe symptoms of illness. An accelerated rhythm may excite us. Minor keys reflect a melancholy which may be intensified into a scream of anguish (Figure 6). In the *St Matthew Passion*, Bach employs violent cadences in order to make us feel the lashes of the scourge that tormented Jesus on Golgotha while reproducing the lament of the women in the background. The idea that the syncopated rhythm in the first movement of Mahler's Ninth Symphony reflects the irregular beats of a diseased heart seems somewhat far-fetched.[5] There is more and better support for the notion that the mischievous Haydn created a far from delicate musical expression for a natural body noise by means of a brief solo in the Largo of his Ninety-third Symphony. Having set the stage by a spell of soft music, he suddenly allows two bassoons to trumpet the sought-for bottom

3 The first time this alleged quotation appeared in print was in a dissertation by René Descharmes, entitled *Flaubert, sa vie, son caractère et ses idées avant 1857*, publishedin 1909; see p. 103 n 3. For doubts about the authenticity of this much-quoted phrase, see https://flaubert.univ-rouen.fr/%C5%93uvres/ressources-pour-la-lecture/madame-bovary/madame-bovary-cest-moi-formule-apocryphe.

4 George Steiner, *Language and Silence* (New York: Atheneum, 1967), p. 23.

5 Christopher H. Gibbs, in 'The Music: Symphony No. 9' in *Season 2018–2019: The Philadelphia Orchestra*, says, 'As early as 1912 (and taken up by Cooke and Bernstein

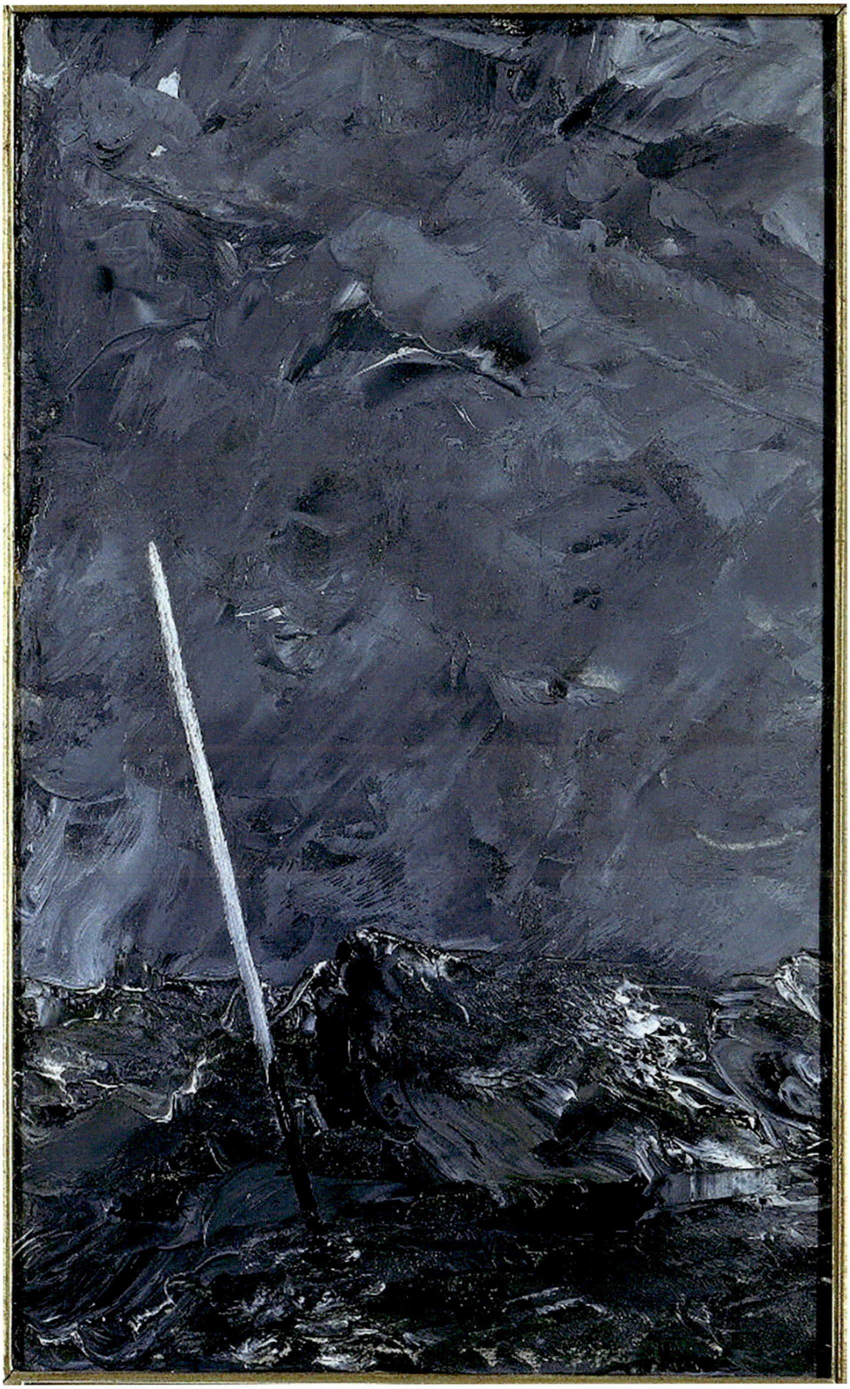

Figure 5 August Strindberg, 'Buoy without a top mark in stormy waters', 1892 (slightly cropped). The author turned to painting when he wished to express turbulent and unrestrained emotion.

C in fortissimo. Delighting in his joke, he then dances away from the smell to the tones of a minuet.

A surfeit of music may depress the spirits, and many people find the intrusive and supposedly entertaining music known as 'muzak' disturbing. A British Member of Parliament regarded it as injurious to health, calling for a ban on it in public spaces.

Carlyle called music 'the speech of angels'.[6] It possesses a special power to loosen inward tensions and thereby dispel 'the spirit of Saul';[7] or, as the eighteenth-century playwright William Congreve put it, 'Music hath charms to soothe a savage breast'.[8] But it may produce excitement as well, an effect which may be recorded in an accelerated pulse and elevated blood pressure. The consequences may be dramatic: von Karajan had to be transported home in an ambulance after conducting *Tristan and Isolde* for the first time.[9]

What about literature and pictorial art in this respect? Do they comprise works able to produce similar physical reactions? It is less than likely with regard to literature: there is no record of a reader's fainting in his or her chair out of sheer ecstasy over a beautiful passage; and if, in a comparable situation, an actor suddenly falls silent, the reason is more likely to be forgotten lines than a sense of being overwhelmed by the beauty of Shakespeare's verse. Even so, Strindberg found it necessary to warn actors not to become so transported by the text that they would lose their presence of mind.[10]

However, poetry occupies a special position owing to its kinship with music. Unlike prose, says Valéry, poetry captures and commands our entire being; through its rhythms, which cause every nerve in our body to vibrate, it has a direct physiologic resonance, eliciting a response in our minds that enhances our sense of being.[11] Otherwise, though, pictorial art may attain higher levels than literature. At the lowest level, that of pornography, simple souls derive greater pleasure from obscene pictures than from written

later), the rhythm was likened to the irregular beating of a diseased heart' (p. 38). (The author did not supply a reference.)

6 Thomas Carlyle, 'The Opera', in *The Keepsake*, ed. by Miss Power (London: David Bogue, 1852), p. 86.

7 The author did not supply a source for this quotation, but the reference appears to be to the evil spirit that inhabited Saul in 1 Sam. 16:14 and was later temporarily dispelled by David's harp music.

8 This is the opening line of Congreve's play *The Mourning Bride: A Tragedy* (1697).

9 Patrick l'Echevin, 'Musique et médecine' (Lille: diss., 1980); the dissertation was subsequently published (1981). A page reference could not be located.

10 From Strindberg's 'Memorandum till medlemmarna av Intima teatern från regissören' ('Memorandum to the members of The Intimate Theatre from the director'), from Strindberg's collected works (*August Strindbergs samlade verk*, Stockholm: Norstedts, 1999), Vol. 64; p. 27 in the Litteraturbanken Open Access file at https://libris.kb.se/bib/13456865.

11 Paul Valéry, *Propose sur la poésie* of 1930. The text is reprinted in Paul Valéry, *Oeuvres: Conférences* (Paris: N.R.F., 1939), pp. 21–22. The relevant passage can be read at https://search.worldcat.org/title/715550476.

descriptions of erotic episodes; and, at the highest, the *beaux arts* possess a power of expression rivalling that of music.

The resulting medical condition has been given a special term, the Stendhal syndrome. This is a kind of collapse which struck the French author on his Italian journey. He describes a day in Florence in the following terms: 'The sibyls of Volterrano gave me the most exquisite delight I ever derived from a painting ... I was dead tired with swollen feet, aching in narrow shoes; that might be a petty sensation, but it would still have prevented me from admiring God in all his glory – but in front of that picture I forgot everything else. O, heavens! How beautiful it is! I found myself in that emotional state where a passionate soul is overwhelmed by the celestial sentiments of art. When I left Santa Croce, I had violent palpitations, I was quite beside myself, and I feared falling to the ground.'[12]

This syndrome, which is caused by an onrush of adrenaline, may not be that uncommon. I pride myself on having experienced a similar attack, shaking legs included, on seeing Cézanne's 'Small bridge', a painting which deserves the same exclamation, 'O heavens! How beautiful it is!'

Just as physical and mental disorders may affect works of art, the opposite may occur: art having an impact on the state of the body. This effect has increasingly been employed for therapeutic purposes in order to promote healing (see pp. 25 and 75).

The similarities in expression between the arts frequently make it possible to increase the appreciation of a particular work of art by means of a comparison to corresponding work belonging to another art form. For example, Gotthold Lessing compared the ways in which Laocoon's lament on being bitten by the snakes has been expressed in the form of sculpture as well as in writing (see p. 154 and Figure 72). In a famous essay, the German philosopher draws a line of demarcation between written art forms and pictorial art. A product of its time, the essay seems pedantic to us: 'Time belongs to the author, space to the artist. To mingle different points in time, and, for example, depict on the same canvas the entire story of the Prodigal Son with his sinful life, his misery, and his return home, as Titian did, constitutes an encroachment by painting upon the domains of fiction and is incompatible with good taste.'[13]

Nobody has repudiated this thesis more firmly than Paul Klee, in words as well as in pictures: 'On closer inspection, this is merely a learned stupidity, for space is a temporal concept as well. For a point to become movement and line, time is required. Like writing, the image is a creative process – the picture is poetry! Only a dead point is timeless. The interest of the observer

---

12 A free translation derived from Stendhal's (Marie-Henri Beyle) *Rome, Naples et Florence*, Vol. 2, 3rd edn (Paris: Delaunay, 1826), pp. 101–102, and supplemented by *The Private Diaries of Stendhal*, ed. and trans. by Robert Gage (London: Victor Gollancz, 1955), pp. 443–444.

13 A free translation derived from Gotthold Ephraim Lessing, *Laokoon, oder Über die Grenzen der Malerei und Poesie*, 3rd edn (Stuttgart: Göschen, 1893), pp. 110–111 (the relevant passage occurs right at the beginning of Part XVIII).

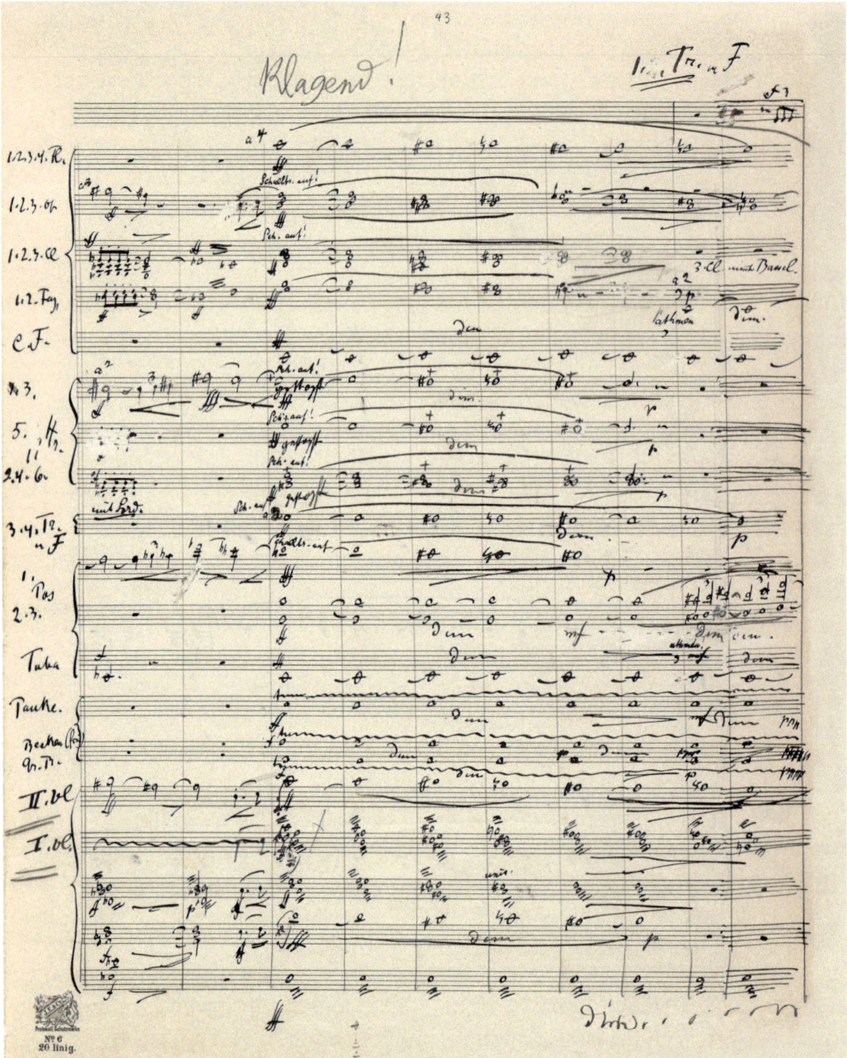

Figure 6 Gustav Mahler, Symphony No. 5, first movement. The composer is complaining!

is time-related as well. Like a grazing animal, his gaze wanders across the work of art' (see pp. 203–206).[14]

During many years of excursions across the varying domains of art, I have collected examples of authors, artists, and composers in whose works

---

14 A free translation from Paul Klee, 'Schöpferische Konfession', in *Tribüne der Kunst und Zeit: Eine Schriftensammlung, XIII: Schöpferische Konfession*, ed. by Kasimir Edschmid (Berlin: Erich Reiss Verlag, 1920), pp. 33–34. The text may be read online at https://de.wikisource.org/wiki/Sch%C3%B6pferische_Konfession:_Paul_Klee. (It should be observed that the exclamation 'the picture is poetry!' is not found in this text locus.)

I discerned evident connections between illness and creation, comparing the effects produced by each disorder on the different forms of art. Since people today do not devote much time to reading, I have aimed for brevity. Nevertheless, I have given special attention to those instances where the creators themselves have attempted to explain the connections; they may not have grasped the situation in its entirety, but they are still entitled to a hearing.

***

With no other guidance than the shallow traces left by a human being after departing this life, it may be hard to determine the particular illness from which a historical personage suffered. To an experienced clinician, however, the history of a person's illness supplies solid points of reference; and, in the cases mentioned here, the relevant diagnosis may be said to be reasonably certain. There are a few exceptions, though; it is, for instance, unlikely that Chopin's slowly progressing lung disease was tuberculosis. Another, and striking, exception is Van Gogh. Over a hundred diagnoses have been proposed as the reason for his mental disturbance, from syphilis to Ménière's disease (pp. 97–98).

I have made no attempt to compile a complete catalogue of human suffering in the arts (an impossible task) but limited myself to a collage of fragments, put together from many different sources – a subjective rhapsody in black, interspersed by bright glimpses supplied by fortitude and joy in creation found in some great writers and artists. Consequently, I make no claim to providing statistically persuasive evidence. As an illustrious physicist once told me, that would have called for two control groups for comparison: one comprising sick artists who had created seemingly healthy works, and the other healthy artists who had produced works that appear to originate in ill health. In the absence of such groupings, I am quite satisfied with the evidence of the Humanities scholar: conviction based on personal experience. The 'two cultures' are still happily distinct.

This study does not aspire to present any scholarly-scientific theory regarding the connection between creativity and illness; but I hope it may contribute to a greater understanding of the creative process by means of demonstrating, and discussing, the ways in which many great authors, artists, and composers have been influenced by ill health in the creation of their works.

I believe such a study may be of value even to those who share George Bernard Shaw's contention that ill health is of no interest, and that there should be a general agreement to pass by the topic in silence.[15] John Updike agrees, arguing that there are aspects of life that do not interest readers – to be sure, illness and pain are of overwhelming interest to those who suffer from them; but an account bores the reader even after the first

15 'Crime, like disease, is not interesting: it is something to be done away with by general consent, and that is all about it'; preface to *St Joan* in Shaw's *Bernard Shaw's Saint Joan, Major Barbara, Androcles and the Lion* (New York: Modern Library, 1956), p. 51.

couple of lines.[16] He comes close to proving his point with a lengthy account of his skin disorder, psoriasis, but maintains the reader's amused interest by describing how this alien presence co-occupies his body, singling him out from the 'happy herds of normal mankind'.[17] It is actually possible that his illness preserved a major writer for us, as Updike regarded himself as unsuitable for tasks calling for personal presence, remaining a 'worker in ink' who could hide himself and send out a 'surrogate presence'.[18] It is intriguing to see how both authors changed their minds when they themselves fell ill. Shaw developed a great and aggressive interest in his osteomyelitis (p. 175), and Updike wrote a delighted account of his operation for appendicitis;[19] with advancing age, as he approached his own final rest, his thoughts – like those of his alter ego – dwelt increasingly on mortal illness.

A cynical view of human suffering was represented by Nietzsche, who observed that a malicious interest in the misfortunes of others is a prominent feature of human nature.[20] A more benevolent interpretation is found in the words of Goethe, who argued that our own pains teach us to share the misery of our fellow human beings: it is through pain and suffering that we find common ground with them. It may be hard to realise that there are grounds for shared happiness, but pain is something we readily comprehend, though we may not understand it completely.[21]

***

The meaning of human suffering has hardly ever been analysed with greater profundity than in the Book of Job. '[For there is] none like him in the earth, a perfect and an upright man, one that feareth God, and escheweth evil' (1:8). Nevertheless, the Lord robbed Job of both family and property and afflicted him with 'sore boils from the sole of his foot unto his crown' (2:7). In his own words, '[m]y bones are pierced in me in the night season: and my sinews take no rest ... My skin is black upon me' (30:17, 30).

Cursing the day of his birth, Job in his despair asks the ancient, indeed eternal, question: Why must human beings suffer so much? 'Wherefore is light given to him that is in misery, and life unto the bitter in soul; Which

16 John Updike, 'The Future of the Novel', in *Picked-Up Pieces* (New York: Random House, 2012; first published in 1975), pp. 16–22 (p. 18).
17 John Updike, 'At war with my skin', *The New Yorker* 61.28 (2 Sept. 1985), republished in *Self-consciousness: Memoirs* (New York. Random House, 1989), p. 42.
18 John Updike, *Self-consciousness*, p. 48.
19 John Updike, 'The City', first published in *The New Yorker* in 1982; also published in John Updike, *Trust Me* (New York: Random House, 2014), pp. 33–53.
20 Friedrich Nietzsche, *Die fröhliche Wissenschaft* (Chemnitz: Ernst Schmeitzner, 1882), p. 23.
21 From a poem dated 'Weimar, den 17. März 1785' in Johann Wolfgang von Goethe, *Goethes Werke*, Vol. 4 (Weimar: Hermann Böhlau, 1891), p. 120: 'Unglück bildet den Menschen und zwingt ihn sich selber zu kennen, / Leiden gibt dem Gemüt doppeltes Streben und Kraft. / Uns lehrt eigener Schmerz der andern Schmerzen zu teilen.'

long for death, but it cometh not?' (3:20–21). His friends, as friends will, assume that it was all a punishment from God and that Job must have sinned. But Job, who knew himself blameless, revolted against the injustice of it all and was incensed that his question remained unanswered: 'Oh that one would hear me! behold, my desire is, that the Almighty would answer me' (31:35).

In the original, stern, and persuasive version of the tale, Job remains a great blasphemer who refuses to accept his fate. But a later version adds a meek supplement to the Book of Job. It maintains that suffering is not necessarily a punishment, but more of a cleansing process and an exhortation to humility as a prerequisite for the exaltation of the soul: 'He delivereth the poor in his affliction, and openeth their ears in oppression' (36:15). Job now bends to the will of the Almighty: 'I have heard of thee by the hearing of mine ear: but now mine eye seeth thee. Wherefore I abhor myself, and repent in dust and ashes' (42:5–6).

In this equally happy and improbable ending, Job is rewarded for his submission. He is not merely cured of his afflictions; he has his property restored to him and is even provided with a new family: 'And in all the land were no women found so fair as the daughters of Job' (42:15)! As one of the first in a long tradition, Job also experienced the effects of suffering on our modes of expressing ourselves: 'My harp also is turned to mourning, and my organ into the voice of them that weep' (30:31).

***

Through the ages, many wise men have urged those affected to evince humility when afflicted by ill health and unsettled by the thought of the uncertain plight of human beings in a world full of hazards. We come across many of them during the Renaissance. One such man is Robert Burton, who wrote the following reflections in *The Anatomy of Melancholy*: 'Sickness, diseases trouble many, but without a cause. It may be 'tis for the good of their souls ... the flesh rebels against the spirit; that which hurts the one must needs help the other. Sickness is the mother of modesty, putteth us in mind of our mortality; and, when we are in the full career of worldly pomp and jollity, she pulleth us by the ear, and maketh us know ourselves ... Princes, Masters, Parents, Magistrates, Judges, friends, enemies, fair or foul means, cannot contain us, but a little sickness (as Chrysostom observes) will correct and amend us.'[22]

A similarly humble attitude to suffering was displayed by the genius Blaise Pascal, who unreservedly accepted health and disease, good and evil, as gifts from God. He himself suffered a surfeit of ill health, his life and his work constituting a continuous victory of the spirit over the ailments of the body. From his eighteenth year onwards, he did not know a day without

22 Democritus Junior [Robert Burton], *Anatomy of Melancholy* (London: Thomas Tegg, 1845), p. 380. (The work first appeared in 1621.)

abdominal pain and headaches; it has been presumed that he suffered from intestinal tuberculosis as well as migraines.[23]

The great scientist, a ground-breaking mathematician and physicist, was also a deeply religious man, guided by his realisation that human reason on its own is not enough to resolve the fundamental existential issues. Pascal discussed his faith and his doubts in his famous *Pensées*, demonstrating how strong faith may help human beings not merely to endure suffering with dignity and equanimity but also to accept it with gratitude and confidence: 'Yet I live with joy, whether in the prosperity which it pleases Him to bestow on me, or in the adversity which He sends for my good, and which He has taught me to bear by His example.' His gratitude does not exclude a natural pessimism; 'it is well to accustom one's self to gain advantage from evil, since that is so common, while goodness is so rare'.[24]

In words reminiscent of Job's, Pascal's 'Prayer for the Right Use of Sickness' states his position: 'Thou alone knowest what is needful for me; thou art my Sovereign Master; do with me as seems good in thy sight. Either give or take away; but at all events, conform my will to thine, so that, in humble and unreserved submission, and in holy confidence, I may prepare myself to receive the allotments of thy eternal Providence, and receive with equal gratitude whatever comes from thee. ... I know not which will be most for my advantage, health or sickness, riches or poverty, nor any other worldly object.'[25]

Pascal's contention that illnesses are meaningless if we cannot believe that they were sent to us by a heavenly Father presaged the Enlightenment, when humanity began to 'venture to know' in earnest as increasing numbers ceased to believe in, or even hope for, a hidden meaning. The idea of an endless universe, so frighteningly different from religion's harmonious picture of the world, had filled Pascal with horror. Suffering was now divested of its ties to religion, as diseases and death became natural processes and rational medical intervention became the best means of, as

23 Lucien Jerphagnon, *Le charactère de Pascal* (Paris: Presses Universitaires de France, 1962), p. 51; the text may be read at https://gallica.bnf.fr.ark:/12148/bpt6k3404181k/f17.image.r=Lucien%20Jerphagnon?rk=236052;4.

24 The first quotation is from *Pascal's Pensées*, translated by W. F. Trotter with an introduction by T. S. Eliot (New York: E. P. Dutton, 1958), p. 223. (The original French text, from Chapter XIV section XIX, runs, 'je vis cependant avec joie, soit dans les biens qu'il lui plaît de me donner, soit dans les maux qu'il m'envoie pour mon bien, et qu'il m'a appris à souffrir à son exemple'.) The second quotation comes from Blaise Pascal, *Thoughts on Religion and Philosophy*, trans. Isaac Taylor (London: Simpkin, Marshall, Hamilton, Adams & Co., 1894), p. 175; the French original text reads, 'il est bon de s'accoûtumer à profiter du mal, puis qu'il est si ordinaire, au lieu que le bien est si rare'.

25 Pascal, *Thoughts on Religion and Philosophy*, p. 222. The French original calls this prayer 'Prière pour demander à Dieu le bon usage des maladies' (*Oeuvres complètes de Blaise Pascal*, Book II (Paris: Hachette, [1871]), pp. 33–34.

Descartes put it, improving health, extending life, and banning the scourges of old age.[26]

* * *

Ever since Antiquity, artistic creation has been thought to be related to physical infirmities. Superhuman exploits have been regarded as indissolubly connected with suffering.[27] In Greek mythology we find the peerless archer Philoctetes, whose snakebite suppurated with a stench so horrible that his companions left him behind on a desert island. According to Sophocles, Philoctetes says, 'I would have remained thoughtless and carefree as an animal if it had not been for my wounds – when pain takes hold of me, I know that I am human.'[28] In André Gide's version of the story, Philoctetes adds that he has learnt to express himself better since he stopped associating with other people: 'I took to telling the story of my sufferings, and if the phrase were very beautiful, I was by so much consoled; I even sometimes forgot my sadness by uttering it.'[29]

'A poet', says Sören Kierkegaard, 'is an unhappy creature whose heart is torn by secret sufferings, but whose lips are so strangely formed that when his sighs and cries escape them, they sound like sweet music.'[30]

The idea that the artist derives his or her power from a physical ailment – that it is the damaged mussel that yields the pearl – is widely accepted. According to Marcel Proust, 'unhappiness develops the forces of the mind (whereas 'happiness alone is salutary to the body'). An amusing consequence is the notion that Mendelssohn did not develop to his full extent as a composer because there was no great hardship in his life which he might have drawn on.[31]

---

26 See René Descartes, *A Discourse on the Method of Correctly Conducting One's Reason and Seeking Truth in the Sciences*, trans. Ian Maclean (Oxford: Oxford University Press, 2006), pp. 51–51 (a World's Classics edition). The original French title runs, 'Discours de la methode pour bien conduire sa raison et chercher la vérité dans les sciences', first published in 1637.

27 See Staffan Björck, 'Sångaren och plågan: Ett litteraturpsykologiskt motiv och ett dikt-komplex hos Birger Sjöberg', in Birger Sjöberg-sällskapet, *Essäer och samtal* (Vänersborg: Sällsk., 1966), p. 34. (This is a yearbook of the Birger Sjöberg Society; all their yearbooks are listed at https://birgersjoberg.se.)

28 The author supplied the following reference, but the quotation could not be found in it: Edmund Wilson, *The Wound and the Bow: Seven Studies in Literature* (Cambridge, MA: Houghton Mifflin, 1941).

29 Quoted by Wilson, *The Wound and the Bow*, p. 236; for the French original, see André Gide, *Philoctete* (Paris: Edition du Mercure de France, 1899), p. 33.

30 *Enten – eller* (Copenhagen, 1843), p. 3.

31 Marcel Proust, *Time Regained*, trans. Andreas Mayor and Terence Kilmartin, revised by D. J. Enright (New York: Random House, 1993), p. 314 (Modern Library edition). The original reads, 'Le bonheur est salutaire pour le corps, mais c'est le chagrin qui développe les forces de l'esprit'; Marcel Proust, *A la recherche du temps perdu*, Vol. 15: *Le Temps retrouvé*, deuxième partie (Paris: Gallimard, 1927), p. 56.

The English Romantics had different ideas. Both Wordsworth and Coleridge maintained that well-being and good health are prerequisites for the writing of poetry. Here we observe a national distinction, in that the German Romantic school found suffering interesting as well as essential to creation, a thesis which remained a leitmotif for a long time.[32] The notion was already present in Goethe, in *Wilhelm Meisters Lehrjahre* (*Wilhelm Meister's Apprenticeship*): 'About the beginning of my eighth year, I was seized with a blood-cough; and from that moment my soul became all feeling, all memory.'[33] Friedrich Schlegel described how he felt during a life-threatening illness: 'I felt that its mysterious life was fuller and deeper than the common health of the people about me, who struck me rather like dreaming sleep-walkers.'[34]

Novalis, poet of the realm of the dead, who died of tuberculosis at the age of 28, experienced a mystical dimension to his illness, wondering whether disease might be a means of a 'more exalted synthesis' and speculating that the best things originate in illness.[35] (Compare Rilke, pp. 196–197.) Like Pascal before him, Novalis attempted to draw benefit from pathological states: 'Illnesses are certainly a most important aspect of human life, since they are so numerous and every human being has to struggle so much with them. As yet we are most imperfect when it comes to the art of benefiting from them.'[36] His remarkable observation, bordering on masochism, 'the more severe the pain, the more we glory in it',[37] recalls Nietzsche's experience: 'I have never felt happier with myself than in the sickest periods of my life, periods of the greatest pain.'[38] He welcomed suffering as a spur to creating. Most of us, however, would probably prefer to look back on suffering, like Goethe: 'The memory of surmounted pain is pleasure',[39] or feel happy, like Montaigne, at 'that sudden revolution when I pass from the

32 See Hermann Weigand, *The Magic Mountain: A Study of Thomas Mann's Novel* (Chapel Hill: University of North Carolina Press, 1964), p. 39.

33 The origin of the quotation is the beginning of the 6th book of Goethe's *Wilhelm Meisters Lehrjahre*, Zweiter Theil (Stuttgart: Cotta, 1876), p. 78, 'Bekenntnisse einer schönen Seele'; but the author probably found it in Weigand, *The Magic Mountain*, p. 40.

34 Quoted from Weigand, *The Magic Mountain*, p. 41; the origin of the quotation is Schlegel's *Lucinde* (Coburg: Georg Sendelbach, 1868), p. 123.

35 Johannes Hegener, *Die Poetisierung der Wissenschaften bei Novalis* (Bonn: Bouvier Verlag Herbert Grundmann, 1975), p. 476. (The original reference is to Novalis's *Die Enzyklopädie*, VI. Abteilung: Die philologischen Wissenschaften, 2. Poetik (2).)

36 Weigand, *The Magic Mountain*, p. 40.

37 Ibid.

38 'Nie habe ich so viel Glück an mir gehabt, als in den kränksten und schmerzhaftesten Zeiten meines Lebens'; Friedrich Nietzsche, *Ecce Homo* (Frankfurt am Main: Outlook Verlag, 2018), p. 44.

39 'Die Erinnerung überstandener Schmerzen, ist Vergnügen'; from a letter of Goethe's to Ernst Wolfgang Behrisch, of 10. November [1797], in *Goethe-Briefe, Band I: Der junge Goethe 1764–1775*, ed. by Philipp Stein (Berlin: Otto Eisner, 1902), p. 90.

extreme pain of voiding my stone and recover, in a flash, the beauteous light of health'.[40]

These lines of thought culminate in Schopenhauer's *Parerga and Paralipomena*, such a fascinating work in its clear-eyed pessimism. True to his nature, Schopenhauer perceives a positive value in pain owing to the intensity of its modes of expression. Conversely, he attributes a negative value to well-being as being dull and tedious. (I have found that my patients have difficulty appreciating this argument.) Schopenhauer remarks that we usually feel pain much more strongly than we feared we would, whereas pleasure rarely lives up to our expectations. He recommends everyone who believes that joy is a more powerful sensation than pain to compare the feelings of a predator tearing its prey apart with the feelings of its victim, concluding with a statement to the effect that human beings require pain and suffering in order to maintain a steady course, just as a ship needs ballast.

Edvard Munch used a similar metaphor, saying that he would have been like a rudderless ship without illness and anxiety.[41] Angst governs a large portion of his artistic output, sometimes taking over completely, as in his famous 'Scream' (Figure 33).

Pain and suffering have been rendered in music as well. When still a young man, Gustav Mahler declared that pain was his sole consolation, and we hear a great deal of lamentation in his music. In the end, though, he arrived at the conclusion that the ultimate aim of art consists in liberation from pain and a lofty independence.[42]

Let us end this discussion on a lyrical note and listen to the relevant line of thought as expressed by two women poets: first, the youngest and gentlest of the Brontë sisters, submissive Anne (Figure 81), when, dying from tuberculosis, she finds strength in her faith:

> That secret labour to sustain
> With humble patience every blow,
> To gather fortitude from pain
> And hope and holiness from woe.[43]

Brontë's words are repeated in Emily Dickinson's pure and personal, slightly tremulous voice when she was threatened with blindness (see p. 144):

40 Quoted from the Penguin edition of Michel de Montaigne, *The Complete Essays*, trans. and ed. by M. A. Screech (London: Penguin, 1991), p. 1241; the French original, from Book III, Ch. xiii of Montaigne's essays, runs 'cette soudaine mutation, quand d'une douleur extreme je viens, par le vuidange de ma pierre, à recouvrer, comme d'un esclair la belle lumiere de la santé' (quoted from the 1969 Garnier-Flammarion (Paris) edition of Montaigne's *Essais*, p. 304).

41 Ragna Stang, *Mennesket og kunstneren Edvard Munch* (Copenhagen: Politikens Forlag, 1978), p. 24.

42 It was not possible to locate this reference.

43 'A dreadful darkness closes in', written in January 1849; Edward Chitham (ed.), *The Poems of Anne Brontë: A New Text and Commentary* (Basingstoke: Macmillan, 1987 [1979]), p. 164.

Must be a Woe –
A loss or so –
To bend the eye
Best Beauty's way –
Delight – becomes pictorial –
When viewed through Pain –
More fair – because impossible
That any gain –
My loss, by sickness – Was it Loss?
Or that Ethereal Gain
One earns by measuring the Grave –
Then – measuring the Sun –[44]

The knowledge I have acquired about the lives of creative artists has led me to conclude that few of them were people in perfect health. I am hence inclined to agree with Ernst Kretschmer when he claims that healthy, harmonious persons are apt to lack the spur that impels the demoniac, discontented ones to the heights of genius.[45]

One of 'the demoniac ones' was Lord Byron, who derived some consolation for his disability from the idea that '[a]n addiction to poetry is very generally the result of "an uneasy mind in an uneasy body"[;] disease or deformity have been the attendants of many of our best – Collins mad – Chatterton *I* think – mad – Cowper mad – Pope crooked – Milton blind –.'[46]

Thomas Mann argued that there is a close relationship between illness and artistic creation. In his early novel *Royal Highness*, he let a poet declare: 'My health is poor. I do not wish to say "unfortunately", for I am convinced that my talent is inseparably united with my ill health.'[47] Mann's own big problem was a sexual ambivalence which he reveals in *Death in Venice*; he goes on to explain and excuse himself in the highly informative novel *The Magic Mountain.* Although otherwise healthy, albeit hypochondriac, he finds, oddly enough, that 'disease is a means of acquiring knowledge'.[48] The leitmotifs in two of his greatest works, *The*

44 According to *The Complete Poems of Emily Dickinson*, ed. by Thomas H. Johnson (Boston: Little, Brown & Co., 1960 and subsequent editions), this quotation would seem to be a combination of lines from three of Dickinson's poems: the first stanzas of 'Must be a Woe –' and 'Delight – becomes pictorial –', and the sixth stanza of 'My first well Day – since many ill –'.

45 Ernst Kretschmer, *Geniale Menschen*, 2nd edn (Berlin: Springer, 1931), p. 14.

46 Letter to Leigh Hunt of 4–6 November 1815?, in *'Wedlock's the Devil': Byron's Letters and Journals*, ed. by Leslie A. Marchand, Vol. 4: 1814–1815 (Cambridge, MA: Belknap, 1975), p. 332.

47 'Meine Gesundheit ist zart, – ich darf nicht sagen "leider", denn ich bin überzeugt, dass mein Talent mit meiner Körperschwäche unzertrennlich zusammenhängt'; p. 229 in Mann's *Königliche Hoheit*, 27th edn (Berlin: S. Fischer Verlag, 1911).

48 This seems to be a reference to a lecture delivered by Thomas Mann in Princeton in 1939. The lecture is quoted in David Gallagher, *Metamorphosis: Transformations of the Body and the Influence of Ovid's Metamorphoses on Germanic Literature of the Nineteenth and Twentieth Centuries* (Amsterdam: Rodopi, 2009), p. 325.

Magic Mountain and *Doctor Faustus*, are thus tuberculosis and syphilis; Mann studied the characteristic symptoms of the latter in Nietzsche, who was afflicted by it.

A similar connection interested T. S. Eliot, who suffered from tachycardia (a rapid pulse) and from bronchitis, which was exacerbated by his smoking. Illness, he said, at least had the advantage of '[releasing] him from the general round of works and days'; it was 'his body's way of telling him to stop', and he seemed better able to write during periods of ill health.[49] In his introduction to Pascal's *Pensées*, he pointed out ('it is a commonplace') that 'some forms of illness are extremely favourable, not only to religious illumination, but to artistic and literary composition'.[50]

It should be pointed out that severe illness in the family may leave profound traces in the creative work of artists who are themselves quite well. Before they fell victim to tuberculosis, both John Keats and Charlotte Brontë had acquired detailed knowledge of the disease having witnessed family members sickening for and succumbing to it. Edvard Munch left us an unforgettable and deeply moving memory of his dying sister in 'The sick girl'. Thanks to living closely together with Iris Murdoch as she was developing Alzheimer's disease, her husband was able to supply an unusually thorough account of this ailment (pp. 104–106).

Growing to adulthood in a medical environment may produce the same effect. Being a physician, Gustave Flaubert's father resided on premises in the hospital grounds, and his son grew up in surroundings where illness and death were everywhere. What he saw when playing in the autopsy room made a deep impression on him, contributing to his precociously misanthropic outlook on life: 'As if all the putrescences and infections that preceded our birth and will repossess us at our death were not enough, during our life we are nothing but corruption and putrefaction, successive, alternate, one overrunning the other. Today you lose a tooth, tomorrow a hair, a sore opens, an abscess forms, blisters are raised on you, drains are inserted. Add to all this corns on your feet, bad natural smells of every kind and flavour, and you have a most inspiring picture of the human person. To think that one loves all this! That one loves oneself and that I, for one, have the nerve to look at myself in the mirror without bursting into laughter.'[51]

Ill health may also favour artistic creation by posing obstacles to other activities. Owing to kidney stones with dreadfully painful attacks, Michel de Montaigne had to refrain from travel, which he loved, and was compelled to retire to his chateau where he was able to devote himself wholeheartedly to his essays. Enforced exile provided him with the distance that enabled

---

49 Peter Ackroyd, *T. S. Eliot* (London: Sphere Books, 1988 (originally Hamish Hamilton, 1984)), p. 261.

50 'The "Pensées" of Pascal', in T. S. Eliot, *Selected Essays* (London: Faber and Faber, 1951), p. 405.

51 Letter from Flaubert to Louise Colet, of 13 December 1846. The French original may be read in Gustave Flaubert, *Correspondance*, Vol. 1, ed. by Jean Bruneau (Paris: Gallimard, 1973), p. 418.

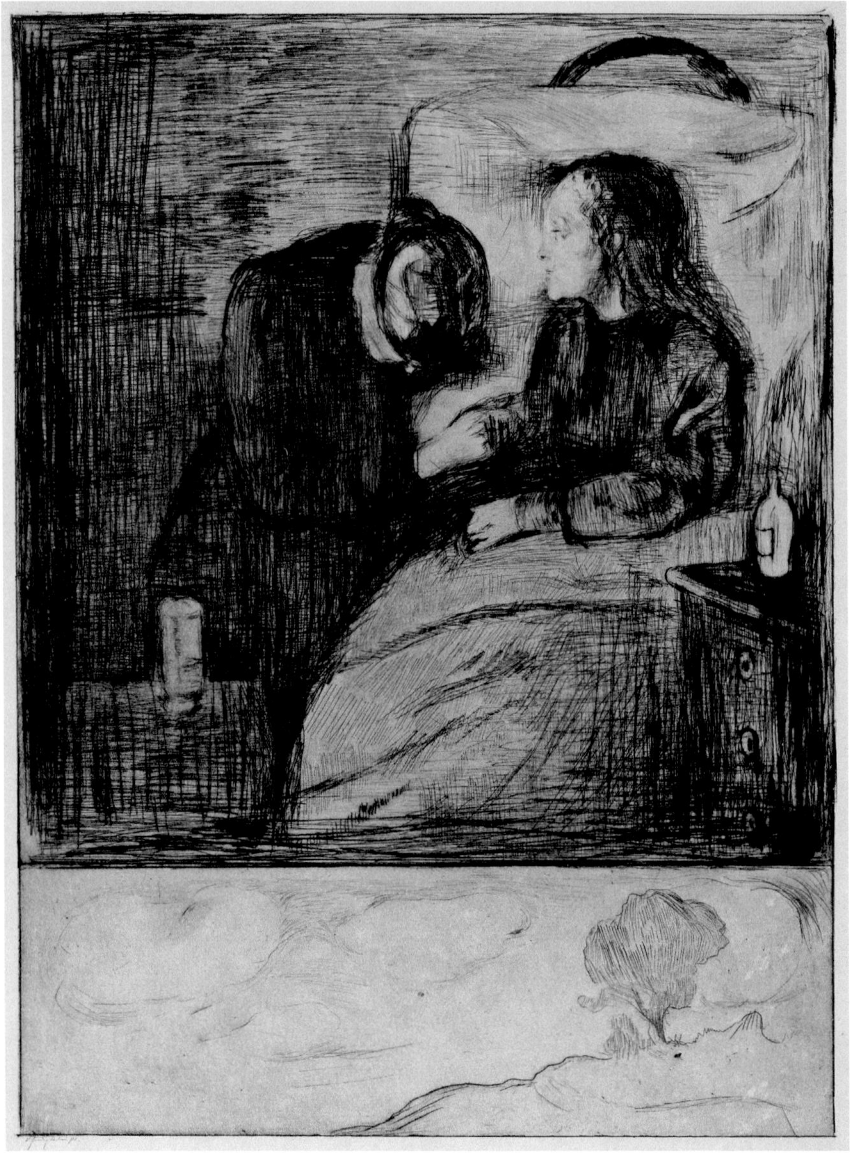

Figure 7 Edvard Munch, 'The sick girl'. Etching. The artist made a portrait of his sister, dying of tuberculosis at the age of 15.

him to ponder human existence free from illusions and prejudice. Calling his kidney ailment a noble and dignified disease, he argued that making a person think about his coming demise meant doing him a favour and observed that his illness gave him a thorough shaking-up for a day or two.[52]

52 Pages 1238, 1240, and 1240–1241 in the Penguin edition quoted in note 41.

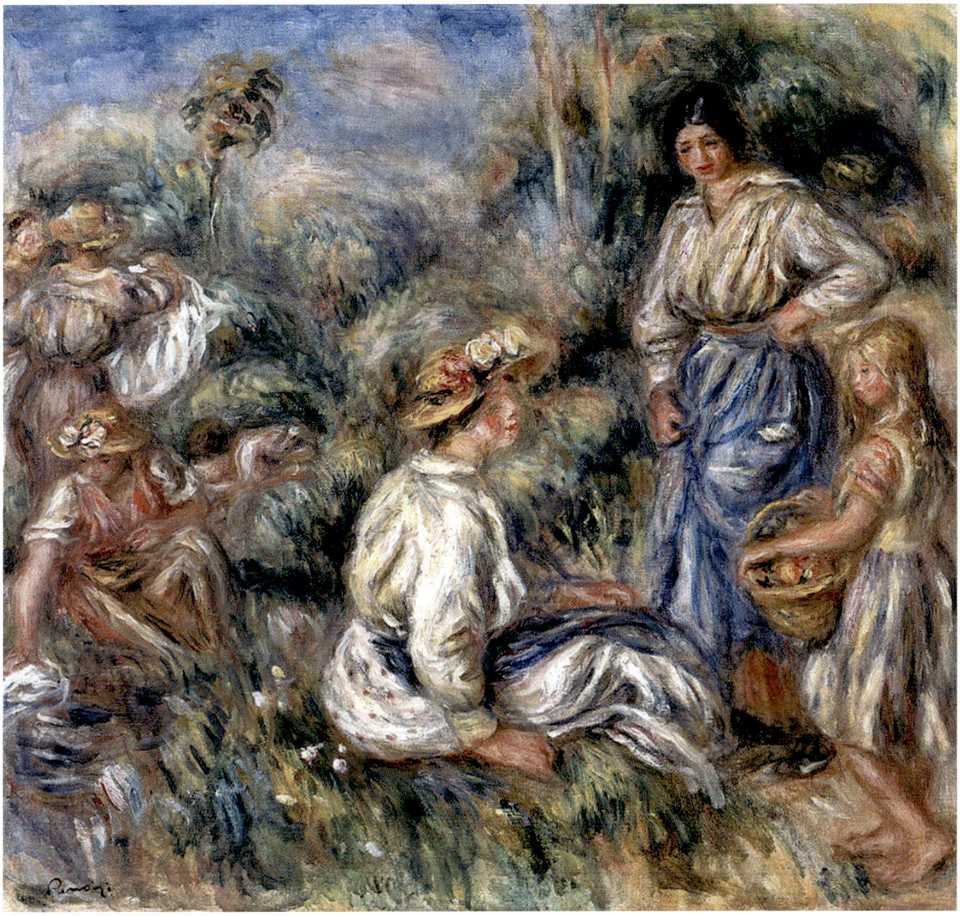

Figure 8 Auguste Renoir, 'Women in a landscape', 1912.

The case of Pierre Ronsard has points in common with that of Montaigne. The famous Renaissance poet was also turned towards a literary life by illness. A brilliant career as a diplomat had lain open for the young aristocrat when sudden deafness put an end to his plans – in the world of whispers, a deaf diplomat is an impossibility. Ronsard returned to the enchanting landscapes and poetic domains of his childhood. In the course of time, the young diplomat became a prince among poets:

I was only fifteen when woods and hills and springs
And brooks delighted me more than the courts of kings.
There, at twilight, I saw the fairies and the fays
Dancing in the meadows in the moonlight rays.[53]

53 'Je n'avois pas quinze ans que les monts et les bois / Et les eaux me plaisoyent, plus que la Cour des Rois, / ... A fin de voir au soir les Nymphes et les Fées / Danser dessous la Lune en cotte par les prées', from 'Hymne de l'Automne', quoted from Pierre

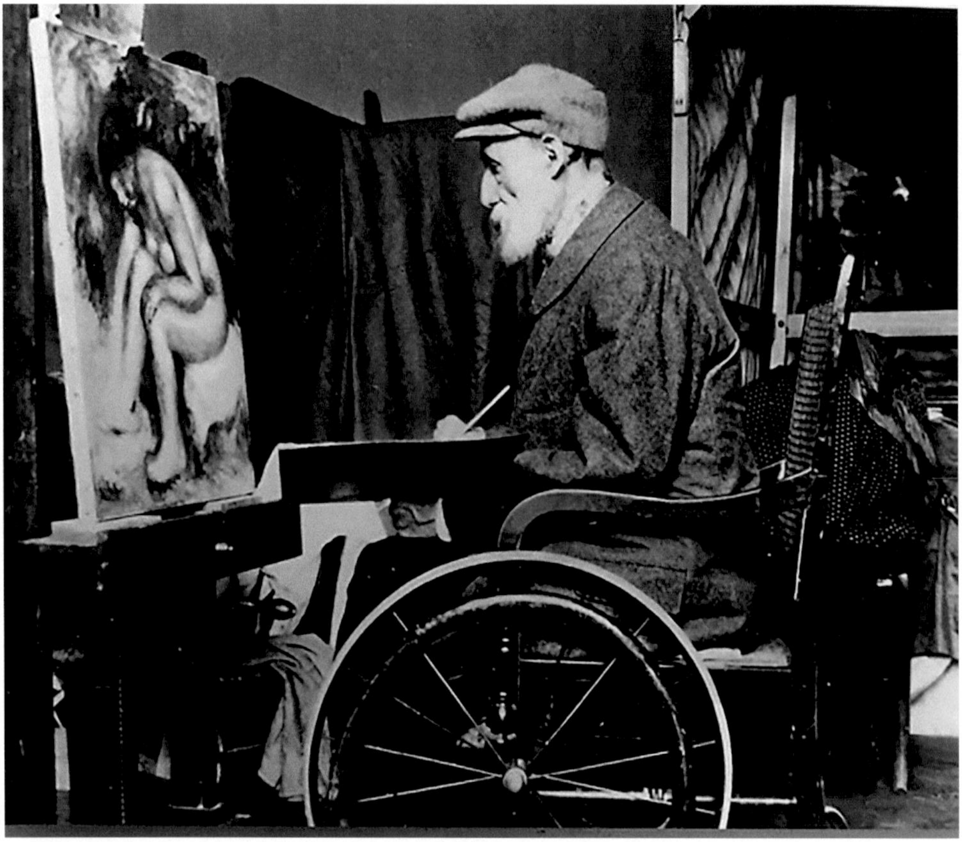

Figure 9 Photograph of Auguste Renoir, approximately 1915. The desire and the effort to preserve a unique personal idea or train of thought for posterity have helped many a great artist to continue with creative work even during periods of grievous ill health. As early as his fifties, Renoir developed a distressing old-age rheumatism which forced him to attach cotton wool to the palm of his hand so that he could hold the brush between thumb and ring finger. Nevertheless, he painted pictures radiating with youthful joy – he loved painting children, young women, and the flowers of spring. In the words of Matisse, who witnessed it, his later life was an extended martyrdom, his finger joints dreadfully deformed, and yet it was at that time that he painted his finest works; while his body was wasting away, his soul seemed to grow stronger, and he expressed himself with ever greater ease.[54]

Towards the end of the nineteenth century, Henri Matisse had already begun a career in law when the direction of his life was radically altered as a result of illness. He developed appendicitis, and, since this happened before surgery had become the common remedy, no operation was undertaken.

Ronsard, *Œuvres complètes*, 2 vols, ed. by Gustave Cohen (Paris: Gallimard, 1950), Vol. 2, p. 240.

54 Jack Cowart and Dominique Fourcade, *Henri Matisse: The Early Years in Nice, 1916–1930* (New York: Abrams, 1986), p. 19. The passage appears to have originated in Frank Harris, *Contemporary Portraits: Fourth Series* (New York: Brentano's, 1923).

The appendix burst, and the ensuing complications including suppuration compelled him to refrain from working for almost a year. In order to pass the time, Matisse attempted to paint and became fascinated. He discovered colour, not, he said, through other painters' work but from the way light revealed itself in nature, and became possessed by painting.[55]

In his own words, Matisse creates a rare opportunity for us to learn how a great master experiences the urge to create: 'When I started to paint, I felt transported into a kind of paradise.' Something drove him, he said, an inexplicable alien force, unlike everything else in ordinary human existence.[56] When Matisse admits that not even he can fully grasp the nature of creativity, how can we solve the mystery?

Matisse soon devoted himself wholly to painting, his work being characterised by intelligence and bold innovation as well as by the finest sensibility. If he had lived now, in a time where appendicitis is treated with surgery and cured in a week, he would probably have become a successful lawyer instead of a pioneer in art.

A new period of ill health, with a severe cough, caused a radical reorientation in Matisse's life. A change of climate was always regarded as beneficial to people suffering from pulmonary disease. Keats was advised to go to Rome, and Chopin found his way to the monastery of Valldemossa on the Mediterranean. Matisse, too, went south: 'I left l'Estaque because of the wind, and I had caught bronchitis there. I came to Nice to cure it, and it rained for a month. Finally I decided to leave. The next day the mistral chased the clouds away and it was beautiful. I decided not to leave Nice, and have stayed there practically the rest of my life.'[57] That entailed leaving his family and abandoning his social responsibilities in order to live entirely for his art. (This did not exclude associating with a number of female friends among his models.)

The change of nature and climate not only benefited Matisse's health; it also brought a profound change in his style of painting, from dashing and radical inventiveness to a new, sensual impressionism. The accusation that he displayed a superficial decorative style can be seen to be false when attention is paid to his highly personal, resplendent colouring and his original approach to composition (see Figure 10).

Matisse also showed how serious illness may leave deep traces even after the patient's recovery. At the age of 70 he developed colon cancer. Reluctantly, he agreed to an operation which was performed by no fewer than three of the most eminent surgeons in France. The patient's life was saved; but he was gravely ill and profoundly shaken. The operation wound became infected, and the infection was exacerbated when the obstinate master painter refused to have his bandages changed. He ended up with a

---

55 It was not possible to locate a reference for this.

56 Lawrence Gowing, *Matisse* (New York: Oxford University Press, 1979), pp. 9 and 32; see also Jack D. Flam, *Matisse on Art* (London: Phaidon, 1973), p. 171.

57 Flam, *Matisse on Art*, p. 134.

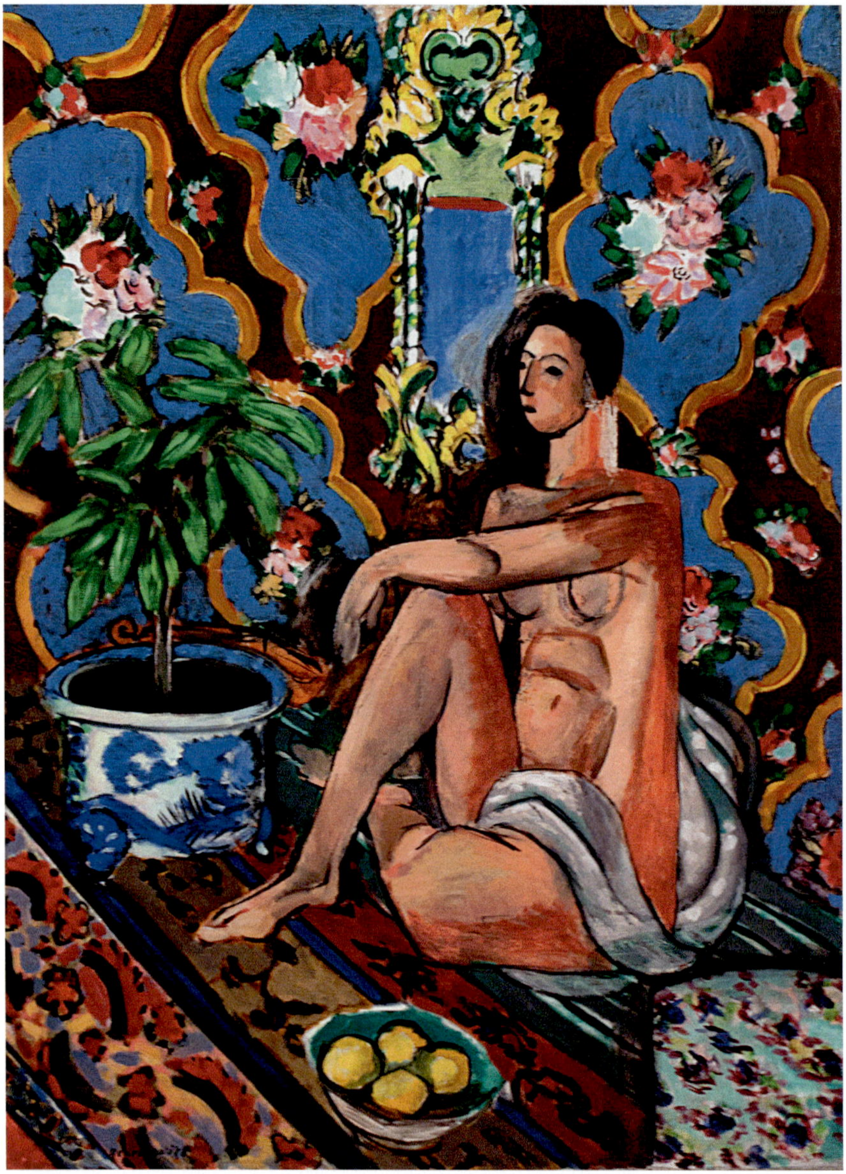

Figure 10 Henri Matisse, 'Decorative figure against an ornamental background', 1927. Wrestling with new problems, the artist attains bold harmonies, never seen before.

large hernia in the scar, which kept him bedridden for most of what was left of his life.

A couple of years after this I had a long conversation with him while he was lying in his bed with a cat at his feet, using a pointer to direct the affixing of his large cut-out pictures on a canvas. He explained to me how his illness had utterly transformed his attitude to life and art and made him wish to fill

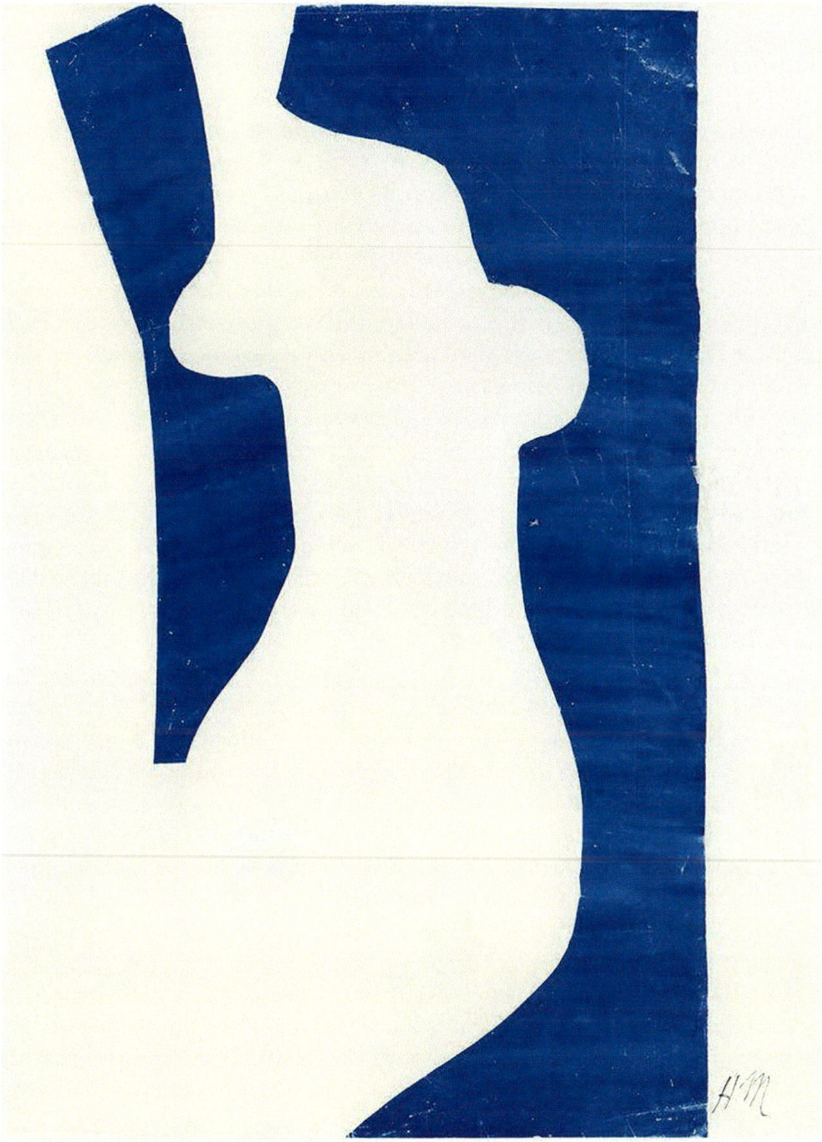

Figure 11 Henri Matisse, 'Venus'. The late collage works radiate a mood of pleasure and relaxed contentment after the artist's recovery from a life-threatening disease.

the new life he had been given with as much happiness as possible. In his earlier years, he had broken new paths for modern art with great labour; now he wished to treat himself to the pleasure of treading these paths again, light of heart and without effort. This mood is apparent in his painting. Many of his earlier works let us observe how hard he struggled against fresh and difficult problems. By contrast, an atmosphere of rest and relaxed contentment after a good day's work characterises his late work. Matisse had begun to paint for pleasure, and that was how he ended. He was so convinced of the beneficial effect of his colours and their healing properties that he took to hanging his paintings around the sickbeds of his friends.

The story of the American abstract-expressionist painter Sam Francis's ill health has striking resemblances to that of Matisse.[58] Like Matisse, Francis had started out in a profession he was forced to abandon as disease afflicted him. At first he studied medicine for two years, but then he joined the US Air Force. During a practice flight, his plane made such a drastic sheer that he broke his back. An X-ray revealed that the reason why moderate violence caused such severe injury, the compression of some lumbar vertebrae, was that they were the location of a tuberculosis which had not been diagnosed before. Owing to the unfortunate combination of injury and illness, he had to be treated while bedridden in a plaster case extending from his shoulders down to his pelvis. Poor Francis felt like the insect in Kafka's *Metamorphosis*.

Francis's treatment had to be extended over a period of three years. Just as Matisse had done, he tried to amuse himself during the dull days confined to bed, and he discovered that the creation of pictures helped him to bear the pain, even to liberate himself from it. His art was thus born out of pain and suffering.

Francis made drawings and painted in watercolours. An arts teacher who saw his pictures became interested in his obvious talent and showed him works by Matisse, Klee, and Miró. 'He brought some actual paintings into my hospital room and ... left them overnight. So, it was a big shock to me. I had never seen anything up close.' Some time later, a visit to a museum in a wheelchair brought on an epiphany. The sight of El Greco's 'Saint Thomas the Apostle', the first masterpiece of art that Francis had seen, made a profound impression. He said that it 'knocked [him] out', and that he would probably have died if it had not been for painting; '[t]he picture by El Greco changed my life'.[59]

From his twenty-third year onward, Francis dedicated himself entirely to painting. According to him, his ailment was the very origin of his art, and it was painting that enabled him to leave the hospital. He claimed that the possibility of painting pictures cured his illness when the doctors had given him up as a hopeless case.[60]

Three years later, Francis's tuberculosis had been halted. At this time, he left figurative art for abstract painting. An intellectual with an original, independent personality, Francis soon gained recognition as a leading member of

58 See William C. Agee, *Sam Francis Paintings 1947–1990* (Los Angeles: The Museum of Contemporary Art, 1999).

59 Ibid., p. 142.

60 The author's exact source could not be located, but the story is told in Gabrielle Selz, *Light on Fire: The Art and Life of Sam Francis* (Oakland: University of California Press, 2021), p. 4.

the school of abstract expressionism and was praised as the most sensuous and sensitive American painter of his generation.[61]

Francis's illness did not only make him an artist; it also left unmistakable marks in his paintings. According to him, painting was the escape that had enabled him to return to life; and in due course, he said, it was more than an escape, it was the path of life itself. Painting was indeed his life during those four years he spent in bed on his back. He did not regard the disease as his enemy, and it did not inflict a sense of death on him; on the contrary, it enhanced his feeling of being alive. His works contain numerous traces of his medical studies and protracted periods of illness, and he claimed that the rendering of rents and slits in his pictures was a product of his own torn and ragged state.[62]

Francis had a special feeling for white, a feeling that may be traced back to the years on his sickbed. He explained that the time spent lying on his back gave him knowledge of the outside world by means of the play of light on the ceiling, the light of dawn and dusk.[63] Many of his pictures are dominated by a rectangular field in the middle, a recovered visual memory (see Figure 12). The white field is surrounded by numerous, vividly coloured small figures which he called 'biomorphic', remembrances from his earlier studies in biology and medicine.

To Francis, colours entailed opportunities to express emotions. He was convinced that colours have healing properties, not just for the artist but also for the beholder, and he articulated his conviction in emphatic terms. In his view, it is apparent that colours constitute forces possessing great strength, a strength we register both in nature and in our souls. If his knee hurt, he said, he would put a strong colour on the canvas, thereby causing the pain to cease.[64]

When Francis was 37 his tuberculosis flared up again, this time in the urinary tract, and it necessitated the sacrifice of one kidney. Once more, he fought the disease through his art. He claimed that his survival was the result of his taking his painting so seriously, and that he had nearly died: his physician had believed that Francis had one last chance, or rather no chance at all.

This experience increased Francis's interest in his own body, and in the course of time his biomorphic figures assumed organic shapes, resembling kidneys and even his own discoloured, swollen scrotum.

Francis's creative joy and power never waned. Towards the end of his life, having developed cancer of the prostate, he suffered a paralysis to the right side of his body but still continued to paint with his unpractised left hand (cf. pp. 46–47). He thus rose above his wretched state, creating luminous paintings in intensively bright and powerful colours.

---

61 By James Johnson Sweeney; p. 9 in Agee, *Sam Francis Paintings*.
62 It was not possible to locate a reference for this statement.
63 See Peter Selz, *Sam Francis* (New York: H. N. Abrams, 1975), p. 34.
64 No reference could be located.

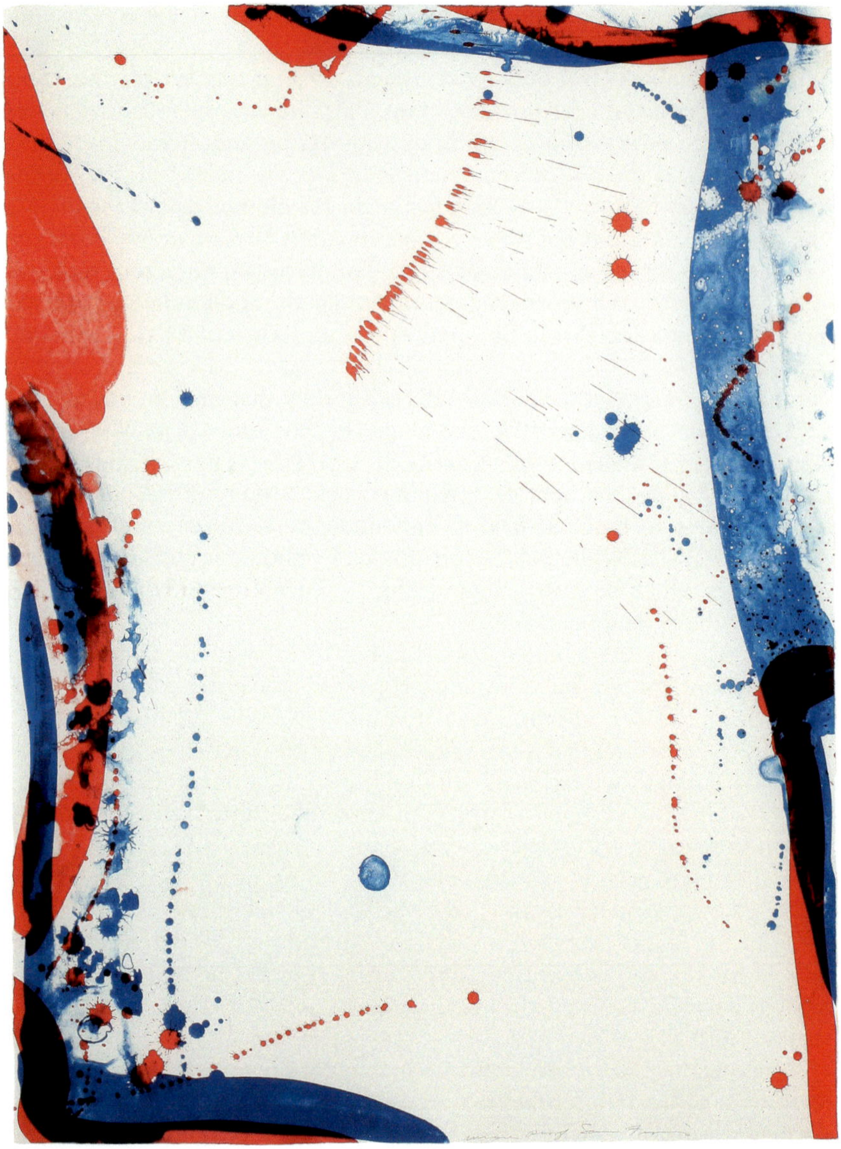

Figure 12 Sam Francis, 'Visual memory', 1968. The Swedish auctioneers Bukowskis refer to this picture as 'Untitled'; see https://www.bukowskis/com/sv/auctions/579/157-sam-francis-untitled?from_language=en.

We are also indebted to an illness for a wealth of wonderful music, namely the asthma which made it impossible for Vivaldi to pursue a career as a priest. He had already been ordained; but, as he was no longer able to celebrate mass, he became a choirmaster instead, appointed to the post of musical director of the Ospedale della Pietà in Venice where composing church music was one of his tasks.

A motor disability gave us another major composer. Robert Schumann's career as a concert pianist was cut short by an ailment affecting his right hand, with paralysis of the long and ring fingers. His condition was exacerbated when, in an attempt to perfect his technique, he tried a mechanical contraption intended to increase mobility in those two fingers, which are hard to control separately.[65]

Schumann lamented to his beloved Clara, telling her that he often felt downhearted, especially when his hand hurt, and that it was getting worse. He would often ask Providence why this had been done to him, saying that he would have had such good use for his hand; 'so much music is alive in me, ready to be expressed, and now I can hardly bring it forth, one finger stumbling over the other. It is dreadful and rather painful.'[66]

Even so, Schumann did not despair, comforting his mother by telling her not to worry about his fingers as he was able to compose music without relying on them, and that he would hardly have been happier 'as a travelling virtuoso' – he could still improvise.[67] We only need to listen to his *Dichterliebe* to realise, in awe, how right he was. (His state of mind is described on pp. 101–103.)

65 R. A. Henson and H. Ulrich, 'Schumann's Hand Injury', *British Medical Journal* 1.6117 (8 April 1978), 900–903 (p. 901).

66 Ibid. The complete translated letter (from Robert Schumann to Clara Wieck, of 3 December 1838) is found in *The Complete Correspondence of Clara and Robert Schumann*, ed. by Eva Weissweiler, trans. by Hildegard Fritsch and Ronald L. Crawford, 3 vols (New York: Peter Lang, 1994), Vol. 1, p. 318.

67 Henson and Ulrich, 'Schumann's Hand Injury', 901.

Chapter 2

The salient characteristics of creative personalities

Examples of illnesses that exert a decisive influence on the works of artists are to be found across the whole spectrum of pathology, mental as well as physical; 'each pain has its own particular cry, but health stays mute'.[1] I begin with mental illnesses, where we may expect to find the most obvious instances considering the profound changes in the personality that may result from mental aberration.

The first question we ask ourselves is whether the creative human being is to be regarded as mentally normal in the first place, a question already part-answered by the proverbial notion that 'there is no cure for genius'. At any rate, the proportion of individuals whose mental constitution borders on the abnormal is very high among original creators.[2] Mental characteristics that deviate from the norm and would be regarded as pathological among ordinary people may contribute to what is felt to be distinctive and appealing in the context of artistic creation; indeed, they may form its actual origin. If these peculiar characteristics increase, crossing the border between normal and abnormal, they may come to form symptoms of mental illness (see pp. 75–107). That boundary, often a fluid one, may be transgressed, temporarily, repeatedly, or permanently. This circumstance has given rise to the question of whether certain creative individuals, such as Byron, Strindberg, Van Gogh, and Schumann, may always be considered entirely normal. The proportion of creative persons with such a hard-to-define mental constitution has been said to be as great as 80 per cent.

Mental illness has sometimes been regarded as a particular asset in creative work. That notion has made for faulty conclusions; one of the most amusing ones has been reproduced by Robert Brittain, editor of *Poems by Christopher Smart*: 'Knowing that Smart had been confined for madness for

1 A translation of a line from the poem 'Odalbonden' ('The Yeoman') by the Swedish poet Erik Gustaf Geijer (1811).

2 The author refers to Kay Jamison, *Mood Disorders*, supposedly published in London in 1989 [1973]. No such publication was identified, but there are two articles either of which – or both – may be Sandblom's source(s): Kay Jamison, 'Mood Disorders and Patterns of Creativity in British Writers and Artists', *Psychiatry* 52.2 (1989), 125–134, and Kay Redfield Jamison, 'Manic-Depressive Illness and Creativity', *Scientific American* 272.2 (1995), 62–67.

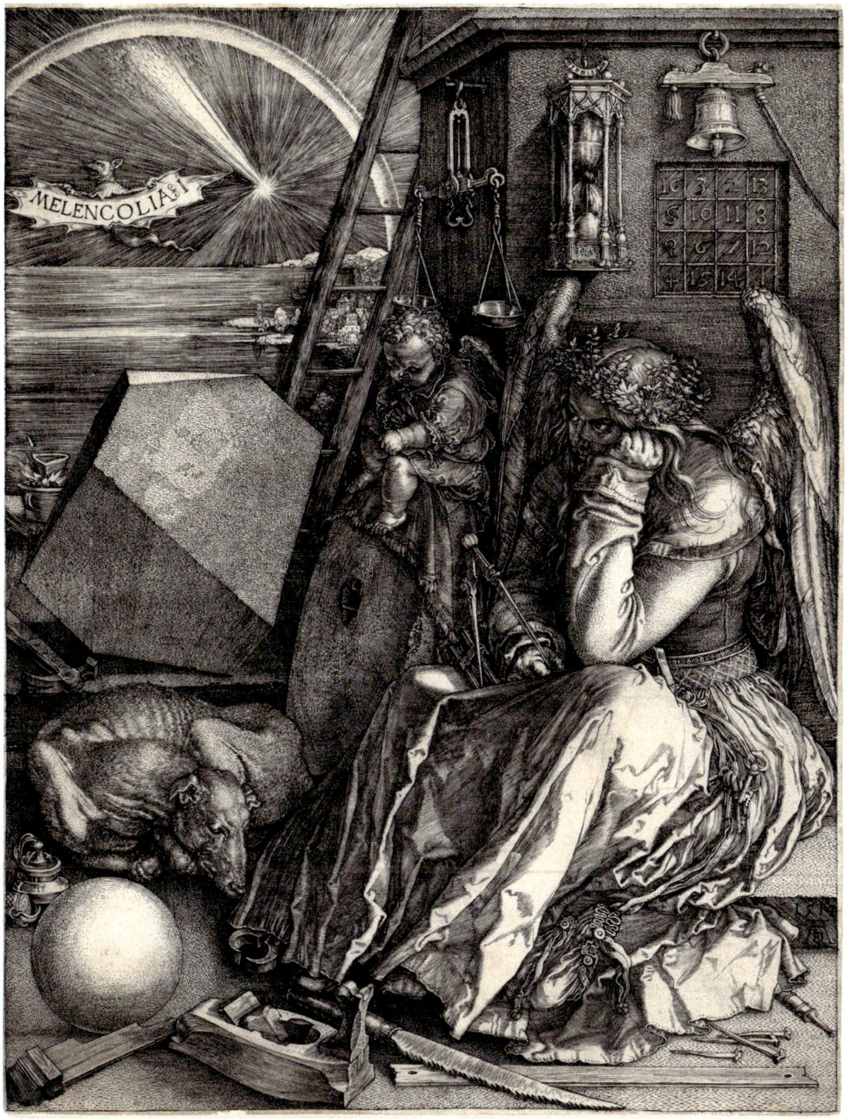

Figure 13 Albrecht Dürer, 'Melencholia', 1514.

several years just before [*A Song to David*] was published, [Robert] Browning [in "Parleying with Christopher Smart"] jumped to the natural but quite erroneous conclusion that the great lyric was a miracle of insanity ... It was an exciting theory: a mediocre poet laboriously grinding out reams of dull and uninspired verse suddenly loses his mind, and in a burst of insane genius scrawls upon the walls of his cell a superb lyric ode worthy to be ranked with those of Milton and Keats; then sanity returns, genius departs, and the sobered poet resumes his patient production of trash. How such nonsense could impose itself on a mind as intelligent as Browning's can only be understood if one remembers the limited evidence he had at his disposal.'[3] In fact, the poem was written after Smart had recovered from his mental illness – it was hence not produced under its influence, but possibly enriched by experiences during that period. 'Even if, half crazed, in the end, he loses sight of his visions, he has seen them!' was Rimbaud's consolation.[4]

No, 'one is not a genius because one is mad' – but it may help, to the extent that the powers of the imagination may be liberated and sharpened in the manner described by Charles Lamb to his friend: 'Dream not Coleridge, of having tested all the grandeur and wildness of Fancy, till you have gone mad.'[5]

Creative work may form a happy way for gifted individuals to resolve the internal conflicts and tensions that accompany all human life. Heinrich Heine expressed it as follows in one of his poems:

Krankheit ist wohl der letzte Grund
Des ganzen Schöpferdrangs gewesen;
Erschaffend konnte ich genesen,
Erschaffend wurde ich gesund.[6]

Even so, he did know that there is a sweeter remedy (see the poem on p. 102).

Graham Greene elaborates: 'Writing is a form of therapy; sometimes I wonder how all those who do not write, compose or paint can manage to escape the madness, the melancholia, the panic fear which is inherent in the human situation.'[7] Here, Greene is stating essential symptoms of the two psychopathological temperaments that frequently occur in creative individuals: melancholy in the manic depressive, angst in the schizophrenic. A common factor in artists of both categories is the attempt to strengthen their endangered self-esteem by claiming independence and originality. Otherwise they differ profoundly, especially in terms of their relationships with the outside world.

---

3 Robert Brittain, *Poems by Christopher Smart* (Princeton: Princeton University Press, 1950), pp. 3–4. Browning's poem is called 'With Christopher Smart' in the collection *Parleyings with Certain People of Importance in Their Day* (London: Smith, Elder, & Co., 1887), pp. 79–95.

4 From a letter of Rimbaud's to Paul Démeny, 15 May 1871, quoted in Barnaby Conrad, *Absinthe: History in a Bottle* (San Francisco: Chronicle Books, 1988; Conrad mistakenly states the year as being 1872), p. 26. The French original, presumably translated by Conrad, runs, 'Il arrive à l'inconnu, et quand, affolé, il finirait par perdre l'intelligence de ses visions, il les a vues!'

5 The first quotation is a translation of the title of a poem by the Swedish poet Johan Henric Kellgren (1787). The quotation from Charles Lamb comes from a letter to S. T. Coleridge, begun on 8 June 1796, in *The Works of Charles and Mary Lamb*, ed. by E. V. Lucas, Vol. VI: *Letters, 1796–1820* (London: Methuen, 1905), p. 17.

6 'Illness is likely to have been the ultimate origin of the whole urge to create; creating, I was able to recover and regain my health.' Heinrich Heine, 'Schöpfungslieder VII' in *Neue Gedichte*, 3rd edn (Hamburg: Hoffmann und Campe, 1852), p. 129.

7 Graham Greene, *Ways of Escape* (London: Vintage, 1999), p. 275 (originally published by Bodley Head in 1980).

The depressed have a great need for good contacts with their fellow humans and wish to be liked and acknowledged; but they are held back since they regard themselves as unworthy of being loved, or even liked, for their own sake. In their fear of rejection, depressed artists instead attempt to achieve appreciation for the works they create, which makes them highly vulnerable. Virginia Woolf, who was over-sensitive to criticism, was thus beside herself with anxiety about the reception of a newly published book, her depression ultimately leading to suicide.

Aristotle maintained that all great artists have been melancholy. Many people have agreed with him, especially and emphatically Lord Byron: 'We of the craft are all crazy. Some are affected by gaiety, others by melancholy, but all are more or less touched.'[8] Though Byron's insanity is not established, Kay Jamison argues that he is a classic, indeed an inspiring, example of the ways in which manic-depressive illness influences creative ability, frequently even increasing it during manic phases.[9] Byron sometimes displayed the conflicting traits simultaneously, in a manner reminiscent of Van Gogh who, in his painting 'Wheatfield', displayed manic and depressive features at the same time. (On Van Gogh, see further pp. 96–99.)

As often happens with sick artists, Byron was himself quite aware of his unusual condition: 'Though I feel tolerably miserable, yet I am at the same time subject to a kind of hysterical merriment.'[10] When that merriment became excessive, it could turn into its opposite, a manic fury which he called 'the mind's canker in its savage mood'.[11]

Michelangelo, a melancholy man – solitary, inaccessible, *terribile* – wrote sonnets about his depressed state of mind. His depression is also reflected in his pictorial art; in 'The Day of Judgment', he lets St Bartholomew, who was flayed alive, display Michelangelo's own stripped skin with a tragically hanging head (Figure 14).

Manic-depressives rejoice in lively activity during their manic phases but fall silent when they turn depressed; for instance, Robert Burns claimed that he hung his lyre on the willow trees except for brief and bright moments.[12] Increased activity during the manic stage may be an attempt to escape subsequent depression. Handel composed *Messiah* during three weeks of hectic creation, his mania supplying him with the requisite creative urge and power: 'I did think I did see all Heaven before me, and the Great God Himself.'[13]

---

8 Margaret Gardiner, Countess of Blessington, *Conversations of Lord Byron with the Countess of Blessington* (London: Henry Colburn, 1834), p. 192.

9 Kay Jamison, *Touched with Fire* (New York: The Free Press, 1993), passim.

10 Ibid., p. 171.

11 Ibid., p. 149 (this is the title of Jamison's fifth chapter, about Byron).

12 Quoted in Jamison, *Touched with Fire*, p. 249.

13 Quoted in Christopher Hogwood, *Handel* (London: Thames & Hudson, 1984), p. 168. (It should, however, be pointed out that Hogwood himself is quite dismissive of this 'legend' with its 'excess romanticism'.)

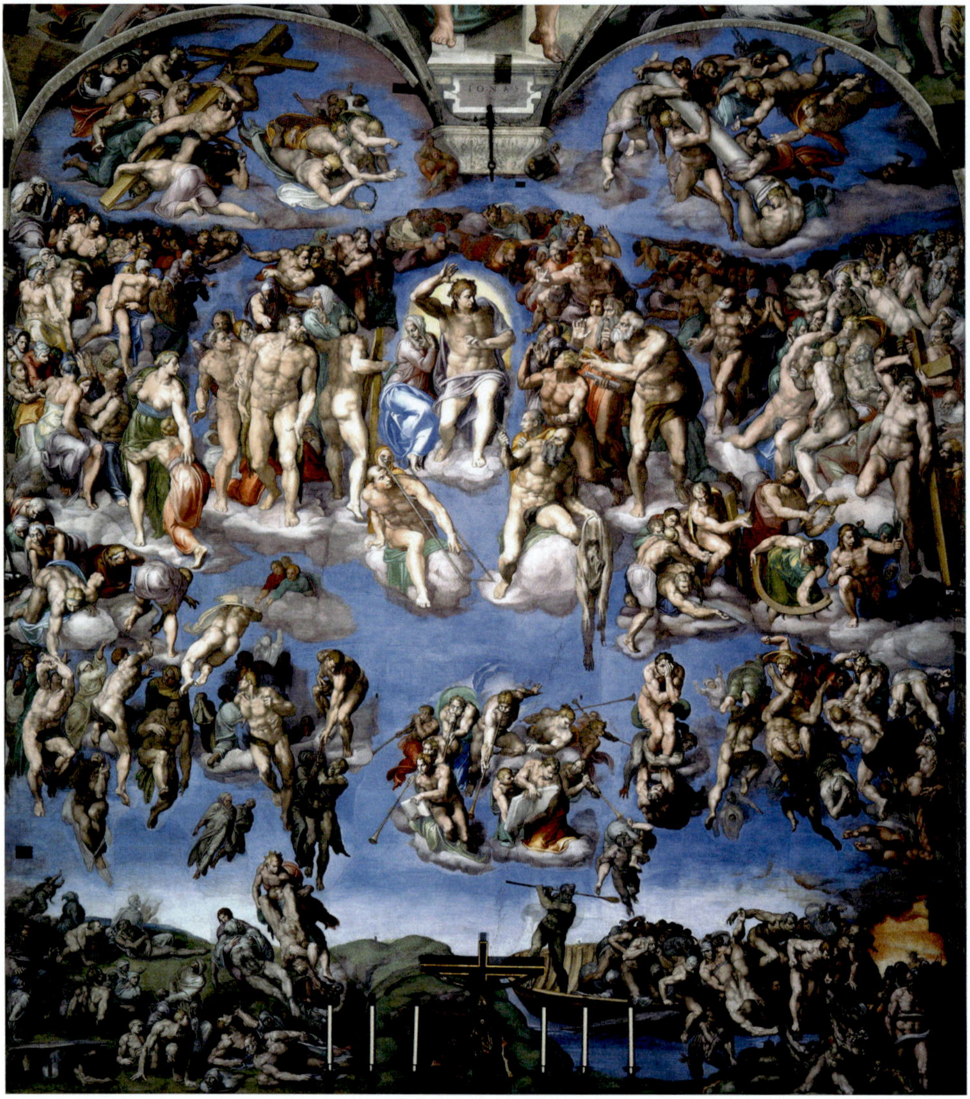

Figure 14 Michelangelo Buonarroti, 'The Day of Judgment', 1536–41. The depressed artist depicts himself as a flayed martyr.

During the last 25 years of his life, Rossini composed only small pieces for his own amusement, calling them the sins of his old age and giving them bizarre titles which suggest his hypochondria, such as 'Asthmatic Etude' and 'My Morning Hygiene Prelude'. Beset by depression and self-reproaches, he said, 'Many would, in my situation, commit suicide – but I am a coward and dare not.'[14] When he began to feel better, he dedicated a

14 Sandblom refers to John O'Shea, *Music and Medicine: Medical Profiles of Great Composers* (London: Dent, 1990), which does have a chapter on Rossini; but the

couple of songs to his wife 'as a simple testimonial of gratitude for the affectionate, intelligent care of which she was prodigal during my overlong and terrible illness', adding that the Faculty of Medicine ought to be ashamed of itself.[15]

In contrast to the manic-depressive, the schizoid individual is characterised by a reluctance, even an inability, to establish human contacts. The schizophrenic seeks that meaning of life which normal people find in human communities in his or her created works. When he or she succeeds, that may be experienced as a re-established link to a lost world. The feeling of alienation, which may be intensified into a dread of fellow human beings, is clearly expressed in the novels of Franz Kafka, where social structures come across as incomprehensible and inexplicably malicious.

The etching made by Charles Meryon of 'The mortuary' (Figure 37) fascinates and moves us with its schizophrenic mood. With his paranoia, August Strindberg casts a spectral light over his hated female characters; he believed that he could ward off the threat of insanity by incorporating them in his fiction.[16] Ezra Pound's outbursts of antisemitism might also be explained as manifestations of a schizophrenic paranoia.

I am not qualified to assess, and still less appreciate, Sigmund Freud's thesis that all artistic creation constitutes a sublimation of remaining infantile sexuality with its '"pregenital" oral, anal, and phallic impulses'.[17] It has led some of his disciples into trains of thought that appear peculiar and even repugnant to someone who is a non-psychoanalyst, for instance the idea that Van Gogh unwittingly equated his painting with masturbation. According to this notion, the anal component in the artist's suppressed infantile sexuality was expressed in his painting, the consistency and pungent odour of the paint reminding him of the excrement he longed to poke about in. That supposedly caused him to paint with his fingers now and then, under the pretext of pursuing a particular visual effect.

There is certainly nothing average about the creative geniuses; they differ from us ordinary mortals in a variety of ways. Like curious children, they perceive with innocent eyes, as if they saw everything for the first time or, in Baudelaire's words, 'genius is nothing more nor less than childhood recovered at will'.[18] Their unique experiences and personal observations are stored and mature in the depths of consciousness, joining their works

---

quotation appears to derive from Emilia Branca Romani's description of a visit to Florence in 1854, on which occasion she called on Rossini. The tribute is quoted in Herbert Weinstock, *Rossini: A Biography* (New York: Limelight Editions, 1987), p. 257.

15 From the dedication to Olympe Rossini of a manuscript headed 'Musique Anodine', quoted in Weinstock, *Rossini*, p. 269.

16 Olof Lagercrantz, *August Strindberg* (Stockholm: Wahlström & Widstrand, 1979), p. 220. The relevant passage may be consulted on Litteraturbanken, https://urn.kb.se/resolve?urn=urn:nbn:se:lb-lb7280408-faksimil.

17 Anthony Storr, *The Dynamics of Creation* (New York: Atheneum, 1972), p. 5.

18 Charles Baudelaire, *The Painter of Modern Life and Other Essays*, trans. Jonathan Mayne (London: Phaidon, 1964), p. 8.

in due course. Strindberg said that when he did not grasp what was going on, he left his mind inactive while waiting for 'the powers' to do their work; and Rainer Maria Rilke, who knew a great deal about silence, wondered 'whether it is not during the days that we are forced to inactivity that we are productive in a deeper sense'.[19] 'In his between-times', said Elizabeth Bowen, 'the writer needs to re-charge his batteries by private living, in any one of several possible forms – well does one recognise the dimming lights in the work of the writer who does not'.[20]

In addition, creative people characteristically experience more powerful moments of ecstasy, keener associations, and clearer perceptions of human situations and peculiarities than the rest of us. Above all, they are impelled by a desire to search for new, more personal ways of expressing themselves, ways that enable them to form closer connections to human beings able to appreciate their fresh creations and share their inmost feelings – the process that Katherine Mansfield described as the terrifying need for establishing contact.[21] This urge to get one's message across may manifest itself in touching ways; for instance, Carl Fredrik Hill, one of the great Swedish artists, who was incarcerated in his room owing to mental ill health, would throw his drawings down to passers-by in the street below.

When gifted creative artists encounter something unexpected in their lives, such as serious illness, they are driven to pursuing knowledge of its nature, sharing their experience with others, and explaining their feelings. When Anatole Broyard fell victim to prostate cancer, he meditated on this urge to communicate: 'Like anyone who has had an extraordinary experience, I wanted to describe it. This seems to be a natural reflex, especially for a writer. ... I wanted ... to tell people what a serious illness is like, the unprecedented ideas and fantasies it puts into your head, the unexpected qualms and quirks it introduces into your body. For a seriously sick person, opening up your consciousness to others is like the bleeding [that] doctors used to recommend to reduce the [blood] pressure.'[22] It is vital that this description be made without delay, for as the well-informed Marguerite Yourcenar explains: 'Just as the secrets of life that we learn through the intimacies of love are rapidly obscured in our memory, so does the convalescent lose contact with the mysterious realities of a disease happily survived.'[23]

---

19 It was not possible to find a source for this quotation.

20 Elizabeth Bowen, *Why Do I Write? An Exchange of Views between Elizabeth Bowen, Graham Greene & V. S. Pritchett* (London: Percival Marshall, 1948), p. 57.

21 Sandblom has not supplied a reference, but the source may be Katherine Mansfield's notebooks; see *The Katherine Mansfield Notebooks*, complete edition, ed. by Margaret Scott (Minneapolis: University of Minnesota Press, 2002), p. 231 (21 or 22 July 1920): 'There is something profound & terrible in this eternal desire to establish contact.' However, the context has nothing to do with creativity.

22 In 'Good books about being sick', *The New York Times Book Review*, 1 April 1990.

23 Sandblom refers to Marguerite Yourcenar, *Le Cerveau noir de Piranèse*; but the source would seem to be Yourcenar's *Mémoirs d'Hadrien*, 1951, p. 22 in the Gallimard edition of 1974. The English translation by Grace Frick, published by Farrar, Straus &

Only those who have themselves been seriously ill and experienced the agony of the body and the deep despair of the soul can fully understand the feelings of blissful relief that accompany recovered health. Many poets, artists, and composers have voiced their gratitude over the joy of regaining the richness of life, the beauty of nature, and the delight of creative work. However, it is significant that this gratitude has seldom been expressed in relation to the medical care they received; in that respect eulogies are rare but reproaches abundant. Monet, Goya, and Rachmaninov form exceptions to this rule, though. Monet and Goya mixed praise and blame, and Rachmaninov dedicated his Second Piano Concerto to a physician who had used hypnosis to cure him of a depression brought on by the failure of his First Symphony.

The melancholy English seventeenth-century poet George Herbert, best known for his religious poetry, devised convincing metaphors for his depression and the alienation of his heart:

> Who would have thought my shrivel'd heart
> Could have recover'd greennesse? It was gone
> Quite under ground; as flow'rs depart ...[24]

Once recovered, and sheltered from the storms of anguish, he is overjoyed to observe the small wonders of nature and recapture the pleasure of writing:

> And now in age I bud again.
> After so many deaths I live and write;
> I once more smell the dew and rain,
> and relish versing: O my only light,
> It cannot be
> That I am he
> On whom Thy tempests fell at night.

A similar feeling of bliss after the restoration of health is seen in the work of Georges Braque after his recovery from severe injuries sustained during the First World War. His friends celebrated his resumption of creative work in 1918 by throwing a party.

Before the war, Braque had developed Cubism in collaboration with Picasso, using the forms of ordinary objects to create intricate geometric compositions in restrained colours, 'loving the rule that corrects the emotion', as Braque put it.[25] Now their paths separated. Picasso explored new fields in bold forms and colours, whereas Braque pursued harmonious, classic still-life pictures in a rich yet subdued colour scale. It would seem as if his newly rediscovered joy in life, having been so close to death, increased

Giroux as *Memoirs of Hadrian* in 1954 and subsequent editions, refers to the law 'which ordains that the convalescent, once cured, ceases to understand the mysterious truths laid bare by illness' (p. 14).

24 From 'The Flower', 1633.

25 'J'aime la règle qui corrige l'émotion'; Georges Braque, 'Pensées et réflexions sur la peinture', *Nord-Sud* 1.10 (December 1917), 3.

his interest in the everyday things which he had formerly only studied intellectually, but now depicted with sensual attentiveness. His emotion took command, 'to correct the rules', while still permitting occasional deformities for the sake of the composition. Support for this contention may be derived from a comparison of the rigid monochrome structure of the fruit bowl from 1913 (Figure 15) with the lovingly reproduced shape and colour in the painting of the pipe from 1929–30 (Figure 16). Coleridge had maintained that it

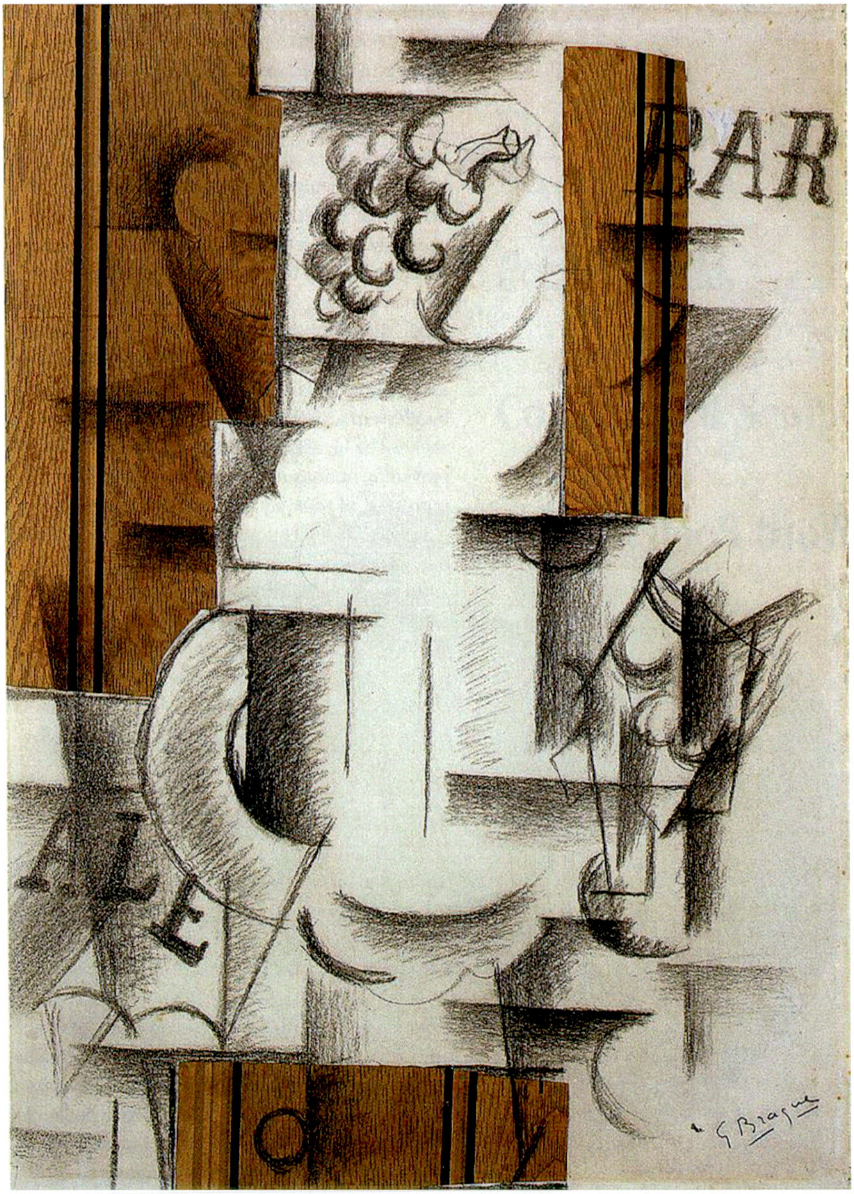

Figure 15 Georges Braque, 'Fruit dish and glass', 1913.

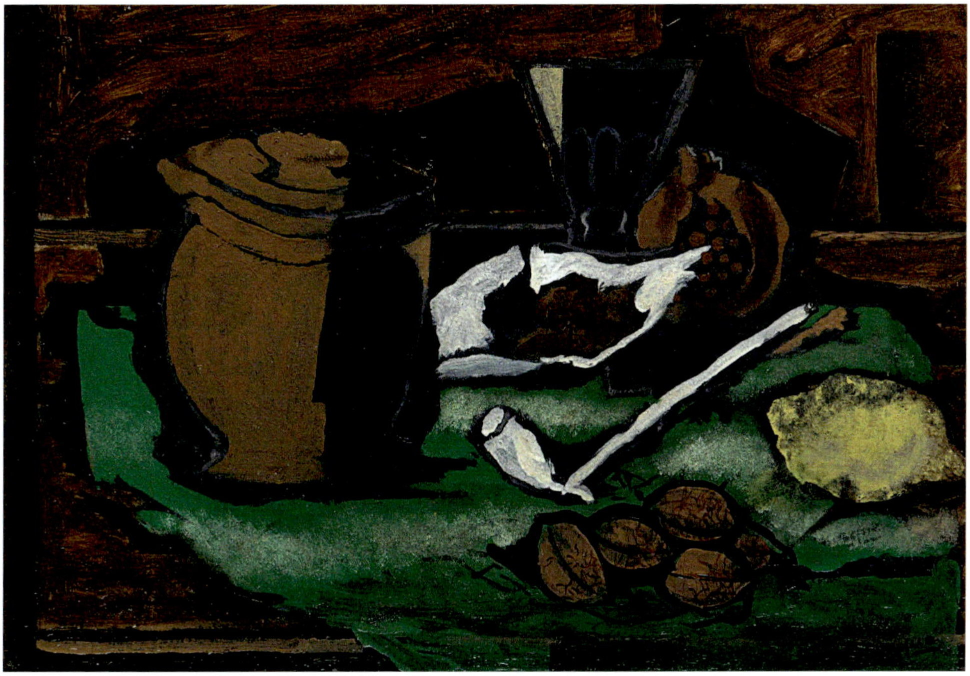

Figure 16 Georges Braque, 'Still life with pipe', 1929–30.

is the convalescent who sees the world in its true colours, but they may not always be as appealing as Braque's perceptions in still-life paintings such as this one.[26]

It is generally believed that François Couperin created his powerful Allemande 'La Convalescente' in order to express his thankfulness for the joy of being able to sit down by his harpsichord again after a period of illness had prevented him from composing music.[27] Maybe the piece contains a suggestion of his illness: '*La Convalescente* is pervaded by an indefinable heavy quality, beginning with the descending arpeggio of the initial theme and lasting until the phrases in lute style transformed in the closing fragments into an asthmatic sort of panting that lands heavily on the bass line. This heaviness is felt consistently, beginning with the *ports-de-voix-coulés* which carry along other notes that make pathetic attempts to make the melody ascend, and ending finally on the restful yet hesitant descent.'[28] The same writer has raised the question of whether this noble and moving Allemande might be compared to Beethoven's

26 The author did not supply a reference, and no original context could be found.

27 Sandblom refers to Wilfrid Mellers, *François Couperin and the French Classical Tradition* (London: Faber, 1987); but the source is more likely to be Philippe Beaussant, *François Couperin*, trans. by Alexandra Land (Portland: Amadeus Press, 1990), p. 336; the original French version of *François Couperin* appeared from Fayard in Paris in 1980, where the relevant passage is on p. 492.

28 Ibid.

fifteenth string quartet, but observes that Couperin never used such intense language as Beethoven and did not aim as high as he did.[29]

While the ageing Beethoven was working on that quartet he was interrupted by illness, jaundice caused by liver damage owing to alcohol abuse, a grave reminder of his fragile health. When he began to improve, albeit not fully recovered, he expressed his relief and gratitude in ethereal music of rare beauty. He called the piece 'Heiliger Dankgesang eines Genesenen an die Gottheit in der lydischen Tonart' ('Holy song of thanksgiving to the Deity from a convalescent, in the Lydian mode'). This autobiographical comment, rare in Beethoven's output, forms the third movement of the quartet. It consists of variations on two strongly contrasted themes. One is a sombre chorale, where Beethoven utilises an archaic church mode to attain an atmosphere of transcendental solemnity which cannot be expressed in words – even his own, 'mit innigster Empfindung' ('with the deepest, most intimate feeling'), pale in comparison. The serene tranquillity of this theme contrasts with the rhythmic variety of the ensuing one, called 'Neue Kraft fühlend' ('Feeling of new strength'). In this lively interlude of a more worldly and robust character, Beethoven praises the return to physical well-being and life's flow of simpler pleasures: 'The movement in a single bar [is brought] out of church into the sun, from the stillness of a devout recollection into the tingling activity of the dance.'[30]

***

A genuine artist must remain a pioneer and run the risk of becoming a pathfinder without companions or followers. Some artists break down under the lack of appreciation and cease doing innovative work; others, stronger souls like Cézanne, indefatigably pursue their solitary course far from the madding crowd. 'Solitude is the school of genius', said Gibbon.[31]

Interestingly, there is a danger that such artists lose their foothold if they achieve general acclaim. Mark Rothko found himself in an intolerable situation when he was suddenly successful after many years of struggle to find a personal style. With the feeling of inferiority that characterises the melancholic, he was afraid he was overrated or at least misunderstood and sank into depression, for which – as ever – alcohol was a poor cure. Having borne adversity, he broke down under success and died by suicide.[32]

29 Ibid.

30 Martin Cooper, *Beethoven: The Last Decade, 1817–1827* (London: Oxford University Press, 1970), p. 364. Sandblom refers to the continuation of this quotation, in Cooper's text '... of the dance, but David's solemn dance of thanksgiving before the Ark'.

31 Edward Gibbon, *The Decline and Fall of the Roman Empire*, ed. by J. B. Bury, 2nd edn, Vol. V (London: Methuen, 1929), p. 360.

32 James Ravin et al., 'Mark Rothko's Paintings ... Suicide Notes?', *Ohio State Medical Journal* (February 1978), 78.

A Swedish example is the poet Birger Sjöberg, who suffered from extreme levels of self-criticism. In his own words, he was tormented by the disease known as lack of self-confidence, channelling his agony into a poem where the creation of a carefully burnished toy horse, 'Konstruktissa', amounts to a tribute to lifeless futility.[33]

The individuality of the human creator is obvious. Plato may have exaggerated in calling inspiration a 'divine mania', but it often resembles a spring gushing forth out of the unknown depths of the personality. In his *Confessions*, Jean-Jacques Rousseau supplies a famous account of such a moment. On a hot day in summer, walking from Paris to Vincennes, he glanced through a copy of *Mercure de France* which he had taken along on his walk and noticed a prize question formulated by the Academy of Dijon: 'Has the progress of the sciences and arts tended to corrupt or purify morals?'[34]

The reaction was instantaneous and dramatic: Rousseau's soul was suffused by a radiant light, and he was overwhelmed by a cascade of new ideas. It was succeeded by confusion, as in a state of intoxication, and with a palpitating heart he sank to the ground. That critique of the condition of society which had been germinating inside him for years was suddenly channelled into thoughts characterised by clarity and vigour. On recovering consciousness after about half an hour, he found that his coat was wet with tears. In the course of this brief moment, he had prepared for the role he would come to play in the transformation of society, with ideas that would lead to the French Revolution.

Even so, it is rare for inspiration to flow freely and continually; it is rather the case that, as incisively formulated by Thomas Mann, '[a] writer is one to whom writing comes harder than to anybody else'.[35]

***

Gustave Flaubert pushed worship of the aesthetic to an almost superhuman height, claiming that he would rather 'die like a dog' than hurry by a single second a sentence that is not ripe.[36] His endeavours were not helped by his

---

33 Called 'Ej för lagrar löpa!', the poem is included in Sjöberg's best-known volume, *Kriser och kransar*, 1926.

34 From Book VIII of Rousseau's *Confessions* (1749). The original French runs, 'Je pris un jour le *Mercure de France*, et tout en marchant et le parcourant, je tombai sur cette question proposée par l'Académie de Dijon pour le prix de l'année suivante: *Si le progrès des sciences et des arts a contribué à corrompre ou à épurer les moeurs*'; a recent modern French edition of *Les Confessions* is the 2009 one by Gallimard, where the quoted passage is on p. 430.

35 Thomas Mann, *Tristan, sechs Novellen* (Berlin: Fischer, 1919): 'wer ihn sah, mußte zu der Anschauung gelangen, daß ein Schriftsteller ein Mann ist, dem das Schreiben schwerer fällt, als allen anderen Leuten' (p. 70).

36 Thus translated by Francis Steegmuller in the 1981 edition from of *The Letters of Gustave Flaubert 1830–1857* (London: Faber and Faber), p. 161. French original: 'Que je crève comme un chien, plutôt que de hater d'une seconde ma phrase qui n'est

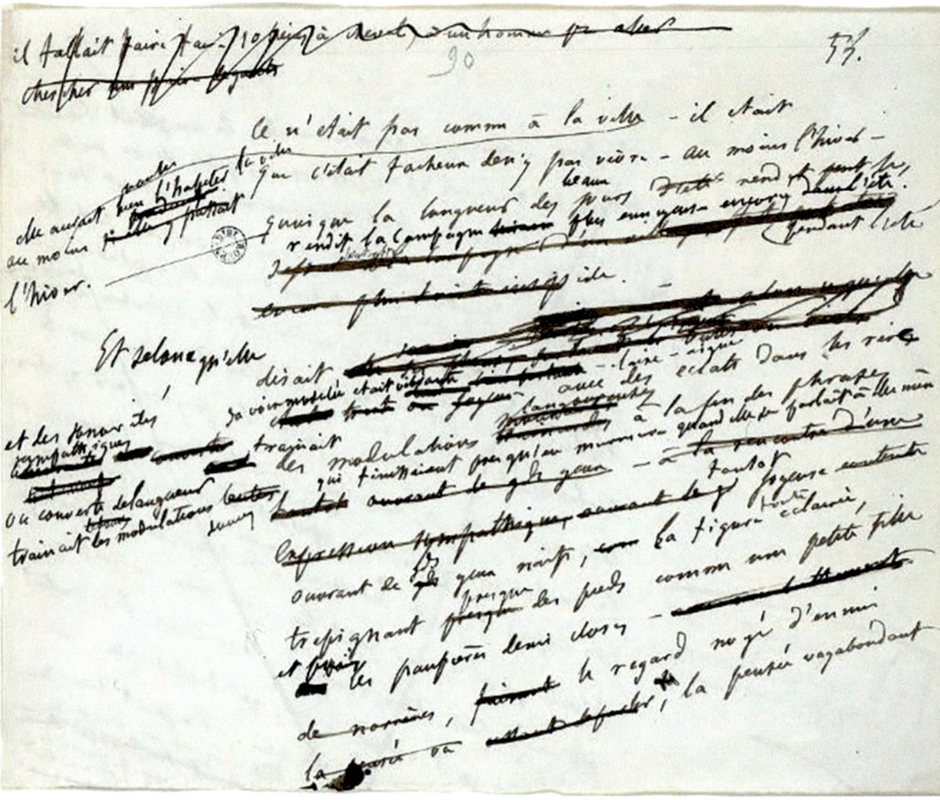

Figure 17 Gustave Flaubert, *Madame Bovary*, MS excerpt. The author lamented over the waste of paper caused by so many cancelled passages as every sentence had to be as it were torn from him. Endless toil may thus be concealed behind masterpieces that do not in themselves show as much as a trace of the effort that creative endeavour entails.

epilepsy, which was of a rare kind that causes a vexatious, to an author almost unbearable, difficulty in finding the right words. Hence, the deletions in his manuscripts occupy more space than the retained text (see Figure 17).

Flaubert's successful struggle against his difficulties forms a beautiful illustration of the way in which the summit of artistic ability, the art of handling words, paints, and tones without noticeable effort, is achieved by those who had to labour harder than others to acquire the requisite technical skills, or those who were hindered by illness. Kant knew that from his own experience, arguing that a human being may achieve incredible things through willpower even while suffering, and that suffering might in fact be the only means of obtaining that height of willpower.[37]

pas mûre'; quoted from *Lettres choisies de Gustave Flaubert*, collected and introduced by René Dumesnil (Paris: Jacques et René Wittmann, 1947), p. 61.

37 The exact source of this assertion could not be found.

When the author Robert McCrum, still a young man, was afflicted by a stroke resulting in right-side paralysis, he decided to keep a diary. With the aid of that diary, he succeeded – despite the split between speech and writing – in finding the right words in *My Year Off* to describe his new, humiliating experiences: 'being an incontinent carcass, quite unable to make any sense of his body'.[38] The continuous recording of his self-observations gave him a good insight into the ways in which his mental and spiritual existence developed following the stroke: 'I eagerly monitored the tiny external changes that constitute convalescence – my confidence, however, remained shot to pieces.'[39]

The French writer Jean-Dominique Bauby's self-confidence was not shattered; rather, it was in fact reinforced when he survived and acquired control over the disastrous situation created by a stroke followed by virtually total paralysis. The sole mobility that remained to him was located in his right eyelid, maybe so as to invest him with the possibility of winking at us with a feeling of pride in his willpower, which would have impressed Kant as well as us (see pp. 157–158).

In emotional terms, Bauby describes his immense disappointment when, after his return to consciousness, his hope of soon being able to regain his powers was dashed; and it was to take a long time before he could obtain nourishment without a feeding tube and breathe without a respirator. Bauby discovered a convincing metaphor for his utter isolation: he felt as if shut into a diving-bell or a bell jar, experiencing a case of 'locked-in syndrome', as the medical term has it. But his thought was a butterfly in free flight, and in the end it would help him escape. With the aid of a skilful speech therapist, and utilising the only remaining mobility he had, he invented a system of communication. The letters of the alphabet were numbered, and when the succession of numbers was read out to him, he was able to designate the letter he wanted. In that way, he was able to combine them into words and sentences. Finally, in the only book ever written with an eyelid, *The Diving-bell and the Butterfly*, he was able to describe the difficulties of the body and the strength of the soul.

Bauby presents an account of the nightmarish sensation of having his clothes roughly pulled over his inert limbs, as heavy as lead and now merely a source of torment, while the saliva gushed forth from his mouth. Occasionally he would break down in despair, as when suffering a wave of grief over his inability to tousle the hair of his small son, sitting there so quietly, and to embrace his soft little body. Strength suddenly abandoning him, tears would course down his cheeks, and his pharynx would emit a wheeze which caused the child to wince.[40] Bauby conducted a comprehensive correspondence with

38 Robert McCrum, *My Year Off* (New York: W. W. Norton, 1998), p. 10.

39 Ibid., p. 71.

40 See Jean-Dominique Bauby, *The Diving-bell and the Butterfly* (London: Harper Perennial, 2008), p. 79. The original French version may be read in Jean-Dominique Bauby, *Le Scaphandre et le papillon* (Paris: Robert Laffont, 1997), p. 77.

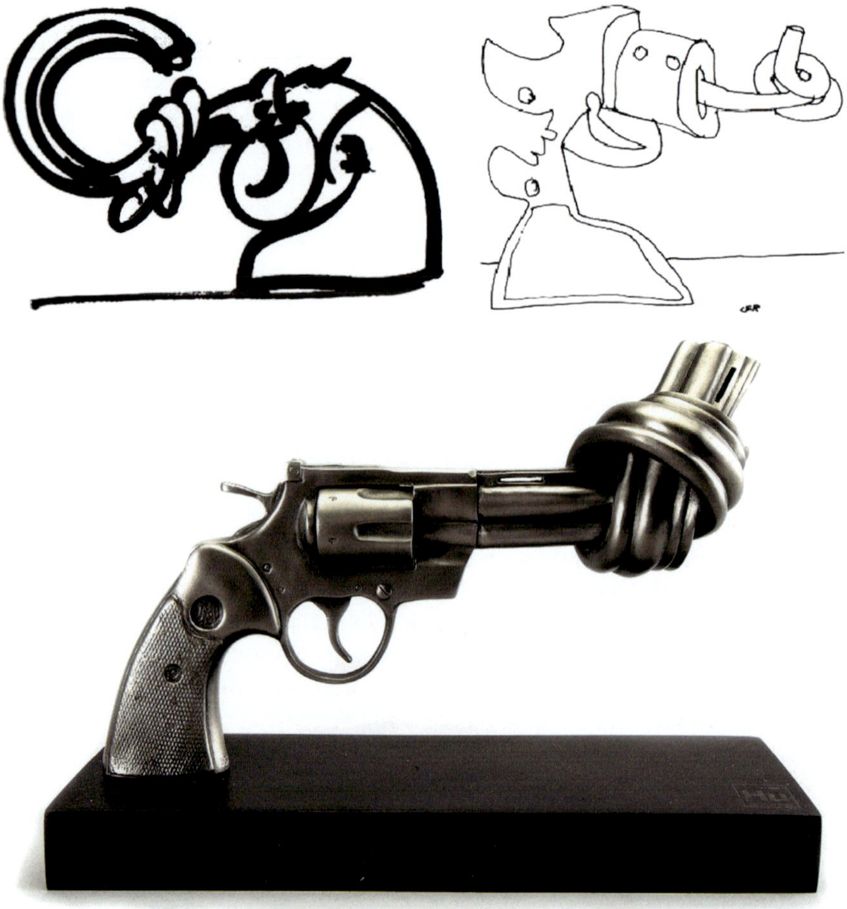

Figure 18–20 C. F. Reutersward, 'Non-violence', a sculpture for the United Nations building in New York. The drawings testify to the skill of the right hand before the stroke (above left) and the playfulness of the left hand after it (above right). A reproduction of the sculpture is seen underneath.

many people eager to be in contact with an outstanding personality for the mutual exchange of thoughts and experiences. The butterfly had found a way out of the diving-bell – an incredible achievement which breeds profound respect for human willpower and intellectual capacity.

Lovis Corinth painted his best pictures with a hand that trembled after apoplexy. Another impressive example is supplied by the Swedish artist Carl Fredrik Reutersward, who was also afflicted by a stroke at the height of his powers, suffering paralysis to the right half of his body and the loss of both the ability to speak and his skill as a draughtsman. Speech therapy enabled him to learn to speak again; but the fact that he regained his artistic capacities is entirely due to his own efforts. With exceptional willpower and creative zest, he forced his unpractised left hand to work for him. The former virtuoso, who had been so sure of his ability, suddenly had to fumble in pursuit of a fleeting line; however, that line was enlivened by a fresh vitality. As Reuterswärd's creative genius was transferred from the intellectually dominated left half of the brain to virgin territory in the emotionally dominated right hemisphere, his personality changed: the penetrating sarcasms and witty eloquence were replaced by a playful, kind-hearted simplicity. In a renaissance of creativity, he began to create original left-hand drawings.

Reuterswärd's new personality is apparent in a series of sketches for the 'knotted gun' – his famous sculpture named 'Non-violence', which stands in front of the United Nations building in New York. Before his stroke, the lethal weapon had been put out of action by means of firm, vigorous lines; afterwards it looks more like an amusing doodle, a toy pistol which was never intended to kill anyone. 'You're mistaken', says the artist; 'there's still a resolute significance behind those playful lines.' He is trying to persuade us that crude violence is best counteracted with warm humour and irony.

Creative difficulties may be self-imposed. Demosthenes put pebbles in his mouth when practising oratory, and in our own time Samuel Beckett wrote *Waiting for Godot* and many of his other works first in French, sharpening his attentiveness by means of employing a foreign language. Degas despised the facile performance of the ignoramus, saying that the art of painting is a simple thing before one knows how, but hard once one has learnt it.[41]

George Sand tells the story of how inspiration could come over Chopin quite unexpectedly. During a walk, for instance, a piece of music might suddenly pop into his head, and he had to hurry home in order to get the musical idea down on paper. A downright heartbreaking activity might ensue, according to Sand; the composer might shut himself into his room for days, sometimes in tears, walking back and forth across the floor, breaking his pen into pieces, altering a bar hundreds of times, cancelling it, writing it out again, and struggling with a single page with desperate pertinacity. In the end, he might decide to stay with the original draft.[42]

***

An artwork is both art and a work, art revealed through invisible labour; at least that is what the artist attempts to make spectators believe.[43] Although cultural masterpieces are often conceived in transports of passion and sometimes created in a feeling of profound joy, they are hence usually born in pain after hard labour. John Kenneth Galbraith expressed the contrast as follows: 'All writers know that on some mornings they are touched by the wand – are on intimate terms with poetry and cosmic truth. I have

41 This view has very often been attributed to Degas, but it has not been possible to identify the actual source.

42 George Sand, *Story of My Life: The Autobiography of George Sand: A Group Translation*, ed. by Thelma Jurgrau (Albany: State University Press of New York, 1991), p. 1108.

43 Cf. what is said about Flaubert above.

experienced those moments myself. Their lesson is simple: It's total illusion. And the danger in the illusion is that you will wait for those moments. Such is the horror of having to face the typewriter that you will spend all your time waiting.'[44] Not many authors join Susan Sontag in enjoying the final stage of writing: 'For three years I worked twelve hours a day in a delirium of pleasure.'[45]

Hard work alone is not enough, however. Artists who lose their drive and creative power run dry, falling into repetition and mannerism. Instead of singing new tunes like blackbirds, they keep repeating the same old melody like cuckoos or doves with embarrassing monotony, and their works degenerate into soulless items smelling of mediocrity.

It remains a mystery why a certain artist's works may stir our innermost being while another's leave us cold and unmoved. Plato says that '[i]f any man come to the gates of poetry without the madness of the Muses, persuaded that skill alone will make him a good poet, then shall he and his works of sanity with him be brought to naught by the poetry of madness, and behold, their place is nowhere to be found.'[46] I venture to adduce F. Scott Fitzgerald after *The Great Gatsby* and Chirico after his surrealist period as examples. These artists resemble the lilacs in a Swedish poem, which 'blossom briefly and spend a long time wilting'.[47] Conversely, others who never lacked inspiration – for instance Milton, Titian, and Verdi – recall some words from Anacreon's fifty-fifth Ode, according to which the pleasing old age of the roses retains the fragrance of youth.

There are many poignant expressions for the deep despondency that artistic sterility produces, often aggravated by painful pangs of conscience over the mechanical reiteration of ideas which have been expressed before, and better. The outcome may be long periods of inactivity. George Gissing supplies a heart-rending account in *New Grub Street*. This vocational illness, a state of frozen impotence entirely opposed to the fever of eager creativity, may sometimes be temporary and transient, sometimes tragically incurable.

Not even such a richly gifted author as Joseph Conrad was unaffected. On one occasion, he laments that 'the work of the last three months makes a miserable show – as to the quantity. And I have sat and sat days and days – It is an impossible existence ... There are moments when I think against my will that I must give up.'[48]

Herman Melville had to give up for good. He was one of those authors who are entirely dependent on their own experiences for their writing and who therefore ultimately run out of material. Having crowned his stories

44 'Writing, typing & economics', *The Atlantic*, March 1978, 103.

45 Leslie Garis, 'Susan Sontag finds romance', *New York Times*, 2 August 1992.

46 Plato, *Phaedrus*, trans. by R. Hackforth (Cambridge: Cambridge University Press, 1952), p. 57.

47 'Syrener' ('Lilacs') by Edvard Bäckström, from *Lyriska dikter* of 1895.

48 From a letter to John Galsworthy, 6 January 1908, in *The Collected Letters of Joseph Conrad, Volume 4: 1908–1911*, ed. by Frederick A. Karl and Laurence Davies (Cambridge: Cambridge University Press, 1990), p. 10.

from the sea with *Moby-Dick*, he had also depleted the last remnants of his artistic capital, his seafaring years. In a letter to Nathaniel Hawthorne he mourns his consumed treasure, saying that he feels he has 'come to the inmost leaf of the bulb, and that shortly the flower must fall to the mould';[49] somewhat later, he tells the same friend that he 'had "pretty much made up his mind to be annihilated"'.[50] While his creativity was ebbing, there came a final tidal wave which carried Billy Budd ashore. In this novella, honoured with an opera by Benjamin Britten, Melville paints a marine background for a gruesome story about the never-ending struggle between good and evil.

49 *The Letters of Herman Melville* (New Haven: Yale University Press, 1960), p. 130.
50 Entry for 20 November 1856 in Nathaniel Hawthorne, *The English Notebooks*, ed. by Randall Stewart (New York: Russell & Russell, 1962), p. 432.

Chapter 3
Artificial stimulation of creativity

Owen Glendower: I can call spirits from the vasty deep.
Hotspur: Why, so can I, or so can any man;
But will they come when you do call for them?
William Shakespeare, *Henry IV*, Part 1, III.1.50–52

It is easy to understand that artists desire to restore freshness to the wilting flower, trying to maintain waning inspiration by means of artificial stimulation. The recipe utilised by the Swiss artist Henry Fuseli (Johann Heinrich Füssli) seems innocuous enough; he is said to have been in the habit of eating raw meat in the evening as a way of engendering fantastic dreams which he would then reproduce in peculiar images.

The means employed by Friedrich Schiller was even more harmless; it was the smell of rotting apples, which would transport him into a mood of reverie. Consequently, he always kept a supply of such apples in a desk drawer. That was not always sufficient, though; Goethe claimed that he was able to distinguish those pieces that the poet had composed when tipsy. Even so, Schiller never became an alcoholic, as so many other great spirits have done. It is too bad that we cannot interrogate Goethe over his observations; were those pieces innovative creations, or had the alcohol merely had a deleterious effect on emerging work? The Swedish writer Marika Stiernstedt, who sought refuge in alcohol during a period of overwork and anxiety, later found it easy to trace those sections that had come into being under the influence of drink: they were definitely of inferior quality.[1]

Poets, artists, and composers use alcohol for the same reasons as the rest of us – to stimulate our thoughts and feelings; to reduce tension ahead of major efforts; 'recreational drinking'; and to ease the inhibitions that hold us ordinary people back from living life to the full and prevent creative spirits from giving free rein to their imagination. As Thomas Moore's translation of one of Anacreon's Odes summarises, with evident glee,

If with water you fill up your glasses
You'll never write any thing wise;

1 Marika Stiernstedt, 'Utgående från gamla farbror Jacques', in *En bok om rus och inspiration*, published by the Swedish Writers' Union (*Vintergatan* 1948), pp. 195–207 (Stockholm: Norstedts, 1948).

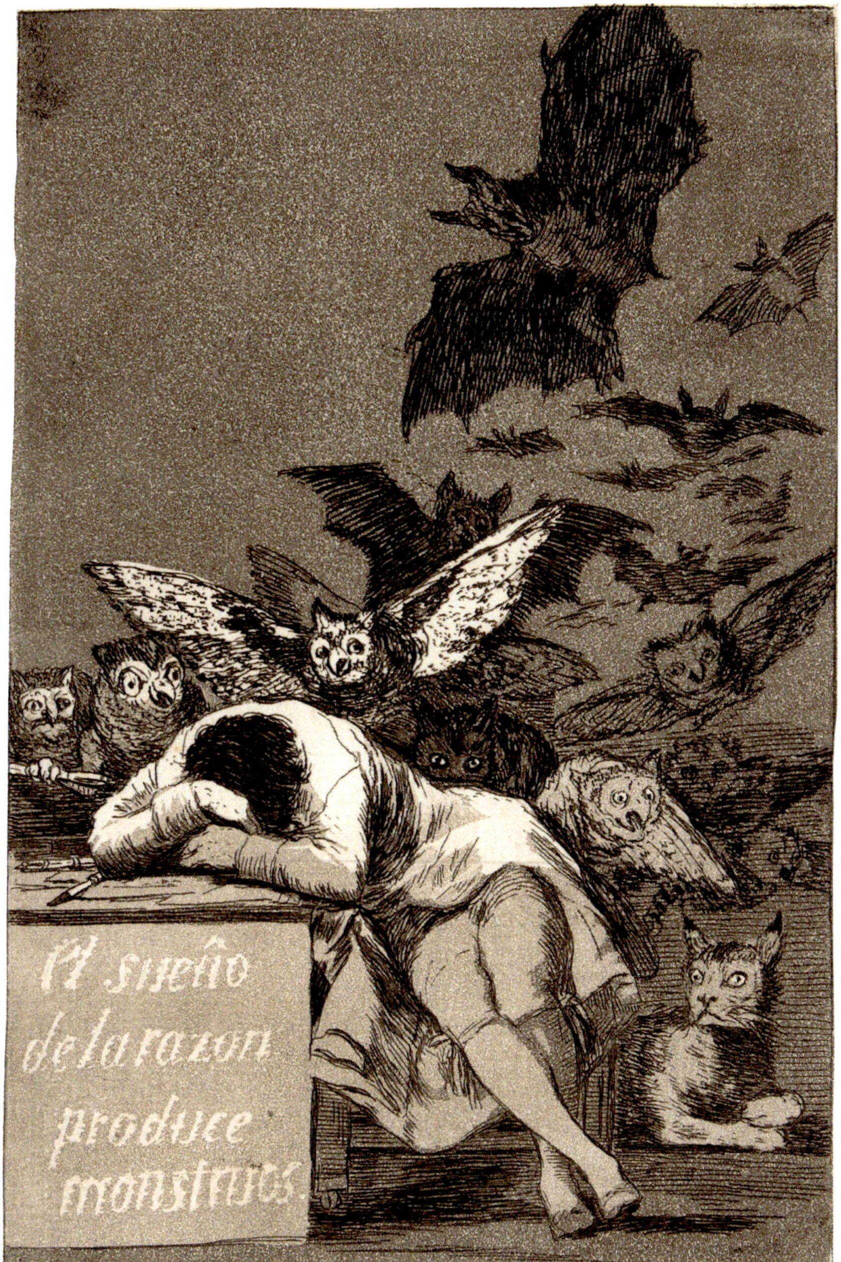

Figure 21 Francisco de Goya, 'El sueno de la razón produce monstruos'. Goya was in a position to testify that the monsters wake up when reason sleeps.

For wine is the horse of Parnassus,
Which hurries a bard to the skies![2]

Like other drugs, alcohol imparts a peculiar, sometimes schizophrenic character to works of art, producing fantastic images and verbal or visual excesses. William Styron, for instance, wrote that he used alcohol, 'often in conjunction with music', as 'a means to let my mind conceive visions that the unaltered, sober brain has no access to'.[3]

Maybe it was alcohol that stimulated James Joyce into making surprising linguistic innovations. Abuse of it ruined his health; but self-discipline enabled him to go on writing – he would never drink until after sunset. In *Dubliners*, on the basis of half-hearted and never completed medical studies, Joyce was able to supply an expert account of that alcoholism with which he was only too familiar. Robert Schumann observed that alcohol in combination with coffee and strong cigars 'would heighten and intensify the auditory sensations which often became the basis of his compositions',[4] and strong coffee was the fuel of Balzac's novelistic machinery.

A particular therapeutic effect of alcohol is that it assuages the depression of manic depressives as well as the anxiety of schizophrenics, thereby tending to encourage over-indulgence. The kindling of creative fire it produces exacts a high price later on, when ashes begin to cover the glowing embers: like all nerve poisons, alcohol damages mental activity in the long term. The category of authors supplies a depressingly large number of examples. The creative ability of Tennessee Williams degenerated from the powerful, original plays of his healthy middle age to the dark and feeble ones written during the last decades of his life, when alcohol abuse imparted a crazed and immoderate character both to the man and to his works. Similarly, Gustave Courbet's artistic vigour is seen to weaken from the monumental works of his mature period to the Swiss pictures of his old age.

Under the influence of wine, young Maurice Utrillo painted exquisite pictures of Paris with subtle nuances in white, greys, and greens. It has been recounted that members of his family would leave him alone with a bottle of wine and a fresh canvas and then come back to collect an empty bottle and an inebriated artist – but also a beautiful painting. As Utrillo became increasingly dependent on alcohol, his creative powers declined and his fine sensibility grew coarse, as is evident in his late works with their facile, garish effects and clumsy execution.

Attacks of *delirium tremens* during the terminal stages of alcoholism, with raging fears and horrible hallucinations, would seem to be a disgracefully high price to pay for past pleasures. Paradoxically, a new dose of the poison takes the edge off the attack. In desperate need of a drink, Malcolm

2 *The Odes of Anacreon*, trans. by Thomas Moore, 8th edn, 2 vols (London: James Carpenter, 1810), Vol. 2, p. 43.

3 William Styron, *Darkness Visible* (New York: Random House, 1990), p. 40.

4 John O'Shea, *Music and Medicine: Medical Profiles of the Great Composers* (London: Dent, 1990), p. 137 in the paperback edition of 1993.

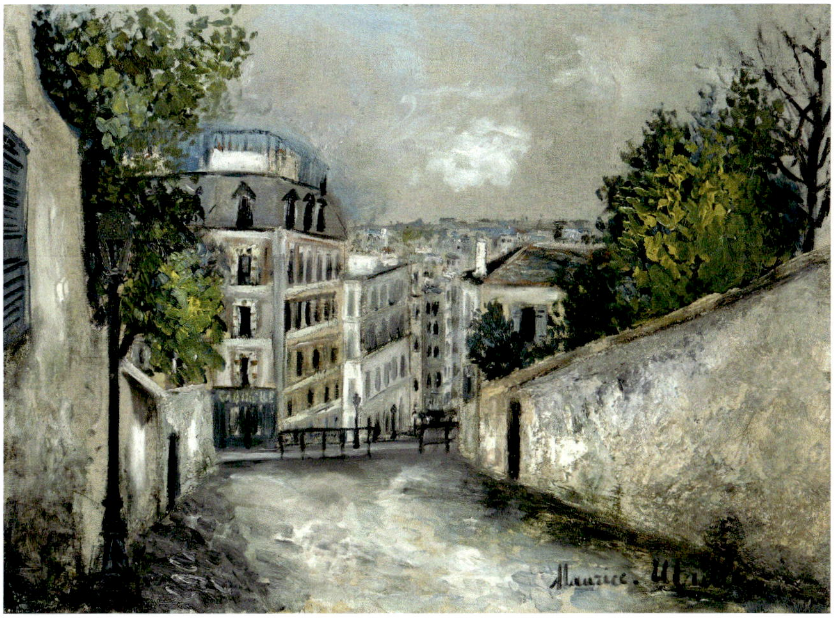

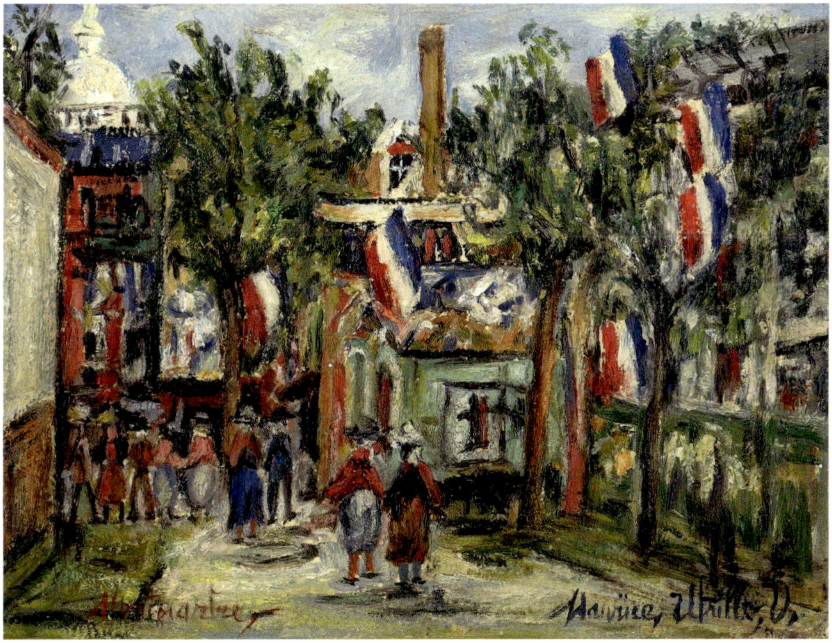

Figures 22 and 23 Maurice Utrillo; above: 'Rue du Mont-Cenis à Montmartre', approx. 1914; below: 'Le 14 juillet à Montmartre', c. 1948. A slight scent of alcohol does not noticeably vitiate the subtly rendered Paris atmosphere of the early work. Forty years later, wine and liquor have moved into the foreground. (The continuous change in aesthetic convention is evident from the fact that some of my young friends prefer this late, awkward painting because of its more expressive approach as compared to the artistic refinement of the early version.)

Lowry suffered hallucinations imbued with surrealism; he described how he saw a huge scorpion solemnly raping a black one-armed woman on a blood-stained bed, and, when his tearful wife appeared and pitied him, she was suddenly transformed into Richard III who sprang forward to smother him.[5]

***

In the nineteenth century, apart from alcohol, the drug of choice was opium. It was especially used by poets in order to stimulate their imagination, make them forget external difficulties, and help them find relief from mental affliction. English Romanticism supplies a number of examples. Samuel Taylor Coleridge saw the palace of Kublai Khan in a vision and sang its praises 'in a sort of reverie brought on by two grains of opium':

> For he on honey-dew hath fed,
> And drunk the milk of Paradise.[6]

John Keats also tried the drug:

> My heart aches, and a drowsy numbness pains
> My sense, as though of hemlock I had drunk,
> Or emptied some dull opiate to the drains
> One minute past, and Lethe-wards had sunk ...[7]

He soon desisted, finding that opium blunted his senses:

> No, no, go not to Lethe, neither twist
> Wolf's-bane, tight-rooted, for its poisonous wine;
> Nor suffer thy pale forehead to be kiss'd
> By nightshade, ruby grape of Proserpine ...
> ...
> For shade to shade will come too drowsily,
> And drown the wakeful anguish of the soul.[8]

Our great Romantic Swedish poet Erik Johan Stagnelius also used opium, and it gave him peace and blissful dreams:

> Kindly night, you are returning again from the land of shades.
> Silence walks beside you, and sleep [wears] a wreath of poppies.[9]

In the mysterious twilight between reality and dreams, where a wreath of poppies is worn, Romantic music is also heard. In his *Symphonie Fantastique*, Hector Berlioz lets an artist sink into a state of intoxication brought on by opium, a state in which he experiences his suffering and his ecstasy in musical

---

5 Malcolm Lowry, *Lunar Caustic*, in *Hear Us O Lord from Heaven Thy Dwelling Place* and *Lunar Caustic* (Harmondsworth: Penguin, 1979 [1963]), p. 299.

6 The last two lines of Coleridge's poem 'Kubla Khan'. The words about opium are quoted from a note written on a manuscript copy of the poem.

7 The first four lines of Keats's 'Ode to a Nightingale'.

8 The first and last lines of the first stanza of Keats's 'Ode on Melancholy'.

9 Lines 2 and 3 from Stagnelius's poem 'Till natten' ('To night').

images. The sentimental programme which Berlioz drew up for his music could have been conceived by one of the Romantic poets: a young composer of delicate sensitivity and passionate imagination has poisoned himself with opium in despair over unrequited love. As the dose was not lethal, it just threw him into a long sleep accompanied by bizarre visions where the spiritualised beloved, like a fixed idea, returns over and over again in a rapturous melody.[10]

The symphony reflects Berlioz's hysterical disposition, which was expressed in his dramatic behaviour. When his beloved betrayed him, he had made advanced plans to shoot her and himself, disguised as a lady's maid – the pistols were already loaded! Having come to his senses again, he coolly commented, a born artist exploiting a truly personal experience: 'It would have been a fine scene. It really is a great pity it had to be dropped.'[11]

We know Berlioz occasionally took powerful medicines, probably containing narcotics, to dispel severe toothache; but there is no reason to suppose that he used drugs for the purpose of intoxication, as Thomas De Quincey did. This candid author of *Confessions of an English Opium Eater* (1821) became enslaved by the craving. As he was, in his own words, 'upon such a theme not simply the best, but surely the sole authority',[12] he was able to give us a masterly, deeply felt personal account of the delights of the addiction as well as of its agonies. He says – not in his defence, because the use of opium was very common at this time and regarded as an innocent pleasure – that it was not 'any search after pleasure, but mere extremity of pain'[13] that first attracted him to the use of opium. De Quincey himself states that his pain was caused by rheumatic toothache; but from his account we may conclude that he actually suffered from something worse, namely trigeminal neuralgia. This disorder is characterised by attacks of piercing facial pain of such severity that they sometimes drive the victim to suicide. Understandably, De Quincey 'began to use opium as an article of daily diet'.[14]

However, pain was not the main cause of his subsequent abuse; the chief reason for his addiction was his discovery of the effect that opium had on his mental and spiritual life. According to his own account, he once sought relief from his toothache by dipping his head in a basin with cold water. That was truly a desperate action, being an almost infallible way of provoking a neuralgic attack. 'The next morning, as I need hardly say, I awoke with

---

10 Robert Clarson-Leach, *Berlioz* (London: Omnibus, 1987), pp. 44–45. The original French version is found in Christian Wasselin, *Berlioz: les deux ailes de l'âme* (Paris: Gallimard, 2002), p. 114.

11 Hector Berlioz, *The Memoirs of Hector Berlioz*, trans. and ed. by David Cairns (London: Victor Gollancz, 1969), p. 185 in the 1970 Panther edition.

12 Page 15 in the Wordsworth Classics edition of De Quincey's *Confessions* (Ware: Wordsworth, 1993 and 2009).

13 Ibid.

14 Thomas De Quincey, *Confessions of an English Opium-Eater and Other Writings*, ed. by Barry Milligan (London: Penguin, 2003), p. 9. (There are different editions of De Quincey's *Confessions*; this reference is from an edition based on the original of 1821.)

excruciating ... pains ... – from which I had hardly any respite for about twenty days. On the twenty-first day ... – I went out into the streets; rather to run away, if possible, from my torments, than with any distinct purpose of relief. By accident, I met a college acquaintance, who recommended opium. Opium! dread agent of unimaginable pleasure and pain! I had heard of it as I had heard of manna or of ambrosia, but no further.'[15]

De Quincey certainly manages to give us such a gloomy background to his discovery that we can easily understand what an overwhelming experience it turned out to be: 'It was a Sunday afternoon, wet and cheerless; and a duller spectacle this earth of ours has not to show than a rainy Sunday in London. ... [On] my road homewards ... – I saw a druggist's shop, where ... I asked for the tincture of opium. ... Arrived at my lodgings ... I lost not a moment in taking the quantity prescribed ... – and in an hour, O heavens! what a revulsion! what a resurrection, from its lowest depths of the inner spirit! what an apocalypse of the world within me. That my pains had vanished was now a trifle in my eyes; this negative effect was swallowed up in the immensity of those positive effects which had opened before me, in the abyss of divine enjoyment thus suddenly revealed. Here was a panacea ... for all human woes; here was the secret of happiness, about which philosophers had disputed for so many ages, at once discovered; happiness might now be bought for a penny, and carried in the waistcoat-pocket; portable ecstasies might be had corked up in a pint-bottle.'[16]

But poor De Quincey soon found that divine joy does not last for ever. His blissful dreams changed into horrific nightmares, which coerced 'suspiria-de-profundis' – sighs from the abyss. His sense of space and ultimately also his sense of time were badly shaken; space swelled and was amplified to an infinite extent. 'This disturbed me very much less than the vast expansion of time. I sometimes had feelings representative of a duration far beyond the limits of any human experience.'[17] He thus acquired a rare, tangible sense of the relativity of space and time. But it came at a high cost: '[These] changes in my dreams were accompanied by deep-seated anxiety and funereal melancholy ... I seemed every night to descend – not metaphorically, but literally to descend – into chasms and sunless abysses, depths below depths, from which it seemed hopeless that I could ever re-ascend. ... The state of gloom which attended these gorgeous spectacles, amounting at last to utter darkness ... cannot be approached by words.'[18]

It has, however, been described in pictures, almost down to the last detail, in the magnificent engravings of Piranesi. His 'Carceri d'Invenzione' engenders the same feeling of despairing hopelessness. In huge mysterious

15 Ibid., p. 140 in the Wordsworth edition mentioned in n. 12 and p. 42 in the Penguin edition mentioned in the preceding note. There are small variations between the two editions regarding this passage.

16 Ibid., pp. 140–142 in the Wordsworth edition; the passage occurs, with small but significant changes, on pp. 43 and 44 in the Penguin edition.

17 Ibid., p. 185 in the Wordsworth edition and p. 76 in the Penguin.

18 Ibid., p. 185 in the Wordsworth edition and p. 76 in the Penguin.

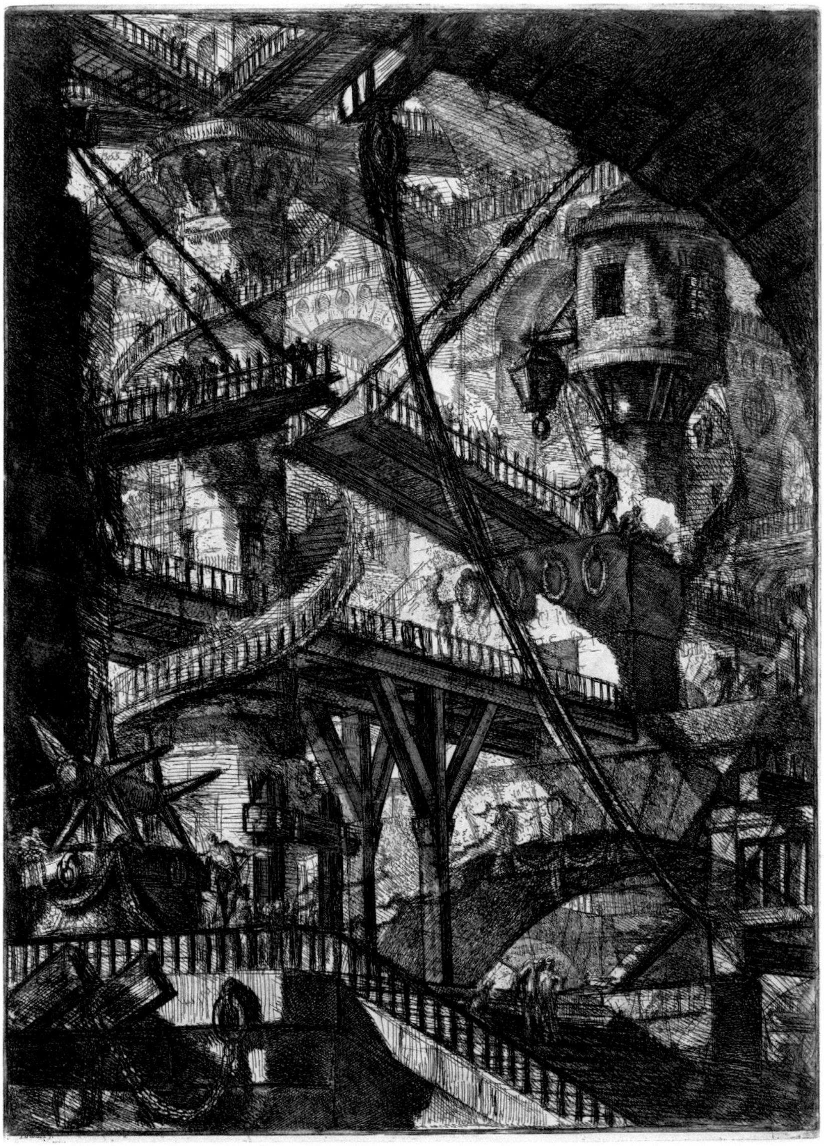

Figure 24 Giovanni Battista Piranesi, 'Carceri d'Invenzione VI', 1745. An imagined prison conveys a feeling of claustrophobia and despairing hopelessness.

buildings with fantastic architecture, small figures lose their way on endless flights of steps and staircases which lead nowhere, except on some occasions when they end abruptly before black chasms. The similarity of expression between these images and De Quincey's narrative is no coincidence; Coleridge once described these fantasy gaols to him in such detail that we can easily identify the relevant engraving.

The similarities have a more profound basis, however, and one that suggests that there is an alignment between states of depression caused by drug abuse and such as originate in other factors. De Quincey is sure to have recognised his own 'deep-seated anxiety and funereal melancholy' in the morose personality that created these pictorial 'suspiria de profundis'. He assumed that they must have been brought on by feverish fantasies, but they are more likely to be associated with a genuine manic-depressive disposition. According to a French scholar in the early twentieth century, Piranesi dwelled on these prisons with such exuberance and frenzy that we must look for their origin in the deepest sources of his nature, in the sombre passion which penetrates his personal life.[19]

Piranesi was extremely irascible, and heated quarrels with his comrades would sometimes lead to blows. On one occasion, he even threatened to kill a doctor who had in his opinion neglected the care of his dying child. In between such episodes, he withdrew in sullen solitude, himself shouting to visitors that Piranesi was unavailable. In his youth, he was attracted to dramatic and cheerless spectacles; for instance, he refrained from studying models in the academy of art, preferring to observe the sick and disabled persons who displayed their misery in Italian churches.

The lugubrious and magnificent imagination which devised the mature and perfected later edition of the 'Carceri', with the most powerful engravings ever made, was obviously that of a depressive.[20] They contain morbid details reminiscent of Meryon's schizophrenic etchings (see Figures 36 and 37). Victor Hugo spoke of Piranesi's 'dark brain' with good reason. The terrifying effect is enhanced by the fact that the mysterious and fantastic architecture is so rational – the endless staircases are solidly constructed and the instruments of torture technically impeccable.

That is the same kind of horror that Edgar Allan Poe allegedly experienced during opium-induced dreams. However, those dreams might have been mere inventions, put about by his enemies. If so, it is likely to have been episodes of alcoholic intoxication in combination with a manic-depressive disposition that opened the dark recesses of his complex mind – the mind that brought forth his fantastic tales, such as 'The Pit and the Pendulum'.[21]

During the last few days of his life, Poe lay unconscious in a hospital after having been found in a gutter, supposedly drunk. But as his symptoms, breathlessness and delirium with hallucinations, were combined with hydrophobia, he is more likely – though no animal bite has been mentioned – to have died of rabies, a more becoming cause of death than dipsomania.[22]

19 Henri Focillon, *Giovanni-Battista Piranesi 1720–1778* (Paris: Henri Laurens, 1918), p. 179.

20 Marguerite Yourcenar, 'Le Cerveau noir de Piranèse' in *Sous benefice d'inventaire* (Paris: Gallimard, 1962).

21 Cf. Carl Fehrman, *Diktaren och de skapande ögonblicken* (Stockholm: Norstedts, 1974), p. 97.

22 R. Michael Bernitez, 'A 39-year-old Man with Mental Status Change', *Maryland Medical Journal* 45.9 (1996), 765–769.

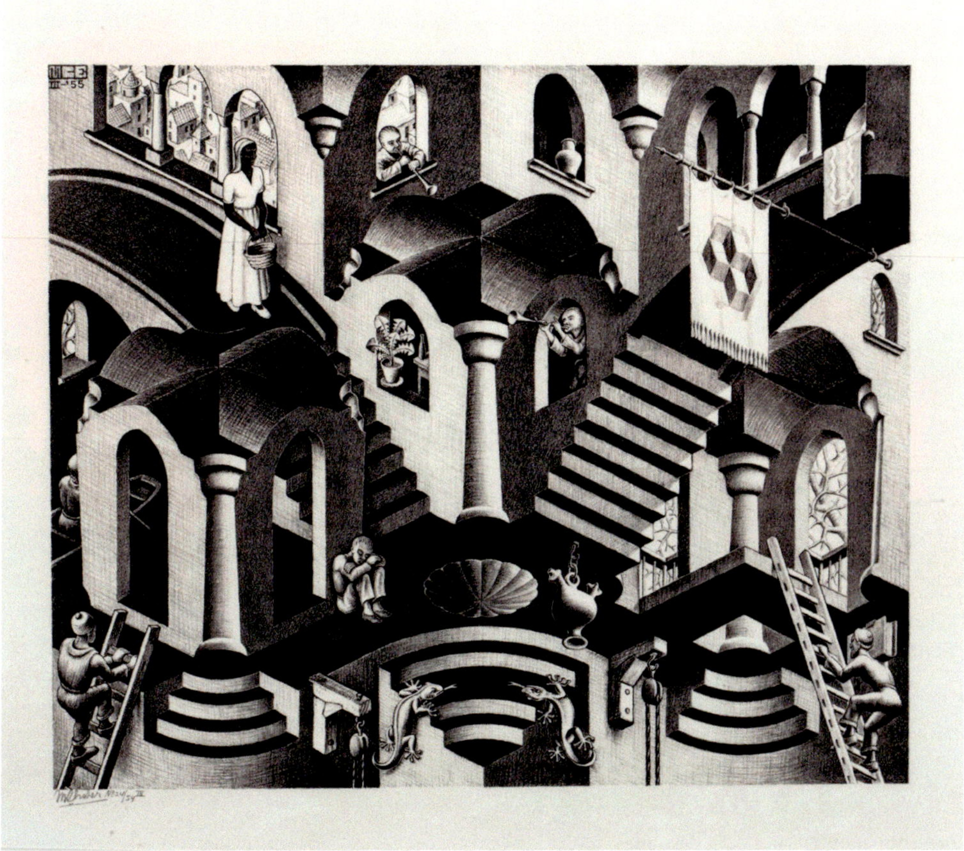

Figure 25 M. C. Escher, 'Hol en bol', 1955 (cropped). Absurd architecture.

The same sense of being lost in a defined space is evoked in M. C. Escher's frightening house, where the spectator's gaze soon loses its way irrespective of which direction it pursues and it is hard to tell what is in or out, up or down. This artist is an example of the fact that it is perfectly possible to create absurd art without being mentally ill. That he used the means at his disposal while clearly being of sound mind does not diminish the disturbing effect of his art.

The poet and artist Jean Cocteau is an opium abuser from our own time. He used the drug in order to restore a sense of balance, saying, 'I preferred an artificial equilibrium to no equilibrium at all'.[23] His self-portrait in *Journal d'une désintoxication* supplies a drastic account of the torment suffered during a detoxification cure, and of how his creative pursuits came

23 Jean Cocteau, *Opium: Journal d'une désintoxication* (Paris: Stock, Delamain & Boutelleau, 1930), p. 18. This work exists in an English translation, *Opium: The Diary of a Cure* (London: Peter Owen, 1957), where the quoted sentence occurs on p. 20.

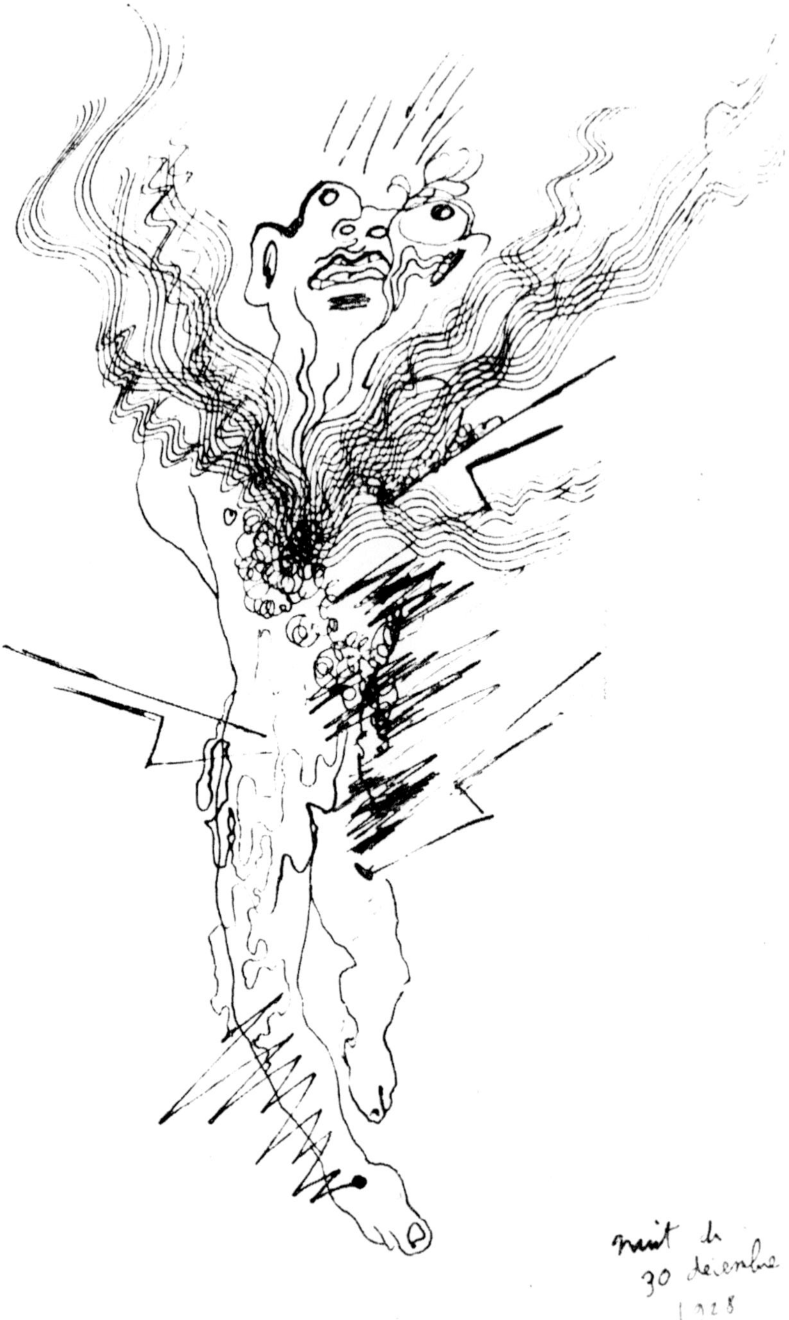

Figure 26 Jean Cocteau, 'Detoxification from opium', 1928. The agonies suffered during a cure.

to his aid: 'Sweat and bile precede some phantom substance which would have dissolved, leaving no other trace behind except a deep depression, if a fountain pen had not given it a direction, relief and shape.' 'After the cure. The worst moment, the worst danger. Health with this void and an immense sadness. The doctors honestly hand you over to suicide.'[24]

* * *

The intensely tragic interest in drugs other than opium and alcohol has also left its mark on the arts, where these agents have been tried in attempts to push the boundaries of human experience and shed light on thitherto impenetrable regions of the soul. In drug-induced hallucinations, a sharpening of the sensations is combined with a dissolution of their borders. Coloured visions may acquire a tactile dimension, and sounds may be perceived as colours. This synesthesia of perceptions yields essential information about the correlations between the different arts. Both Charles Baudelaire and Théophile Gautier, founders of the 'Club of Hashish-smokers' (Club des Hachichins), claimed to be able to hear the tones emitted by green, red, blue, and yellow colours. Gautier described strange experiences during hashish intoxication: it was, he said, as if he had been dissolved into nothing, so distant and liberated from his self – to which he referred as 'that disagreeable witness to everything we do that always haunts us' – that he had a clear conception of angels and souls liberated from the corporeal, something he had never felt before.[25]

Baudelaire experienced the same intensification of vitality, the sensation of being 'high'. In the course of hashish intoxication, he once drew a self-portrait which lends emphatic expression to a feeling of superiority – he is literally twice as tall as the Vendôme column in Paris. While sober, he suffered from disgust and a sense of emptiness, insisting that we must continually intoxicate ourselves – with wine, poetry, or even virtue, whatever we want – if we wish to escape the horrible burden of an existence which crushes our shoulders and presses us to the ground.[26]

24 The two sentences are quoted from the English translation, mentioned in the preceding note, where they occur in two distinct places, on pp. 139 and 93. The corresponding sentences are found on pp. 250 and 162 in the French original.

25 It appears that the text referred to was originally published as an article in *La Presse* on 10 July 1843 (see https://gallica.bnf.fr/ark:/12148/bpt6k4292749/f2.item.r=hachich); posthumously published in the collection *L'Orient*, 2 vols (Paris: G. Charpentier, 1877), pp. 52–53. An English translation by Maurice Stang was published in a book called *Hashish, Wine, Opium* (London: Calder & Boyars, 1972), the authors' names being given as Théophile Gautier and Charles Baudelaire; see p. 60.

26 Charles Baudelaire, 'Be Drunken' in *Poems in Prose from Charles Baudelaire*, trans. Arthur Symons (London: Elkin Mathews, 1913), p. 58. The French original version can be read in Charles Baudelaire, 'Enivrez-vous' in *Petits poems en Prose (Le spleen de Paris)*, ed. by Henri Lemaître (Paris: Editions Garnier Frères, 1962), p. 167.

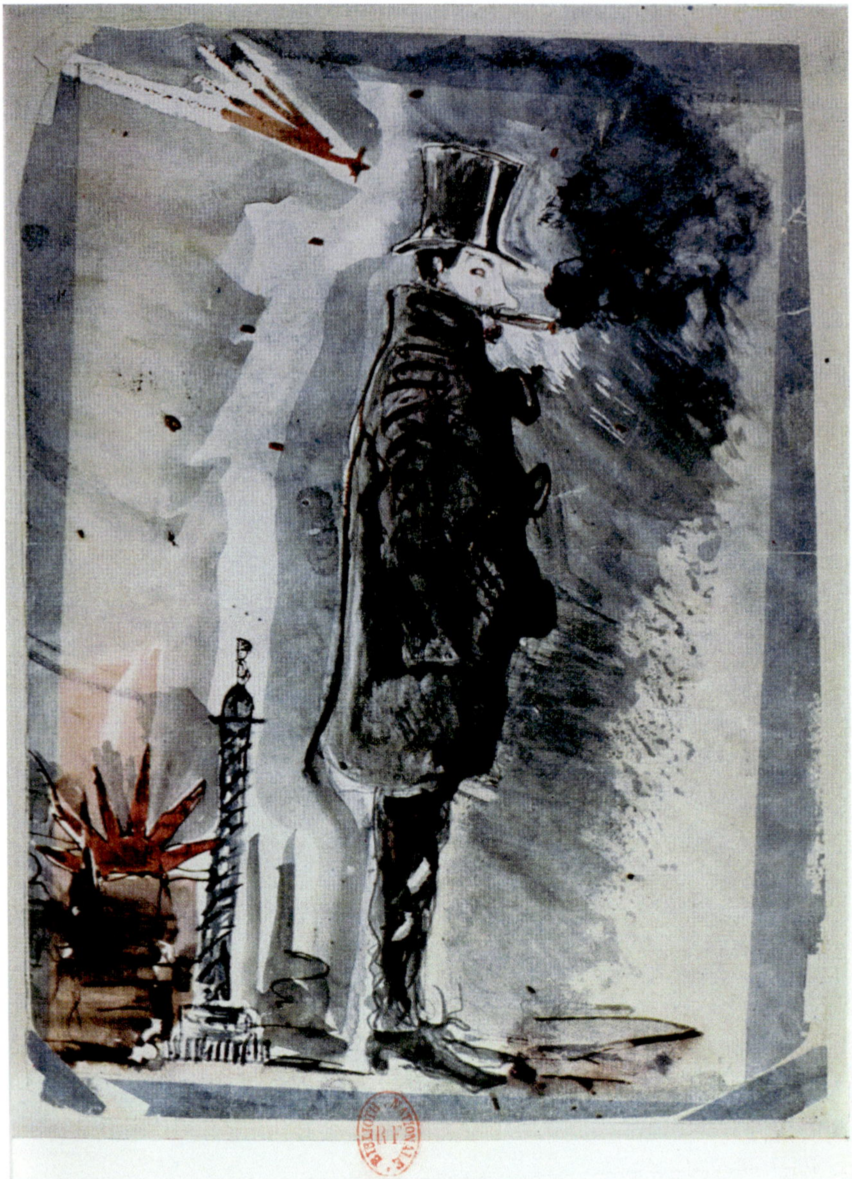

Figure 27 Charles Baudelaire, 'Self-portrait under the influence of hashish'. The artist feels 'high', even in comparison with the Vendôme column.

Under the influence of the powerful hallucinogen mescaline, our conception of things undergoes a peculiar change. To Aldous Huxley, experimenting with this drug was a revolutionary experience which transformed his view of human existence. While admitting that the sensation was verbally incommunicable, he eulogised it as ecstatically as De Quincey did his opium dreams: 'I was seeing what Adam had seen on the morning of his creation – the miracle, moment by moment of naked existence.' 'The flowers ... glowed ... with brighter colours' – 'shining with their own inner light and all but quivering under the pressure of the significance with which they were charged.'[27] Huxley's summary of the experience, in which 'visual impressions are greatly intensified and the eye recovers some of the perceptual innocence of childhood', recalls the great human geniuses' accounts of their heaven-sent moments of creation.[28] It is an experience that resembles the sensation caused by other drugs, but it is not exactly the same. While De Quincey was terrified by the tremendous extension of space, place and distance mattered little to Huxley; and his indifference to space was followed by an even greater indifference to time. A state wholly remote from human aims and ambitions, '[i]t just *is*', 'Being-Awareness-Bliss', '[a] gratuitous grace'. 'The glory and the wonder of pure existence belong to another order, beyond the power of even the highest art to express.'[29]

As is the case with most drugs, the return to everyday existence – so necessary to human life and relationships – is felt to constitute a deplorable surrender, and as such Gautier and Baudelaire have described it. In a similar frame of mind, and almost in the very same words, Huxley laments, 'Most men and women lead lives at the worst so painful, at the best so monotonous, poor and limited, that ... [there is an] urge to escape, ... [a] longing to transcend themselves if only for a few moments.'[30] In order to achieve that aim, Huxley prefers mescaline to other agents, alcohol included; and although he does not share Baudelaire's view that people should intoxicate themselves incessantly, he firmly recommends 'frequent chemical vacations from intolerable selfhood and repulsive surroundings' 'into the world of transcendental experience'.[31] Huxley seems to suggest that such excursions through what H. G. Wells called 'the door in the wall' benefit artists by making them intensely aware of inward and outward reality.

Although some of the changes in human consciousness that accompany mescaline resemble those that are caused by schizophrenia, Huxley did not see faces or human or animal figures. Such hallucinations, however, often occurred in the dreams of the painter and poet Henri Michaux as he drew pictures under the influence of mescaline. In his images, we see how the external world changes during intoxication and fills with frightening creatures. They are reminiscent of some etchings by Goya, who knew that monsters appear when reason sleeps (see Figure 21). There is an even greater resemblance between these mescaline drawings and the works of genuinely schizophrenic artists such as the Swede Carl Fredrik Hill, a resemblance which illustrates the close connection between mental illness and certain forms of intoxication.

27 Aldous Huxley, *The Doors of Perception* (London: Chatto & Windus, 1960), pp. 11, 13, and 12.
28 Ibid., p. 18.
29 Ibid., pp. 12, 58, and 26.
30 Ibid., p. 49.
31 Ibid., pp. 51 and 63.

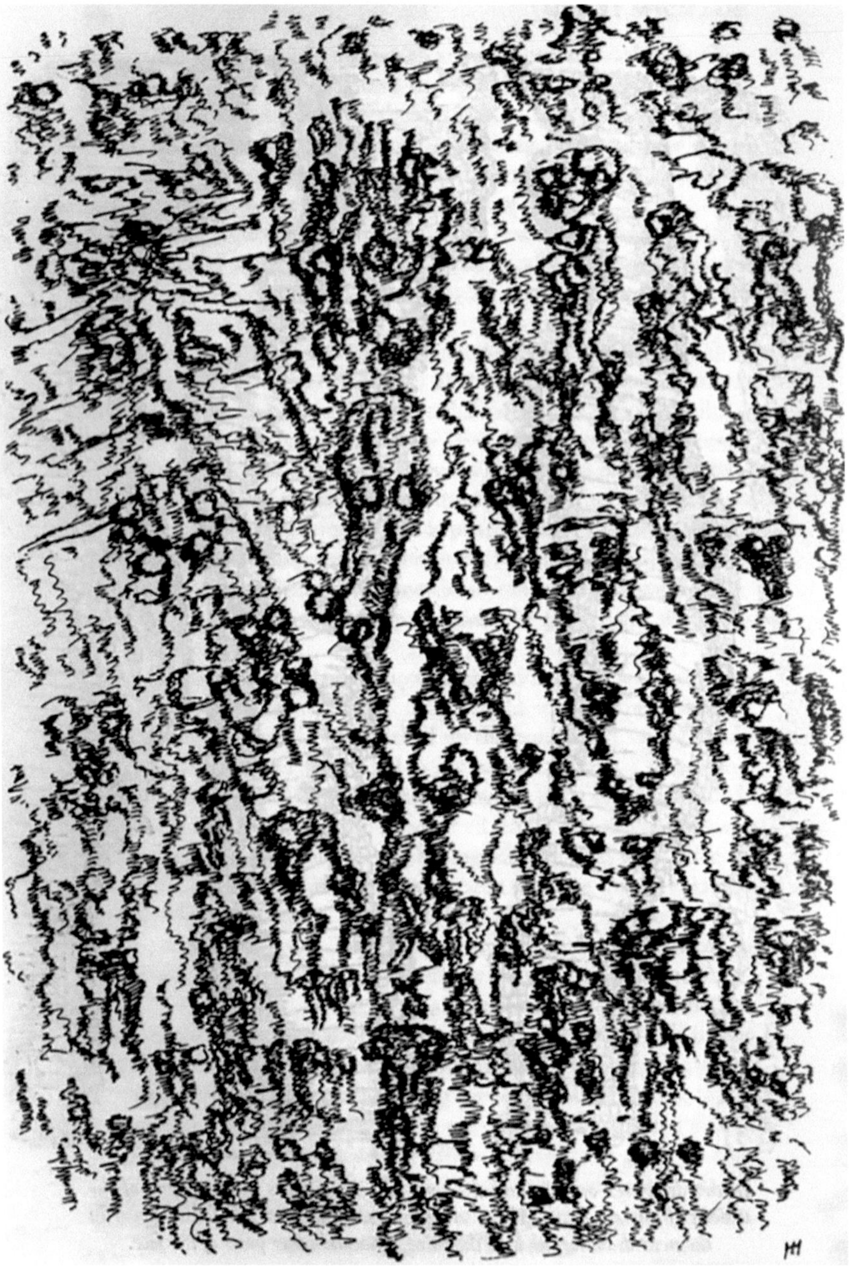

Figure 28 Henri Michaux, mescaline drawing. The world outside is filled with beasts. The endless repetition of signs, called perseveration, is a symptom of schizophrenia.

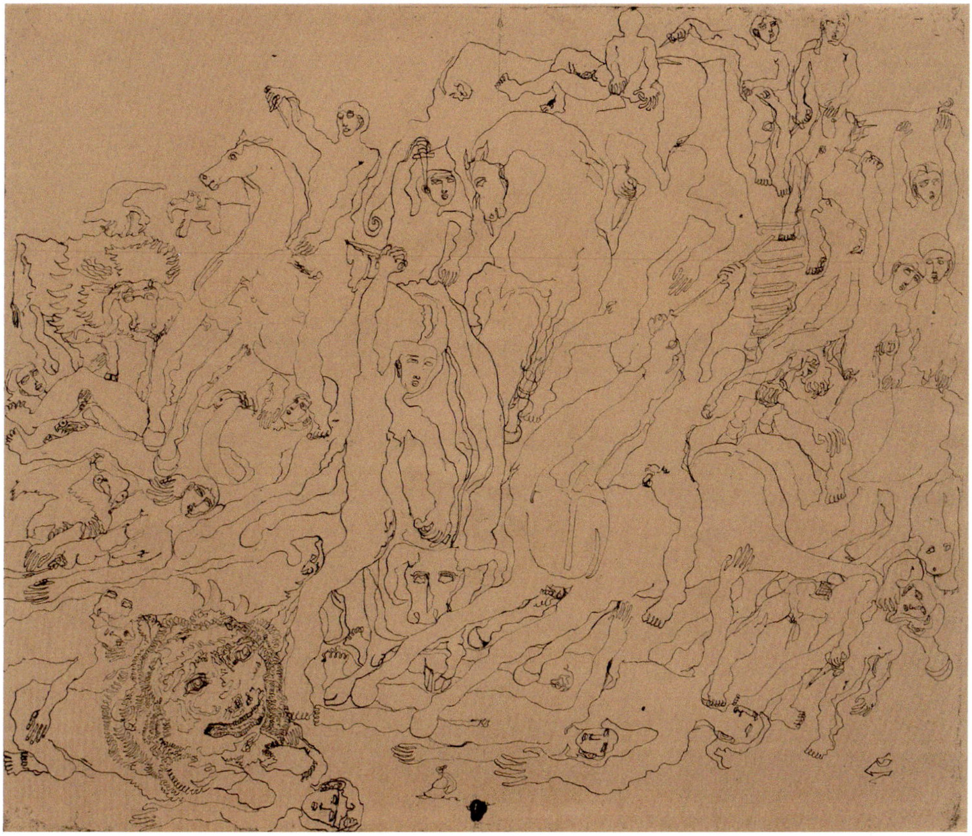

Figure 29 Carl Fredrik Hill, drawing from a period of illness. The monsters seen and reproduced by the schizophrenic artist are astonishingly similar to those drawn by Michaux while intoxicated by mescaline.

These artificial paradises, or rather infernos, form a natural transition to mental illnesses. There is an intermediary stage in a condition we have all experienced, namely the confusion engendered by a high fever as our cells are invaded by toxins which temporarily disturb the functioning of our minds. Aldous Huxley said that the only times when his mental images came to have independent life were when he had a high temperature.[32] Many artists have reproduced their feverish dreams in words or pictures; in 'Hospital Ward II', for instance, the Swedish painter Hilding Linnqvist gives vivid expression to the angst-filled atmosphere, smelling of carbolic acid, where physicians and nurses do their rounds seen as if in a dream. We are reminded of De Quincey's idea that Piranesi's fantastic prisons (Figure 24) must originate in the artist's visions during a spell of feverish delirium.

32 Ibid., p. 10.

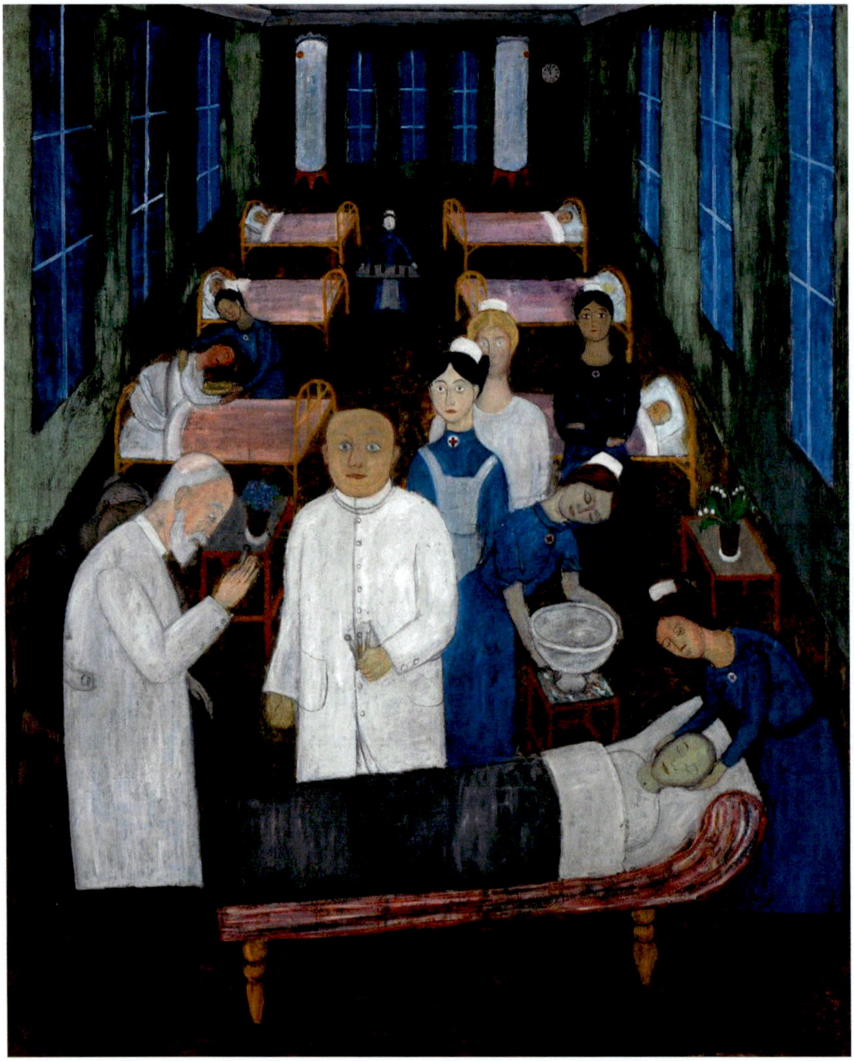

Figure 30 Hilding Linnqvist, 'Hospital Ward II'. The hospital ward is characterised by an atmosphere of anguish caused by illness and fever.

Chapter 4
Neuroses and psychosomatic disorders

Neuroses and psychosomatic disorders are of special interest in the present context, as they frequently have a powerful influence on artistic creation; indeed, they are sometimes the very cause of it. They vary a great deal with regard to their nature as well as their strength. In their mildest form, they may consist in unusual sensitivity to ordinary physical sensations. In their most pronounced manifestations, however, mental tensions may engender actual corporeal manifestations such as asthma. Being of a sensitive disposition, artists easily fall victim to this kind of illness.

The English seventeenth-century preacher and poet John Donne was a hypochondriac who asked himself whether there was a worse disease than the knowledge that we never are, or even can be, well.[1] During a severe illness, he observed the development of his symptoms, evincing great interest in the medical details.

Donne's writings, neglected for two hundred years, are now thought to be among the most beautiful and most expressive works in the English language. They contain an abundance of medical metaphors which derive from experiences during his childhood. His stepfather was a physician, and the boy would occasionally play in the autopsy room where he acquired knowledge of the anatomy, disorders, and degeneration of the human body. Donne spoke of a realm where the inhabitants themselves breed the worms that silently devour it, expressing his despondency in statements about the impossibility of looking in any direction, as misery and impending death cause such anguish.[2] He employed cynically medical terms in his criticism of society, too:

> My bowells are growne muddy, and mine eyes
> Are faint with weeping: and my liver lies
> Pour'd out upon the ground, for miserie
> That sucking children in the streets doe die.[3]

1 From 'An Anatomie of the World: The First Anniversary' in John Donne, *Poetical Works*, ed. Herbert Grierson (London: Oxford University Press, 1964 [1933]), lines 93–94, p. 210.

2 'Of the Progresse of the Soule: The Second Anniversary', lines 117–118, p. 230, and 'Holy Sonnets' No. I, p. 293 in the edition mentioned in note 1.

3 'The Lamentations of Jeremy, for the most part according to Tremelius', lines 129–132, p. 327 in the same edition.

His view of the world brightened, however, and he became an incomparable preacher: 'I have used [the] leisure [of convalescence] to put the meditations had in my sicknesse, into some such order, as may minister some holy delight.'[4]

In the sensitive and misanthropic Jonathan Swift, a mania for cleanliness was intensified into a compulsion, inspiring the aversion to the human body and its excretions that occurs in *Gulliver's Travels*: 'As soon as I entered the house, my wife took me in her arms, and kissed me, at which, having not been used to the touch of that odious animal for so many years, I fell into a swoon for almost an hour. ... during the first year [after my return] I could not endure my wife or children in my presence, the very smell of them was intolerable.'[5]

Marcel Proust's intense interest in the tiniest details of daily life, and his vivid memories of them, form the basis of his great autobiographical work *A la recherche du temps perdu*. But they are also responsible for his neurotic disposition in respect of physical sensations; he suffered from allergic asthma from childhood. His ill health was very troubling to his parents. The experience of unceasing medical care generated a profound interest in illness in Proust, providing him with a large number of those metaphors that are so characteristic of his literary style. They reveal remarkable knowledge of medical matters: 'He would not let her go, but sat there like a surgeon who waits for a spasm to subside that has interrupted his operation but need not make him abandon it.'[6]

After the death of his mother, on whom he had a great, childlike dependence, Proust withdrew more and more from social life and interactions. His asthma grew worse, compelling him to step up his consumption of powerful medicines – opium, veronal, and heroin – in order to find relief. Proust went so far as to line his bedroom with cork in order to insulate himself from noise and disturbance. An ever-increasing proportion of his waking hours was moved to nighttime, and his great novel came into being during long working hours in his bedroom in an almost autonomous process; his failing health caused him to fear that he would not be able to finish his work.

Proust himself claimed that '[a]ll the greatest things we know have come to us from neurotics. It is they and they only who have founded religions and created great works of art. Never will the world be conscious of how much it owes to them, nor above all of what they have suffered in

4 John Donne, 'To the Honourable Knight, Sir Robert Karre', in *Letters to Severall Persons of Honour* (London: Richard Marriot, 1651), p. 249.

5 Jonathan Swift, *Gulliver's Travels*, ed. by Peter Dixon and John Chalker (Harmondsworth: Penguin, 1967 [1726]), p. 339.

6 Marcel Proust, *Swann's Way*, trans. C. K. Scott Moncrieff (New York: Modern Library, 1956), p. 521. The French original reads, 'ne la lâchant pas, comme un chirurgien attend la fin du spasme qui interrompt son intervention, mais ne l'y fait renoncer'; Marcel Proust, *A la recherche du temps perdu, II: Du Côté de chez Swann* (Paris: Gallimard, 1954), p. 185.

order to bestow their gifts on it. We enjoy fine music, beautiful pictures, a thousand exquisite things, but we do not know what they cost those who wrought them in sleeplessness, tears, spasmodic laughter, rashes, asthma, epilepsy, a terror of death which is worse than any of these.'[7] As death eventually drew near, Proust commented, 'A stranger has taken her abode in my mind. – I was surprised at her lack of beauty. I had always thought Death beautiful, how otherwise should she get the better of us?'[8] In a book called *Creative Malady*, George Pickering surmises that Proust, realising that creation calls for solitude, sought refuge in his illness in order to safeguard the seclusion necessary in order to attain a superhuman achievement.[9]

Gustave Flaubert would probably have found himself in a similar quandary after his father sent him off to study law; his disgust and boredom, along with the comfort he sought in the bottle, contributed to an attack of epilepsy, the consequence of which was that he was permitted to return home to the atmosphere of reverie, reading, and writing, his passion in life. After his father's death, his epileptic attacks having had their desired effect, they very conveniently subsided, only to increase again when Flaubert, aged 50, saw his home occupied by the Prussians.

* * *

An example of how a neurosis may develop into a mental obsession is provided by the Swedish natural scientist and Professor of Theology Samuel Ödmann, one of Linnaeus's favourite disciples. He was so afraid of catching cold that the mere thought of a draught made him shiver. He himself admitted that he, 'your otherwise sensible friend', became half-mad the moment he turned the doorknob.[10] To be on the safe side, he took to his bed at the age of 43 and stayed there for another 40 years, until he was consigned to the most sheltered resting-place of all.

The Swedish poet Erik Gustaf Geijer wrote that Ödmann had only lived in the bosom of Nature during the years of his youth, whereupon he brought her image into those four walls that formed the boundaries of his world – where he kept it as fresh as if it had been from the day before. Ödmann's confined life was conducive to literary production and lively correspondence; from his pitiful refuge, he exercised a strong influence on the world of international science.

7 Marcel Proust, *The Guermantes Way*, Part One, trans. C. K. Scott Moncrieff (London: Chatto & Windus, 1967 [1925]), p. 418.

8 The source of this quotation could not be located.

9 George W. Pickering, *Creative Malady: Illness in the Lives and Minds of Charles Darwin, Florence Nightingale, Mary Baker Eddy, Sigmund Freud, Marcel Proust, Elizabeth Barrett Browning* (London: Allen & Unwin, 1974), p. 232.

10 Undated letter from Samuel Ödmann to Carl Peter Thunberg, quoted in Henning Wijkmark, *Samuel Ödmann* (Stockholm and Uppsala: Svenska kyrkans diakonistyrelses bokförlag, 1923), p. 64.

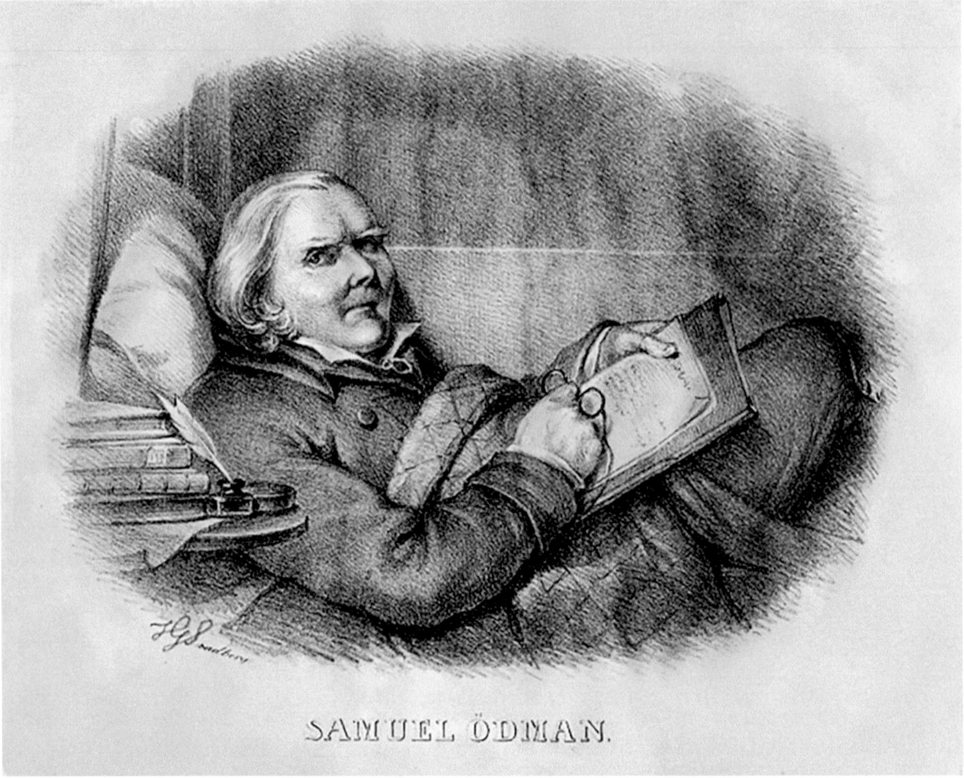

Figure 31 J. C. Sandberg, 'Samuel Ödman'. To protect himself against draughts and colds, the neurotic author Ödmann stayed in bed for 40 years, wearing his coat and wrapped in blankets.

The painter Piet Mondrian provides an example of a milder kind of neurosis.[11] This master of purist, abstract art had a lifestyle characterised by exaggerated orderliness; he was pedantic, sometimes pernickety.

Mondrian's neurasthenic disposition was noticeable in everything he did. He was, for instance, fond of dancing and danced according to all the rules, but his movements were rigid and angular. He kept his studio meticulously clean, never a grain of dust, everything gleaming white, sparse, and immaculate. These personality traits were fundamental to Mondrian's distinctive art. His colours were absolutely pure and finally reduced to the primary ones on the spectrum: red, yellow, and blue. One has the impression that when he occasionally mixed white and black to form a pleasing grey, he was half-frightened at having made himself guilty of something so

11 Piet Mondrian's writings are collected in his *The New Art – the New Life: The Collected Writings of Piet Mondrian* (London: Thames and Hudson, 1987), available on the Internet at https://archive.org/details/newartthenewlife0000mond_c0g8/page/288/mode/2up.

audacious (see Figure 1). The strictly vertical and horizontal lines are subtly arranged, distributed according to some unknown principle, and the rectangles are lovingly balanced with a transcendent harmony of which he was himself aware; he was convinced that he was passing on a very particular message.

***

Gilles de la Tourette's syndrome surely contributed to the prose of the famous lexicographer Dr Samuel Johnson, and probably also to Mozart's music. This baffling disorder is characterised by involuntary spastic twitchings or tics, especially in the face, often combined with the emitting of inarticulate sounds.

What interests us more, though, are certain mental symptoms. They arise owing to an accelerated inner rhythm manifested in restlessness and an irresistible craving for action, with unexpected, surprising initiatives. In addition, there are some more peculiar symptoms: a kind of playfulness expressed in practical jokes, puns, and verbal games, preferably obscene ones, and a childish preoccupation with urine and faeces.

If Tourette's syndrome appears in creative individuals, one would expect the symptoms to be noticeable in their output, maybe contributing to the very design of their works. The neurologist Oliver Sacks, a leading expert on the disorder, expressed the connection in clear and persuasive terms: 'phantasmagoric Tourette's syndrome ... can hardly fail to touch, to interact with, a person's character and creativity and even to lend that person some of its own striking "character"'.[12] Truly, it is remarkable that a biological dysfunction may express itself in creative work. Now that doctors have learnt to 'cure' these and similar conditions, they might be robbing us of multiple masterpieces at the same time!

Samuel Johnson suffered from pronounced Tourette's. His tics were so intrusive that he had to abandon his plans to be a schoolteacher – his strange demeanour and grotesque movements provoked merciless laughter from his pupils. His mental symptoms were of better use to him. A legendary memory, which enabled him to recite literary texts for hours – texts always present in his thoughts – came in useful in his work on his dictionary. The ready wit and facetiousness recorded by Boswell may well have derived from his impulsive mental hyperactivity.

The Tourette's diagnosis is less certain in respect of Mozart, but advocates of this hypothesis have drawn attention to several characteristic traits.[13] Many of Mozart's contemporaries observed his restlessness, especially during composing, a restlessness occasionally accompanied by

12 Oliver Sacks, 'Tourette's Syndrome and Creativity', *British Medical Journal* 305 (1992), 1515.

13 Lars Gunne, 'Hade Mozart Tourettes syndrom?', *Läkartidningen* 88.50 (1991), 4325–4326.

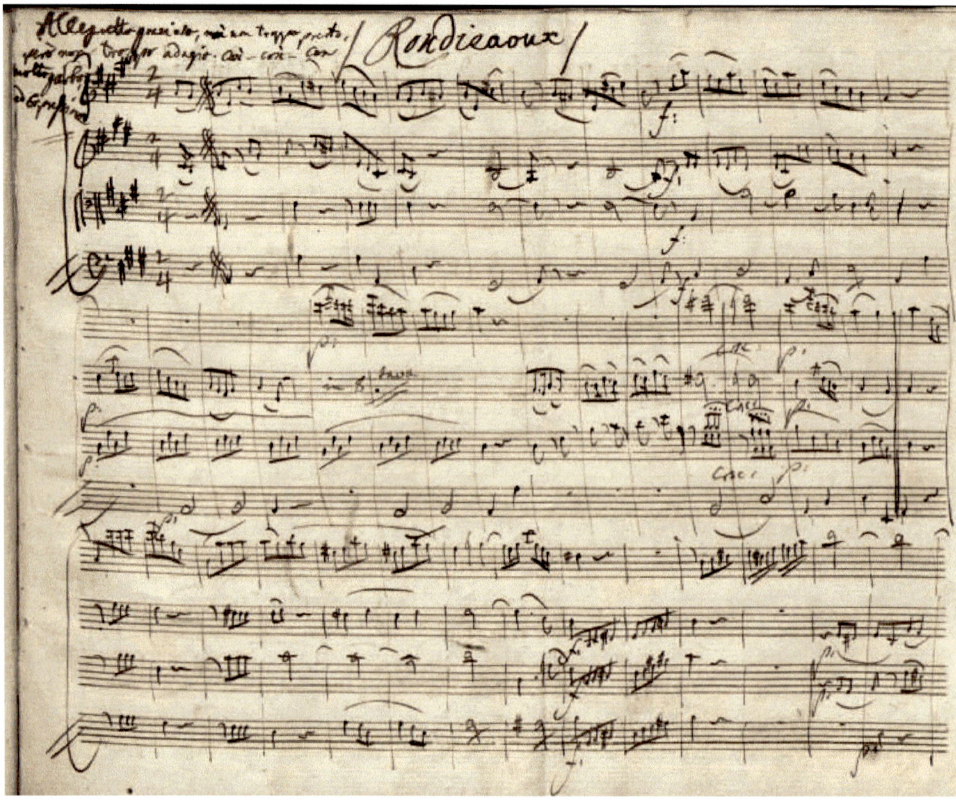

Figure 32 W. A. Mozart, Flute Quartet No. 4 (K.298), 'Rondieauox'. Symptoms of Tourette's syndrome?

exaggerated movements, somersaults, and pirouettes. His language, especially in letters to his family, was strikingly obscene even when regarded in the context of the outspokenness of the time, with an inclination to anal humour. Consequently, there is reason to speculate about the possibility that the syndrome may also have influenced Mozart's music. His composing ought to have been facilitated by his lively intellect with its inventiveness and sudden whims, and by the way in which his mind was always occupied with music, whatever he was actually doing – he composed all day long.

Mozart's roguish playfulness was expressed in bold improvisations and in comical canons, often with scatological texts by Mozart himself. A pretty example of his play on words and topics is found in the tempo notation for the last movement in a flute quartet (K. 298) called 'Rondieaoux': 'Allegretto grazioso, ma non troppo presto, para non troppo adagio, così – così – con molto garbo, ed expressione' ('Allegretto grazioso, but not too quick, and not too slow either, like that – like that – with much sweetness and expressiveness'). At this time he frequently amused himself by meowing like a cat, even in his music (K.625). Perhaps Papageno's melodic sallies in *The Magic Flute* constitute more refined manifestations of his Tourette's?

***

Gustav Mahler's fear of death and his hope for an afterlife, which form such a powerful current in his music, had a medical origin.[14] During an early casual examination, a physician had found that Mahler had a heart murmur and diagnosed a harmless congenital valvular defect. This finding had serious consequences for Mahler's life, and it had a considerable impact on his *oeuvre*. His wife Alma relates, 'Mahler was lying on the sofa and Dr. Blumenthal had been kneeling beside him. "Well, you've no cause to be proud of a heart like that," he said in that cheery tone doctors often adopt after diagnosing a fatal disease. This verdict marked the beginning of the end for Mahler.'[15]

It is shocking to see how a physician's imprudent remarks may be enough to quench a sensitive patient's zest for life. With the best of intentions, he does more harm than good when prescribing lifestyle changes that prevent the patient from cultivating his essential interests: '[Professor Kovacs] forbade [Mahler] to walk uphill, or bicycle, or swim; indeed he was so blind as to order a course of training to teach him to walk at all; first it was to be five minutes, then ten, and so on until he was used to walking; and this for a man who was accustomed to violent exercise!'[16]

Such a prescription would have been sufficient to make anyone downhearted, and it turned Mahler into a fearful hypochondriac. His wife describes his neurasthenic reaction as follows: 'We avoided strenuous walks owing to the ever-present anxiety about [his] heart. Once we knew he had valvular disease of the heart we were afraid of everything. He was always stopping on a walk to feel his own pulse; and he often asked me ... to listen to his heart and see whether the beat was clear, or rapid, or calm. ... [Mahler] had a pedometer [step-counter] in his pocket. His steps and pulse-beats were numbered and his life a torment.'[17]

The Mahlers had lost a small much-loved daughter, and Mahler was heartbroken. 'This summer was the saddest we had ever spent or were to spend together. Every excursion, every attempt at distraction was a failure. Grief and anxiety pursued us wherever we went. Work was his one

14 See N. P. Christy et al., 'Gustav Mahler and His Illnesses', *Transactions of the American Clinical and Climatological Association* 82 (1971), 215.

15 Alma Mahler, *Gustav Mahler: Memories and Letters*, trans. Basil Creighton (New York: The Viking Press, 1946), p. 110. The German-language original has the doctor exclaim 'Na, auf dieses Herz brauchen Sie aber nicht stolz zu sein!'; Alma Mahler, *Gustav Mahler: Erinnerungen und Briefe* (Amsterdam: Allert de Lange, 1940), p. 151.

16 Page 110 in the English translation mentioned in the preceding note; p. 151 in the German-language original.

17 Page 129 in the translation and p. 175 in Alma Mahler's German-language original.

resource.'[18] In composing, he found consolation in his grief and an escape from his angst, transforming his anxiety into distinctively personal strains and harmonies.

When we listen to *Das Lied von der Erde, The Song of the Earth*, which he composed at this time, bearing these circumstances in mind, our hearts fill with compassion for the great composer, but also with gratitude for his ability to transpose his sorrow into the most beautiful music (see pp. 207–209 and Figure 6).

18 Page 129 in the translation and p. 175 in the original.

Chapter 5
Mental illnesses

Sunt verba et voces, quibus hunc lenire dolorem
possis et magnam morbi deponere partem.

Words will avail the wretched mind to ease
and much abate the dismal black disease.

Horace, *Epistles, Book 1*

The connection between mental illness and creativity is so comprehensive that it constitutes an independent research discipline with an abundant literature. This chapter is restricted to a small number of examples.

A mental illness exercises a profound influence on creative activity. Autobiographies by psychotic authors (see p. 00) //99// and pictures made by sufferers from mental illness have provided important information about several forms of psychosis. In certain cases, indeed, they may also contribute to the formulation of a diagnosis. In addition, artistic creation such as poetry, painting, and music may have a favourable therapeutic effect.[1] For instance, there are distressing conditions where, as a result of mental illness, a patient has been apathetic and withdrawn, incapable of contact with fellow human beings. If such patients can be encouraged to draw, paint, or make music, the barrier may be removed so that they resume contact with their surroundings, a change they perceive as an intense relief. This is one of the similarities between psychiatric and normal art; for, even in the latter, one of the most urgent incentives is the artist's desire to connect with fellow humans, experiencing a feeling of personal contact with them and liberating himself or herself from suffering by means of creative effort.

An example: an apathetic woman was completely inaccessible, without any kind of contact with her surroundings. Given a pencil and paper, she drew something that is somewhat difficult to understand. In the view of an expert, she drew herself, torn between some odd figures she had seen in her hallucinations. She continued to draw, and in her next drawing she was better able to portray both herself and those evil spirits that threatened her.

---

1 See Gunnar Berefelt, 'Notiser om psykopatologiskt bildskapande', *Forskning och praktik* 4.7 (1972), 73–82 (pp. 73–74).

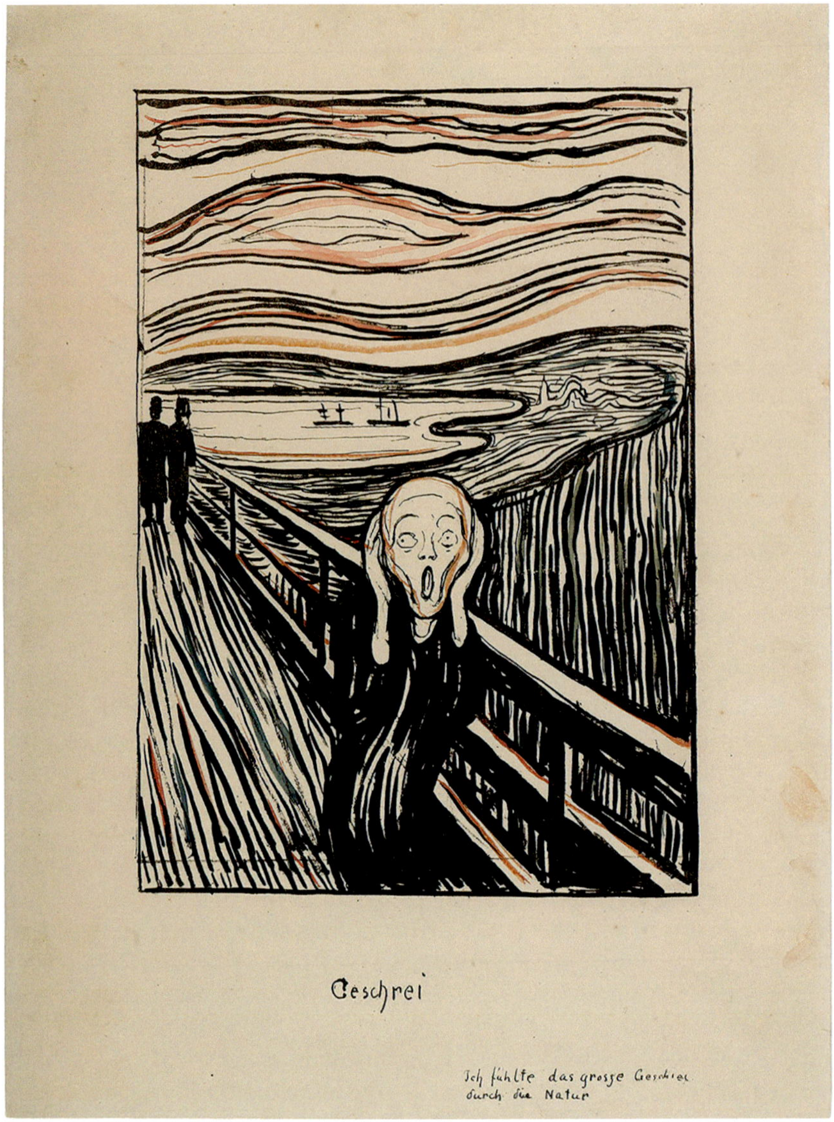

Figure 33 Edvard Munch, 'The scream', 1896.

Patients who have been thus induced to communicate what goes on inside them to their doctor will often be more amenable to treatment. In her last drawing, the woman patient made a self-portrait but erased half of her face, as is typical of patients with her illness, schizophrenia. The patient herself experiences a split in her personality and illustrates it by cutting her face in half. Closely resembling some of Picasso's portraits, her drawing tells us about otherwise opaque phenomena in the life of the soul.

* * *

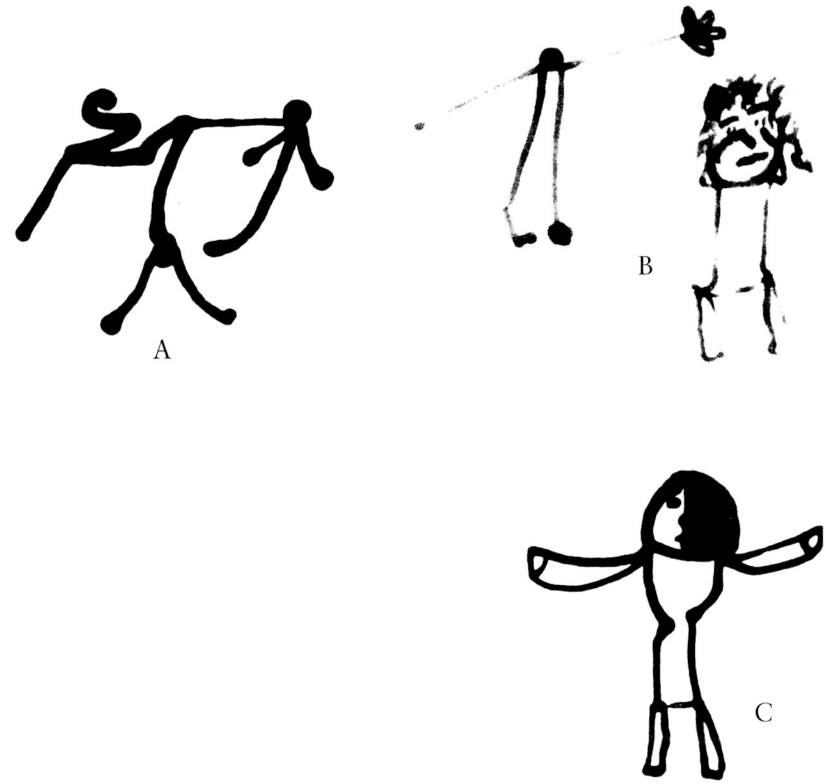

Figure 34 Unknown, schizophrenic drawings by a hallucinating patient. A refers to a representation, hard to understand, of a hallucination; B shows how the improved patient is better able to reproduce the hallucination of a frightening monster; and C expresses the split personality by means of the half-erasure of the face.

Many sufferers from mental illness experience a spontaneous urge to create, and their art evinces features characteristic of their particular disorder. Drawing on congenital artistic talents, some of them have evolved into true revolutionaries in art. Their works have given us insights into their inner world, a fantastic place quite unlike our own environment, sometimes charged with anxiety, at other times tinged with a strange humour (Figure 36). This so-called *art brut* has aroused the interest of psychiatrists as well as art historians; it has even been honoured with a special museum.[2] Healthy artists have received impulses from the art of their sick comrades, which has thereby influenced the development of art in general – those that are lost sometimes happen upon new paths.

2 Michel Thévoz, *Art Brut* (New York: Rizzoli International, 1976).

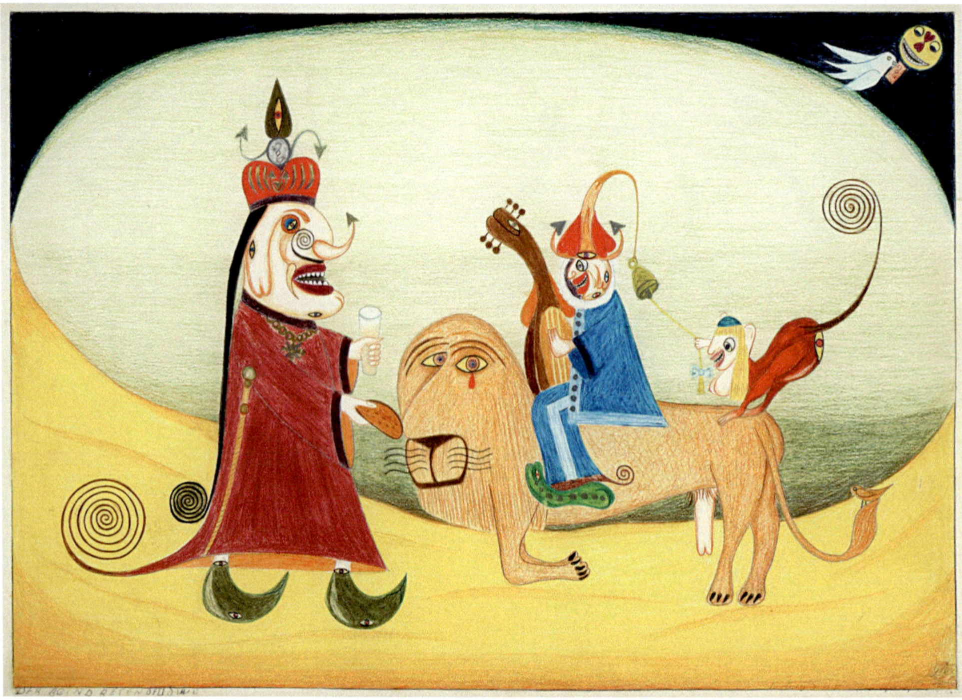

Figure 35 Friedrich Schröder-Sonnenstern, 'Der blinde, betende Löwe' ('The blind praying lion'), 1952. The artist led an adventurous life, in and out of mental hospitals. He declared, 'I am unique – there is no double. The King of animals must receive bread and wine from the King of men, he must let the jester ride on his back while the monkey, the link between man and beasts, rings the jester's bell.'[3]

Quite a number of great artists have suffered from fully developed mental illness, usually schizophrenic or manic-depressive. The German Romantic poet Friedrich Hölderlin lauded the ancient ideals lacking in his own time in superbly wrought, musical verse. Aged 32, he fell ill with symptoms typical of catatonic schizophrenia which left marked traces in his work. Even before that stage, there are premonitions of the disease in his personality, a presumptuousness as in the megalomaniac dreams of a paranoid individual alternating with insecurity and self-contempt.[4]

Hölderlin harboured an ardent, or perhaps rather romantic, passion for a young banker's wife whose children's tutor he was. Diotima, as he called her after Plato's *Symposium*, answered his feelings, expressing the purity and strength of their love in moving letters. She became his muse for the four years during which his poetry achieved fullness and maturity.

3 Unfortunately, it was not possible to locate this reference.

4 Michael Hamburger, *Hölderlin: His Poems*, trans. Michael Hamburger (New York: Pantheon, 1952), pp. 71–74. Available on Internet Archive, https://archive.org/details/holderlin0000mich/mode/2up.

> ... Meanwhile we – like the mated swans in their summer contentment
> When by the lake they rest or on the waves, lightly rocked, ...
> Moved and dwelled on this earth. And though the North Wind was threatening
> Hostile to lovers ...[5]

By 'North Wind', Hölderlin meant the menace to their happiness, the fact that their relationship was a fragile one and that the day would come when they would have to part, as the lady's husband was more earthbound – less esoteric, as it were – than the two lovers. The good burgher can hardly be blamed for taking a more down-to-earth view of the situation. To him, the tutor was conducting a clandestine relationship involving petting with his wife, and he was obliged to send the man packing. Thus Hölderlin found himself facing the abyss that separates human destiny from the exalted serenity of the gods.

After the brutal dismissal, Hölderlin's existence was miserable and aimless:

> Desolate is now my house, and not only her they have taken,
> No, but my own two eyes, myself I have lost, losing her.
> That is why, astray, like wandering phantoms I live now
> *Must* live, I fear, and the rest long has seemed senseless to me.[6]

This condition may well have been connected with the insanity that suddenly afflicted Hölderlin. His employment as a tutor in the south of France terminated, he returned home after a couple of months roaming about. His mother and sister were horrified at the sight of him, broken in body and mind, filthy and unkempt, his clothes like those of a beggar. He was totally confused, his eyes were wild, and he frightened the neighbours with outbursts of rage.

Hölderlin's friends tried to help him by arranging a sinecure as a teacher, but that activity had to cease as his pupils once had to save themselves from being thrown out of the window. He spent a short period in an asylum, but subsequently he was able to lodge peacefully with a carpenter's family with whom he lived in seclusion until his death, 30 years later.

It is interesting that the poet was – as is often the case with creative spirits – himself aware of his illness and its effects. Even before tangible

5 From 'Menons Klagen um Diotima' ('Menon's Lament for Diotima'), an unfinished elegy first published in 1802 and 1803. In German: 'Aber wir, zufrieden gesellt, wie die liebenden Schwäne, / Wenn sie ruhen am See, oder, auf Wellen gewiegt, / So auf Erden wandelten wir. Und drohte der Nord auch, / Er, der Liebenden Feind ...' There is an English translation in Michael Hamburger, *Friedrich Hölderlin: Poems and Fragments*, trans. Michael Hamburger (Ann Arbor: University of Michigan Press, 1966), p. 235.

6 'Aber das Haus ist öde mir nun, und sie haben mein Auge / Mir genommen, auch mich hab ich verloren mit ihr. / Darum irr ich umher, und wohl, wie die Schatten, so muss ich / Leben, und sinnlos dünkt lange das Übrige mir'. Both quotations are from the fourth strophe in 'Menons Klagen'.

symptoms appeared, he had a premonition of how his mind and his art would change, first with a schizophrenic dream image in 'Hyperion's Song of Fate':

But we are fated
To find no foothold, no rest,
And suffering mortals
Dwindle and fall
Headlong from one
Hour to the next,
Hurled like water
From ledge to ledge
Downward for years to the vague abyss.[7]

And then, at the time when he first fell ill, his 'The Middle of Life' lent heart-rending expression to the contrast between love and suprasensuous bliss in Nature on the one hand and an increasing feeling of cold and emptiness on the other:

With yellow pears the land
And full of wild roses
Hangs down into the lake,
You lovely swans,
And drunk with kisses
You dip your heads
Into the hallowed, the sober water.

But oh, where shall I find
When winter comes, the flowers, and where
The sunshine
And shade of the earth?
The walls loom
Speechless and cold, in the wind
Weathercocks clatter.[8]

In the poem called 'Mnemosyne', Hölderlin himself observes a couple of symptoms, lack of feeling and alienation:

---

7 'Hyperions Schicksalslied': Doch uns ist gegeben, / Auf keiner Stätte zu ruhn, / Es schwinden, es fallen / Die leidenden Menschen / Blindlings von einer / Stunde zur andern, / Wie Wasser von Klippe / Zu Klippe geworfen, / Jahr lang ins Ungewisse herab.' Hamburger has translated the poem into English; see p. 79 in the collection mentioned in n. 5.

8 'Hälfte des Lebens': 'Mit gelben Birnen hänget / Und voll von wilden Rosen / Das Land in den See, / Ihr holden Schwäne, / Und trunken von Küssen / Tunkt ihr das Haupt / Ins heilignüchterne Wasser. // Weh mir, wo nehm' ich, wenn / Es Winter ist, die Blumen, und wo / Den Sonnenschein, / Und Schatten der Erde? / Die Mauern stehn / Sprachlos und kalt, in Winde / Klirren die Fahnen.' Hamburger's English translation is on p. 371 in the previously mentioned edition.

> A sign we are, without meaning
> Without pain we are and have nearly
> Lost our language in foreign lands ...[9]

Never has the schizophrenic uncertainty about one's identity, the feeling of being an alien to oneself, received more eloquent expression.

Hölderlin's insanity affected his poetry as profoundly as it did his personality and behaviour. To be sure, his writing reached new heights in the early years of his illness; but his creative power suffered from his increasing spiritual exhaustion, and towards the end of his life not a lot of it remained. The large existential perspectives and the emotional intensity were dissolved and vanished. Those short lyrics and fragments that replaced them are saved by his strong feeling for Nature and his infallible sense of rhythm and language.

The Swedish poet, critic, and translator Erik Blomberg has commented on these short pieces in the following terms: 'They shimmer like pure, limpid raindrops after a storm, filled with boundless light ... a harmony, a peace passing all human reason, perhaps precisely because reason has been sacrificed.'[10] The poem 'Spring' serves as an illustration:

> O what a joy it is for mankind! Content
> The lonely walk on riverbanks, peace, delight
> And bliss of healthy vigour bloom, and
> Not far away is kind-hearted laughter.[11]

What a moving sight – the lonely poet rejoicing in the kind laughter of strangers, but surely even more in 'the world's agreeable things', which include the ability to shape language and simple thoughts into poetry:

> The world's agreeable things were mine to enjoy,
> The hours of youth, how long they have been gone!
> Remote is April, May, remote July;
> I'm nothing now, and listless I live on.[12]

However, it is with the great odes, the 'night hymns' written a short time after the onset of insanity and surely influenced by it, that Hölderlin enters

---

9 'Mnemosyne': 'Ein Zeichen sind wir, deutungslos, / Schmerzlos sind wir und haben fast / Die Sprache in der Fremde verloren.' The English translation is by Richard Sieburth in Friedrich Hölderlin, *Hymns and Fragments*, trans. Richard Sieburth (Princeton: Princeton University Press, 1984), p. 117.

10 Erik Blomberg, *Hölderlin: Lyriskt urval* (Stockholm: Norstedts, 1960), p. 35.

11 'Der Frühling': 'oh welche Freude haben die Menschen! Froh / gehn an Gestaden Einsame, Ruh' und Lust / und Wonne der Gesundheit blühet, / freundliches Lachen ist auch nicht ferne.' Translated by Michael Hamburger; see Friedrich Hölderlin, *Poems and Fragments*, 4th edn (London: Anvil, 2004), p. 749.

12 'Das Angenehme dieser Welt': 'Das Angenehme dieser Welt hab ich genossen, / Die Jugendstunden sind, wie lang! wie lang! verflossen, / April und Mai und Junius sind ferne, / Ich bin nichts mehr, ich lebe nicht mehr gerne!' Translation by Michael Hamburger in Friedrich Hölderlin, *Poems and Fragments*, trans. by Michael Hamburger (Ann Arbor: University of Michigan Press, 1966), p. 587.

the circle of the great innovators in poetry. An example is provided by his most visionary poem of this kind, 'Patmos', named after the Greek island where St John, the favourite disciple of Jesus Christ, received his revelations:

Near is
And difficult to grasp, the God.
But where danger threatens
That which saves from it also grows.
In gloomy places dwell
The eagles, and fearless over
The chasm walk the sons of the Alps
On bridges lightly built.
Therefore, since round about
Are heaped the summits of Time
And the most loved live near, growing faint
On mountains most separate,
Give us innocent water,
O pinions give us, with minds most faithful
To cross over and to return.[13]

In this new poetry, Hölderlin also walks across the chasm on flimsy bridges, and it is not surprising that it has been very variously received and assessed.

To begin with, this poetry was thought to be worthless from a literary point of view, and its linguistic peculiarities were regarded as an awkward accumulation of words with convoluted sentence structures – taken altogether a pointless stammer. During the first half of the twentieth century, however, a complete revaluation took place: no longer regarded as meaningless, his text was seen as passionately stammering and endlessly expressive. According to one of his most enthusiastic interpreters, it is only in the works dating from his years of illness that Hölderlin's creative power achieves its entire originality and strength: 'The language, subverted by volcanic eruptions, titanically towering and with dizzying crater depths in the sequence of words, forms full-throated expressions of a boundless innovative joy in creation. ... "Patmos" is by no means, as many appear to believe, a shapeless work of poetry affording glimpses of beauty brought forth by genius; it is not fragmentary and broken into pieces, but conceived as a single breath of inspiration. It has a surreal clarity of rare persistence; and if it seems obscure, it is because it dazzles ... [It] was created in the frightening proximity of madness, not enclosed within it but vibrating with premonitions.'[14]

13 'Patmos': 'Nah ist / Und schwer zu fassen der Gott. / Wo aber Gefahr ist, wächst / Das Rettende auch. / Im Finstern wohnen / Die Adler und furchtlos gehn / Die Söhne der Alpen über den Abgrund weg / Auf leichtgebaueten Brücken. / Drum, da gehäuft sind rings / Die Gipfel der Zeit, und die Liebsten / Nah wohnen, ermattend auf / Getrenntesten Bergen, / So gieb unschuldig Wasser, / O Fittige gieb uns, treuesten Sinns / Hinüberzugehn und wiederzukehren'. The English translation is from the collection mentioned in the preceding note, p. 463.

14 Bertil Malmberg, *Idealet och livet: Klassisk diktning i översättning* (Stockholm: Bonniers, 1951), pp. 9–10.

The assumption of a connection between the work of the poet and his insanity is supported by their parallel development. When the illness erupts, its symptoms manifest themselves in the poetry: the tone becomes agitated and 'passionately stammering', and, as the creator's spiritual impoverishment progresses, his poems turn simple and naive.

In his night hymns, Hölderlin continued to regard himself as the chosen one, prepared to remind the People of past heroic deeds and to summon them to noble exploits. Not surprisingly, the Nazis responded to these ideas.

There can be no doubt that the schizophrenic dream-images bordering on psychosis and the bizarre language together increased the expressive power of Hölderlin's major works and gave his poetry its peculiar power. It has been argued that Hölderlin's musical sense of beauty was not liberated until his cognitive perspectives broke down.[15]

It is a remarkable thing that the whole lyrical development towards greater linguistic richness and liberty, as well as towards bolder images untrammelled by conventional logic, in the work of a great poet originates in a mental illness, or at least in schizophrenic features. Contemplated from this point of view, efforts to save Hölderlin's poetic reputation by making light of his mental illness seem doubly ridiculous.

While reading Hölderlin's late works, the modern reader frequently feels close to the poetry of our own time. Here, too, the metaphors, albeit beautiful, are often hard to understand; and not until we reread them with concentration – perhaps with the aid of interpreters – do they yield fresh and unexpected truths.

In the knowledge of the ways of life adopted by some more recent poets, one cannot but ask oneself if it might have been alcohol that helped them make the transition to those schizophrenic states where linguistic conventions collapse and fantastic dreams appear. Did not Coleridge see the palace of Kublai Khan while intoxicated by opium, and did not the drawings of Michaux turn patently schizophrenic, perseverations included, under the influence of mescaline?

* * *

One of the most outstanding graphic artists of the nineteenth century, the French etcher Charles Meryon, developed schizophrenia and went through all stages of the disease up to the final mental breakdown.[16] His famous series of etchings 'Eaux-fortes sur Paris' offers the rare opportunity to follow the entire course of this mental illness and its connection with creation in works by a major artist. Even the images that precede the emergence of

15 Erik Blomberg, 'Friedrich Hölderlin', *Frihet* 2 (1921), 4, quoted in Pär Hellström, 'Hölderlinporträtt i svensk 1900–talspoesi', in *Läskonst, skrivkonst, diktkonst*, ed. by Pär Hellström and Tore Wretö (Stockholm: Askelin & Hägglund, 1987), p. 116.

16 Lars-Ingemar Lundström, 'Charles Méryon, peintre-graveur schizophrène', *Acta Psychiatrica Scandinavica* 40 (1964), 159–165.

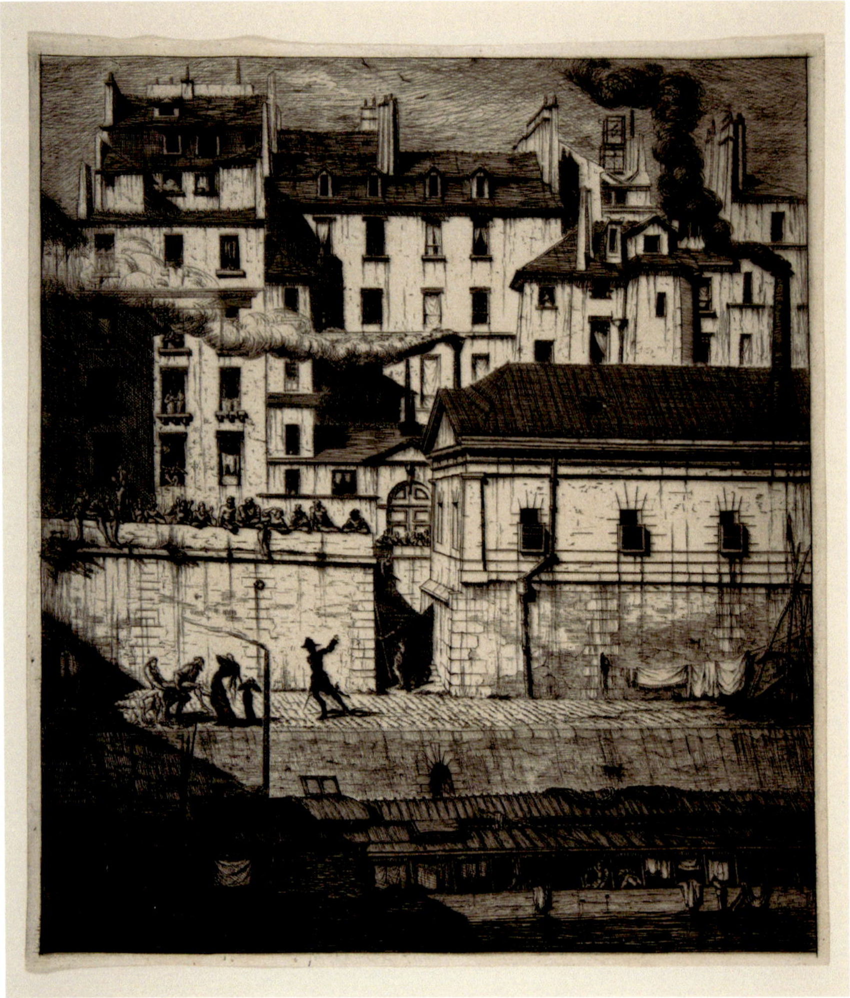

Figure 36 Charles Meryon, 'The mortuary', 1854 (cropped). Morbid details, such as the scene where a dead body is pulled out of the Seine, suggest a schizophrenic personality.

unmistakable signs of illness afford glimpses of a schizophrenic personality, a fact that accounts for their unusual appeal. Victor Hugo noticed it and observed that 'the breath of the universe breathes through all [Meryon's] works, and makes his etchings more than pictures – visions' (in a letter to Philippe Burty); another letter of Hugo's, to Baudelaire, claims that Meryon's 'plates live, shine, and think'.[17]

17 The letter to Burty is quoted in Philippe Burty, *Charles Méryon, Sailor, Engraver, and Etcher: A Memoir and Complete Descriptive Catalogue of His Works* (London: Fine Art Society, 1879), p. 22. For the letter to Baudelaire, see Timothy Raser, 'Capturing

Meryon created his major works after the illness had begun to show clear symptoms. The magnificent etching 'La morgue' features a gloomy corner of the city, with an oppressive atmosphere and morbid details, including the pulling-out of a dead body from the waters of the Seine. In the end Meryon had to be admitted to an asylum, and his art degenerated, though there were lucid intervals. During one of those intervals he created 'Ministère de la Marine', where his original greatness finds expression in the impressive architecture while his confused, dismal imagination produced the monsters he thought he saw in the sky – or are they simply allegorical figures, whose secrets are concealed in the sequestered, deranged mind of the artist?[18]

* * *

Two pictures by the eminent Swedish artist Ernst Josephson allow us to study how artistic greatness changes under the influence of mental illness: one was painted at a time when he was in good health and the other somewhat later, after he had fallen ill. As Josephson wielded the pen with the same mastery as the brush, his pictures sometimes bear devices in his own hand. The small painting 'A summer day in the pine forest', also known as 'Gelly Marcus in the wood at Dalarö' (Figure 38), originates in his last healthy summer; it is a work of Nordic impressionism, where the gentle green of the deciduous trees painted by French artists has been replaced by the darkness of firs.

The sunny clearing is depicted in splendidly Oriental colours which remind us of the artist's Jewish descent. The spontaneous, naive joy of the senses is arresting, although it is still controlled by tight artistic constraints. In this the picture resembles the poem Josephson wrote at the same time, in the collection he called *Lilla Gellys visor* ('Songs for little Gelly'). Composed for his much-loved niece, his model in the painting, it contains the following passage:

> Wearing galoshes and my blue cardigan
> I walked in the grass where wild flowers grow fragrant
> ...
> There was my pine, my rowan tree,
>   my birch with its tender leaves,
> all was just like it used to be, o god, what bliss for me;
> My anthill, my frogs, my angling-worm of old,
> my dragon-fly, my butterfly, my sun with all its gold.[19]

Josephson's disagreements and quarrels with his fellow artists in the Swedish Society of Artists may have been the first symptoms of his schizophrenic mental illness – but they will have contributed to its outbreak, too.

Images: Baudelaire's Account of Méryon's Etchings', *Word and Image* 38.4 (2022), 375–393 (p. 380).

18 Ph. Junod, *Méryon en Icare* (Geneva: Tricorne, 1981). It was impossible to locate a page reference.

19 Free translation from the Swedish language.

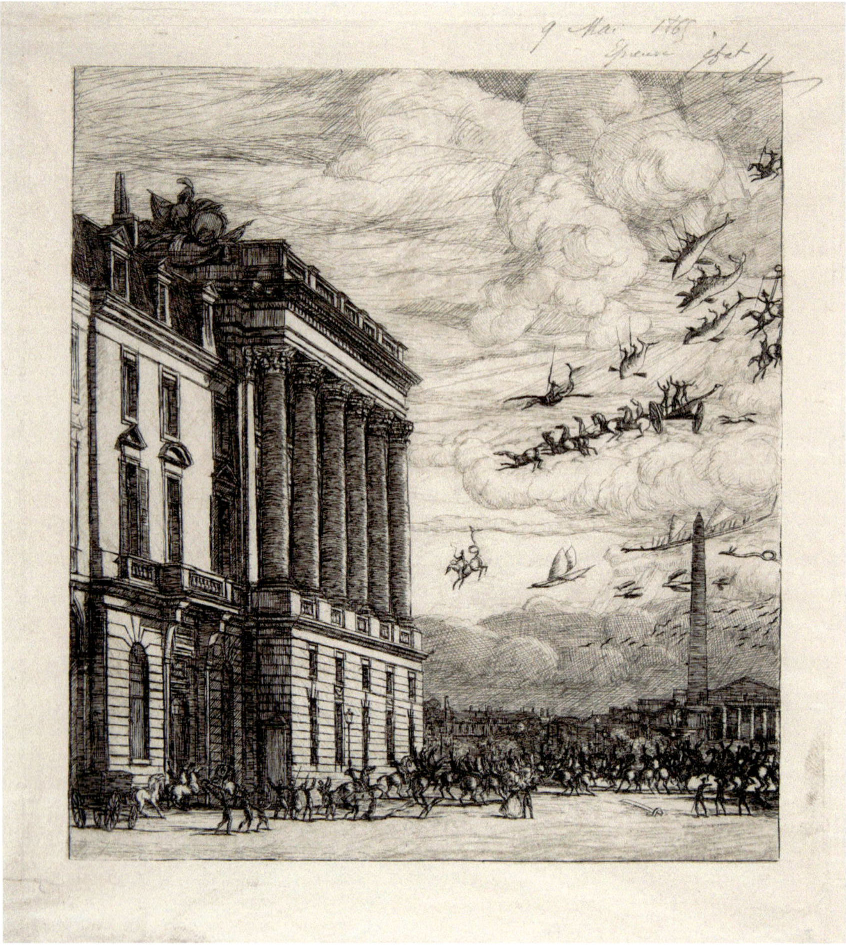

Figure 37 Charles Meryon, 'The Admiralty', 1865 (cropped). In fully developed schizophrenia, the artist is able to supply sharp pictures of the monsters he perceives in the sky.

The severe impact of the illness on Josephson's personality may be studied in his letters as well as his art. The normal mental inhibitions having been dispelled, he lost control over his means of expression so that the artistic balance evaporated.

At the same time, though, the restraints on his creative powers gave way as well, and they erupted with tremendous force, uncontrolled, uninhibited by formal demands for exact drawing and anatomical accuracy; the illness transformed the moderate Impressionist into a savage Expressionist, as seen in his picture of his uncle, the theatre director.

An artist friend observed that it was not until 'Joseph' grew mad that he found his proper self. Josephson himself provided the best account of his experience in a letter to a fellow artist, a letter in which he proposes a journey: 'There we will let our brushes dance in a way hitherto unknown in

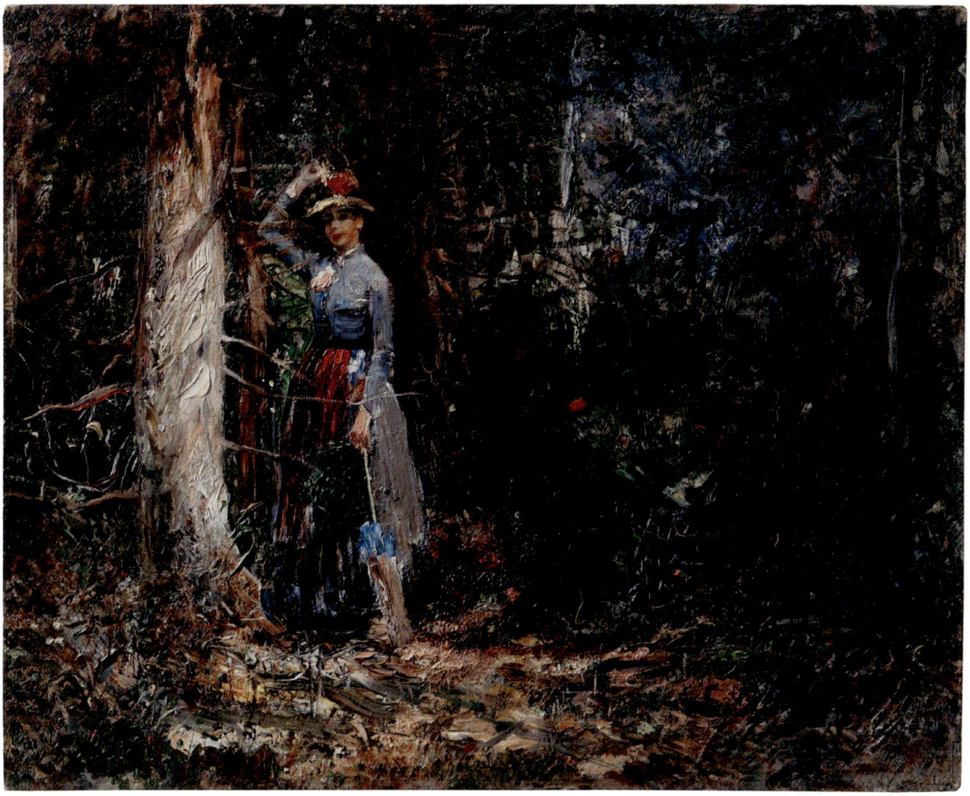

Figure 38 Ernst Josephson, 'A summer day in the pine forest', also known as 'Gelly Marcus in the wood at Dalarö', 1885.

Sweden. Here I haven't a single tube of paint to make splashes with ... Let us challenge Heaven and Hell out of our paint-boxes ... and if that's what it takes, let us paint on the same canvas with our hands and feet. The waves will dance in our pictures, the clouds will drift across our skies, the wind stirring grass and twigs.'[20] The idea of painting with both hands and feet was a revolutionary one at that time; today such excesses are generally accepted.

When Josephson thus allowed colour and emotion to banish exact drawing and reason under the influence of his mental disorder and in a state of savage, unbridled passion, he anticipated European Expressionism. Since he had no immediate followers – Picasso did not study the works created during Josephson's illness until much later – he was no pioneer. The artist who most resembles him is Edvard Munch, whose works were also affected by a pathological, probably schizophrenic, state of mind. In 'The scream', the great Norwegian master lets a frenzied figure, depicted in glowing colours

20 Ernst Josephson, from a letter to Richard Bergh, quoted in Erik Lindorm, *Oscar II och hans tid: En bokfilm*, 2nd edn (Stockholm: Wahlström & Widstrand, 1936), p. 224.

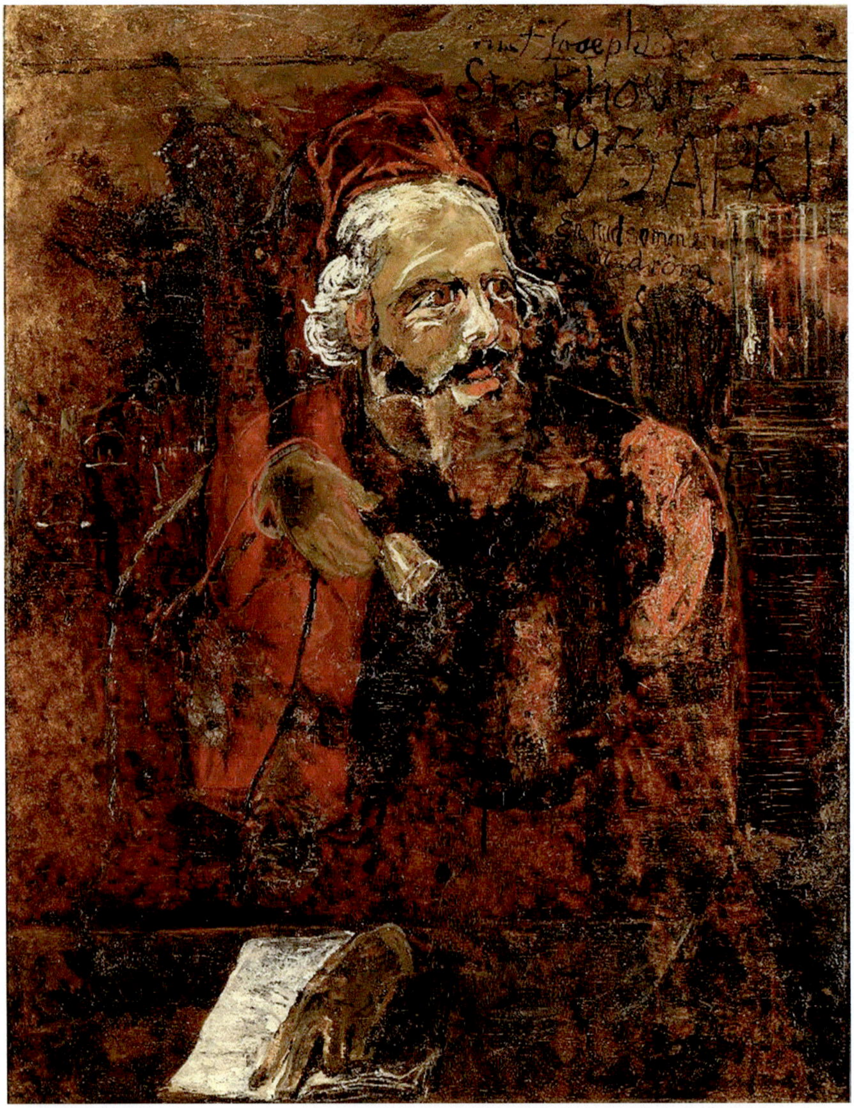

Figure 39 Ernst Josephson, 'Ludvig Josephson, theatre director', 1893. The portrait was painted during Ernst Josephson's mental illness, violent passions finding expression with no thought for precise draughtsmanship. In its darkly resplendent colours, the painting is reminiscent of Rembrandt's late work.

and with agitated brushstrokes, reveal his innermost feelings of anguish and alienation (Figure 33).

* * *

Many creative individuals afflicted by severe manic-depressive illness have been affected by their melancholy in their work, and some have left records of their wretchedness. Virginia Woolf did so in fiction, Sylvia Plath in poetry, and William Styron and Kay Jamison in autobiographies.

Anxious for recognition and vulnerable to criticism, Woolf was close to a mental breakdown every time she finished a book. While working she was able to keep her 'blue devils' at bay and transform her mental agony into fiction. In *Mrs Dalloway* she described, with the merciless candour born of personal experience, how a young man develops a mental illness. There is the typical overweening pride, 'the Lord who had come to renew society', alternating with feelings of guilt and hallucinations of shame and misery: 'the sin for which human nature had condemned him to death; that he did not feel. ... He lay on the sofa and made her hold his hand to prevent him from falling down, down, he cried, into the flames! and saw faces laughing at him ... and hands pointing round the screen ... The whole world was clamouring: Kill yourself, kill yourself' – and so he did, foretelling his author's own suicide.[21]

The manic-depressive Sylvia Plath declared that her sole reason for writing was that there was a voice within her that refused to fall silent.[22] An intense desire for success, in her life and in her work, became fatal when she feared failure. The devising of ingenious metaphors for leave-taking and death gave her solace, at least temporarily, when depression had deprived her of all desire to continue to live, 'quietly / With no attachments, like a foetus in a bottle'.[23] However, no metaphor, no Greek toga, could conceal the inexorable fate, her suicide:

> The woman is perfected
> Her dead
>
> Body wears the smile of accomplishment,
> The illusion of a Greek necessity
>
> Flows in the scrolls of her toga
> Her bare
>
> Feet seem to be saying:
> We have come so far, it is over.[24]

The 'Greek necessity' refers to the notion that suicide constitutes an honourable escape from disgrace.

* * *

21 Virginia Woolf, *Mrs Dalloway*, first published in 1925. The quotations are on pp. 32, 118, 87, and 120 in the Oxford University Press edition of the novel, published in 1998 and edited by Claire Tomalin.

22 Sylvia Plath, *Letters Home: Correspondence, 1950–1963* (London: Faber and Faber, 1975), p. 35: 'I write only because / There is a voice within me / That will not be still'.

23 'A Life', penultimate stanza; Sylvia Plath, *Collected Poems*, ed. by Ted Hughes (New York: Harper & Row, 1981), p. 150.

24 The opening of the poem 'Edge'. Ibid., p. 272.

A seventeenth-century hymn writer, George Herbert (see p. 00), provided a simple poetic account of his depression and his recovery; but it is only through the written testimony of a great writer, William Styron, who had himself come through this illness, that we ordinary souls – who are merely occasionally low-spirited – can even begin to grasp the full extent of the appalling suffering caused by depression in its disastrous, potentially fatal, form. But even Styron complains, in his *Darkness Visible*, of the difficulty in finding apt and sufficiently powerful expressions for it: 'Depression is a disorder of mood, so mysteriously painful and elusive in the way it becomes known to the self – to the meditating intellect – as to verge close to being beyond description.'[25]

Styron searches in vain for examples of situations that are sufficiently horrifying to bear comparisons to the torment he suffers: 'the pain is most closely connected to drowning or suffocation – but even these images are off the mark'. 'It may be more accurate to say that [the] despair ... comes to resemble the diabolical discomfort of being imprisoned in a fiercely overheated room. And because no breeze stirs this caldron, because there is no escape from this smothering confinement, it is entirely natural that the victim begins to think ceaselessly of oblivion.'[26]

Like Saul in the Bible, Styron was saved by music, 'a sudden soaring passage from the Brahms *Alto Rhapsody*'. Realising that he could no longer inflict this outrage on himself, he 'drew upon some last gleam of sanity to perceive the terrifying dimensions of the mortal predicament I had fallen into'.[27]

Consequently, Styron requested close institutional confinement: 'In fact, the hospital was my salvation, and it is something of a paradox that in this austere place with its locked and wired doors ... I found the repose, the assuagement of the tempest in my brain [that I was unable to find in my quiet farmhouse]'.

That which we would most of all wish to have clarified in this context, namely how Styron's writing was affected by his illness, is explained to us in forthright terms: 'after I had returned to health and was able to reflect on the past in the light of my ordeal, I began to see clearly how depression had clung close to the outer edges of my life for many years. Suicide has been a persistent theme in my books, three of my major characters killed themselves. In re-reading, for the first time in years, sequences from my novels, passages where my heroines have lurched down pathways towards doom, I was stunned to perceive how accurately I had created the landscape of depression in the minds of these young women, describing with what could only be instinct, out of a subconscious already roiled by disturbances of mood, the psychic imbalance that led them to destruction.'[28]

25 William Styron, *Darkness Visible* (New York: Random House, 1990), p. 7.
26 Ibid., pp. 17 and 50.
27 Ibid., pp. 66–67.
28 Ibid., 68–69.

Styron found many fellow-sufferers among the great geniuses of the past. Above all, he admired and felt affinity with Dante and with his metaphors:

> I woke to find myself in a dark wood,
> Where the right road was wholly lost and gone.[29]

In Dante's company, too, Styron experienced the relief of recovery:

> [We] Came forth, to look once more upon the stars.[30]

Kay Jamison was another fellow-sufferer, and her *An Unquiet Mind* supplies an equally harrowing image of the torment inflicted by this illness. Like Styron, Jamison admits that '[d]epression is awful beyond words or sounds or images';[31] but when depression takes them to the brink of suicide, the two authors find the same persuasive metaphor for that predicament: a 'murderous cauldron'.[32]

However, it is to Jamison we should turn for the most enlightening as well as the most beautifully written account of the manic phase of bipolar illness, especially its effect on creative activity. Writing as an erudite psychiatrist as well as from personal experience, Jamison possessed dual competence. Her two striking examples are Lord Byron (see p. 35) and herself.

Jamison loves her manic phases: 'When you're high it's tremendous. The ideas and feelings are fast and frequent like shooting stars.' 'I have been aware of finding new corners in my mind and heart. Some of these corners were incredible and beautiful and took my breath away.'[33] This is a marvellous description of the moderate mania that has bestowed flows of ideas and enraptured creativity on so many great spirits throughout the ages. The enhanced mental lightness and originality were useful to Jamison in her academic career as well: 'having fire in one's blood ... is not without its benefits in the world of academic medicine'.[34]

Like Byron, Jamison had experienced exaltation that went out of control: 'The fast ideas are far too fast, and there are far too many; overwhelming confusion replaces clarity.' This sense of becoming 'enmeshed totally in the blackest caves of the mind', in addition to the threat of a depression leading to suicide, called for medical treatment. She had become dependent on the mania, though: 'It was difficult to give up the high flights of mind and mood, even though the depression that inevitably followed nearly cost me my life.' In the end, she gave up: with lithium and psychotherapy, her symptoms receded – but this entailed 'a rather bittersweet exchange of a comfortable and settled present existence for a troubled but intensely

---

29 '[M]i ritrovai per una selva oscura / ché la diritta via era smarrita', *Inferno* I.2–3. The translation is from Dorothy L. Sayers's Penguin edition of 1964 [1949], p. 71.

30 '[E] quindi uscimmo a riveder le stelle', *Inferno* XXXIV.139; p. 289 in the Sayers translation.

31 Kay Redfield Jamison, *An Unquiet Mind* (New York: Alfred A. Knopf, 1995), p. 217.

32 Ibid., p. 114.

33 Ibid., pp. 67 and 219.

34 Ibid., p. 123.

lived past'.[35] By way of a happy ending, Jamison found that a reduction of the lithium dose allowed her to recover some of her previous state of mind.

An affinity similar to that which Styron felt for Dante was experienced by Jamison towards Edna St Vincent Millay, who emerged from the darkness of depression with the poem 'Renascence':

> How can I bear it; buried here,
> While overhead the sky grows clear

Millay moved into clarity and new miracles:

> And all at once the heavy night
> Fell from my eyes and I could see, –
> A drenched and dripping apple-tree[.]

* * *

Hallucinations and illusions connected with epilepsy and migraine have had a great impact on many creative individuals, influencing their work. An association between genius and epilepsy, 'the sacred disease', has been deemed likely since so many creative spirits have suffered from this disorder, among them Petrarch, Pascal, Molière, Byron, Flaubert, and Swinburne. In none of them did the illness cause any reduction of mental capability.

Epilepsy played an essential role in the life of Dostoevsky, and it had a marked impact on his work.[36] From a medical point of view, what he experienced were quite ordinary epileptic fits. What made them extraordinary were his subjective symptoms, described in his fiction – above all the well-known premonition of a coming attack called the aura, a phenomenon rarely described in medical literature.[37]

The aura experienced by Dostoevsky was associated with a feeling of ecstasy which in his view set him apart from other people. It resembles the sensations felt by De Quincey in his opium dreams (see pp. 55–57) and Huxley in his mescaline intoxication (pp. 62–63): '[A]ll his vital forces [seemed to] tense themselves at once in an extraordinary surge. The sensation of being alive and self-aware increased almost tenfold in those lightning-quick moments. His mind and heart were bathed in an extraordinary illumination. All his agitation, all his doubts and anxieties, seemed to be instantly reconciled and resolved into a lofty serenity, filled with pure, harmonious gladness and hope, filled too with the consciousness of the ultimate cause of all things.' In a letter about the same phenomenon, Dostoyevsky wrote, 'for several brief moments I feel a contentedness which

---

35 Ibid., pp. 67, 91, and 211.

36 Shannon Murray and T. J. Murray, 'The Epilepsy of Dostoevsky', *The Nova Scotia Medical Bulletin* 59.3 (August 1980), 90–94.

37 Henri Gastaut, 'Fyodor Mikhailovitch Dostoevsky's Involuntary Contribution to the Symptomatology and Prognosis of Epilepsy', *Epilepsia* 19 (1978), 186–201 (pp. 188–189 about the aura).

is unthinkable under normal conditions, and unimaginable for those who have not experienced it. At such times I am in perfect harmony with myself and with the entire universe. Perception is so clear and so agreeable that one would give ten years of his life, and perhaps all of it, for a few seconds of such bliss.'[38] This aura of bliss was a complete contrast to the feeling of guilt and shame that accompanied the epileptic attacks, represented as the evil and demonic feature of the character Smerdiakov in *The Brothers Karamazov*. That feeling is more closely connected with the fundamental tone of Dostoevsky's fiction, the descent into the darkest recesses of the soul, than with the sense of happiness that preceded his attacks – a sense which nevertheless helped him describe his ideal of goodness and purity, Prince Myshkin in *The Idiot*.

Just after an attack, Dostoevsky would be dejected and listless. As he himself put it, 'the aftereffects of my fits, i.e., nervousness, shortness of memory, an intensified and foggy, quasi-contemplative state, persist longer now than in previous years. They used to pass after three days, while now it may take six. Especially at night, by candlelight, an indefinite hypochondriac melancholy, and as if a red, bloody shade (not color) upon everything. Almost impossible to work during those days.'[39] Even so, he did not experience the kind of writer's block that afflicted Flaubert between attacks (pp. 43–44); on the contrary, he would usually express himself with remarkable ease and rapidity, employing a concise, abundant, and colourful vocabulary. Indeed, he registered an increase in his literary output just before an attack. He drew on his experience of the disease in his novels: no fewer than five of his fictional characters are epileptics, above all Prince Myshkin, and he provides them with the same symptoms that he had experienced himself.

So did Dostoevsky's epilepsy affect his outlook on life as well, and did it form part of the basis for his writing? '"What if it is the illness then?" he decided finally. "What does it matter if it is some abnormal tension, if the end-result, the instant of apprehension, recalled and analysed during recovery, turns out to be the highest pitch of harmony and beauty, conferring a sense of some hitherto-unknown and unguessed completeness, proportion, reconciliation, an ecstatic prayerful fusion with the supreme synthesis of life?"'[40]

* * *

38 The first quotation is from Fyodor Dostoyevsky, *The Idiot*, trans. by Alan Myers (Oxford: Oxford University Press, 1998), pp. 237–238. The second, from a letter to Nicolai Strakhov, is quoted by Henri Gastaut in the article mentioned in the preceding note, p. 188.

39 Fyodor Dostoyevsky, *The Notebooks for* The Possessed, ed. by Edward Wasiolek and trans. by Victor Terras (Chicago: University of Chicago Press, 1968), p. 29.

40 From *The Idiot*, p. 237 in the edition mentioned in note 38.

This kind of perfect harmony has been described as occurring in conjunction with a large number of various conditions, including drug-induced intoxication (see pp. 61–65). Alfred Tennyson experienced it during his well-known 'waking trances'.[41] These spells might occur spontaneously, or they might be evoked by the poet himself when silently repeating his own name until 'the individuality itself seemed to dissolve & fade away into boundless being – & this not a confused state but the clearest of the clearest, the surest of the surest, utterly beyond words – where Death was an almost laughable impossibility – the loss of personality (if so it were) seeming no extinction but the only true life'.[42]

In his early years, Tennyson was very afraid of these waking dreams and tried to keep them a secret, as they could be signs of epilepsy. In his day, that was a shameful disease believed to be caused by masturbation. Not until much later in life did Tennyson speak frankly about his fruitful, mystical visions, convinced that they were unconnected with epilepsy; they were simply referred to as gout, a diagnosis given to a number of different pathological conditions at the time.

Even so, given that epilepsy was common in Tennyson's family, his visions may still have had an epileptic dimension; the absence of convulsions does not preclude that diagnosis. His ability to bring about the condition by means of self-hypnosis indicates an epileptic centre in his temporal lobe. To Tennyson, the condition entailed a 'surge of his poetic imagination', a genuine pathway to suprasensory knowledge.[43]

In 'The Ancient Sage', Tennyson describes the ability to 'escape from self into the Nameless' – an explanation of his dream trances. He transformed his experiences into exalted poetry expressed as visions; in the conclusion of 'The Holy Grail', King Arthur speaks about them to his knights:

> Let visions of the night or of the day
> Come, as they will; and many a time they come,
> Until this earth he walks on seems not earth,
> This light that strikes his eyeball is not light,
> This air that smites his forehead is not air
> But vision – yes, his very hand and foot –
> In moments when he feels he cannot die[.]

During the aura that preceded his attacks of migraine, Lewis Carroll (real name Charles Lutwidge Dodgson) experienced hallucinations in which he felt that his body became distorted in size and shape.[44] *Alice in Wonderland* reproduced its spiritual father's peculiar experiences in words and pictures:

---

41 Robert Bernard Martin, *Tennyson: The Unquiet Heart* (Oxford: Clarendon, 1980), p. 238.

42 Ibid., pp. 28–29 (the quotation comes from a letter of Tennyson's to B. P. Blood, of 7 May 1874).

43 Ibid., pp. 555 ('surge of poetic imagination') and 278.

44 C. W. Lippman, 'Certain Hallucinations Peculiar to Migraine', *Journal of Nervous and Mental Disease* 116.4 (1952), 346–351 (p. 351).

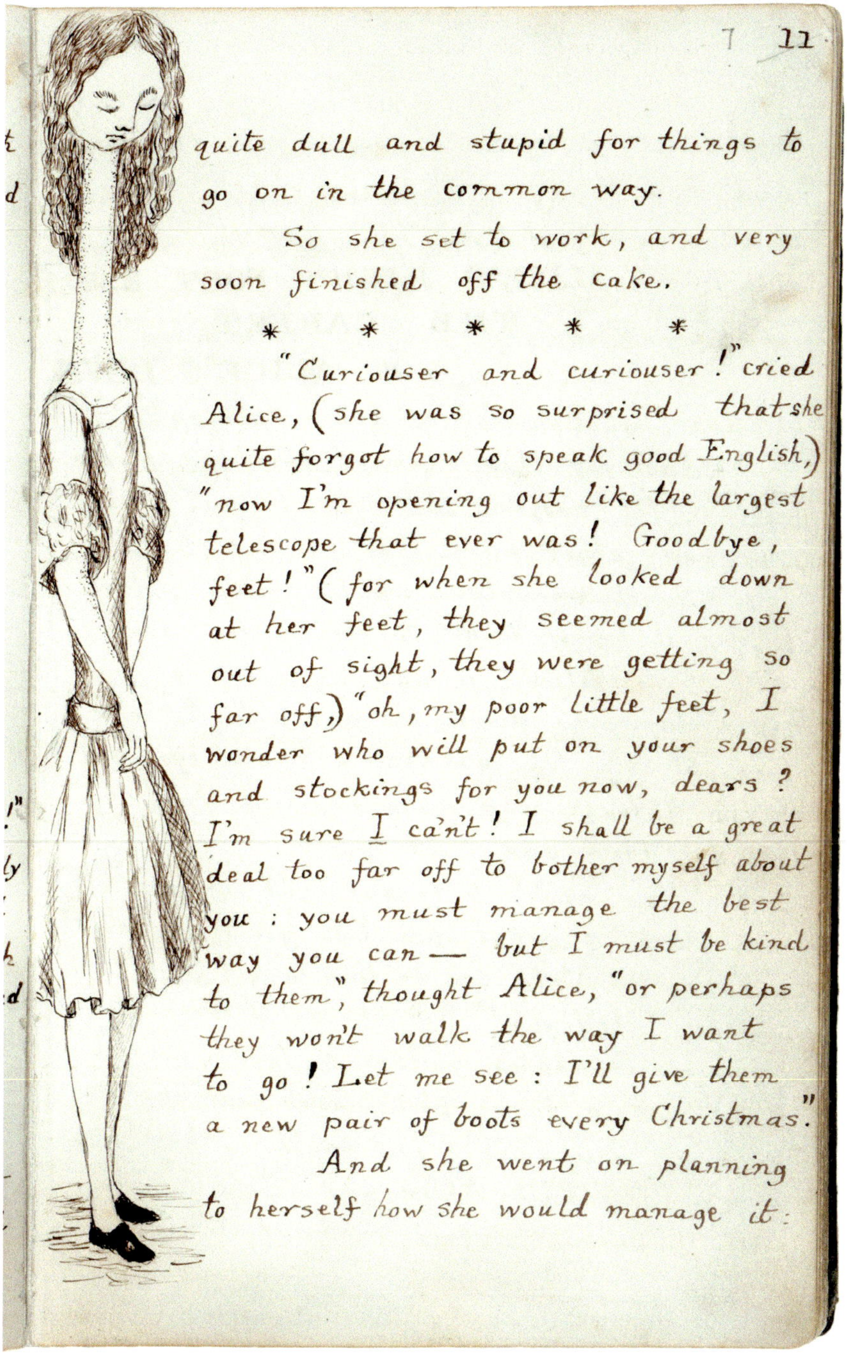
7 11

quite dull and stupid for things to go on in the common way.

So she set to work, and very soon finished off the cake.

* * * * *

"Curiouser and curiouser!" cried Alice, (she was so surprised that she quite forgot how to speak good English,) "now I'm opening out like the largest telescope that ever was! Goodbye, feet!" (for when she looked down at her feet, they seemed almost out of sight, they were getting so far off,) "oh, my poor little feet, I wonder who will put on your shoes and stockings for you now, dears? I'm sure I can't! I shall be a great deal too far off to bother myself about you: you must manage the best way you can — but I must be kind to them", thought Alice, "or perhaps they won't walk the way I want to go! Let me see: I'll give them a new pair of boots every Christmas."

And she went on planning to herself how she would manage it:

Figure 40 Lewis Carroll, *Alice in Wonderland*. This is a page from the manuscript, with the protagonist drawn by the author, not by the famous *Alice* illustrator John Tenniel.

'"Curiouser and curiouser!" cried Alice (she was so much surprised that for the moment she quite forgot how to speak good English). "Now I'm opening out like the largest telescope that ever was! Good-bye, feet!" (for when she looked down at her feet, they seemed to be almost out of sight, they were getting so far off).'[45] This rare disorder has been referred to as the *Alice in Wonderland* syndrome. It would surely have amused the author to have heard a fellow mathematician observe, many years later, that 'the method of condensation is like Alice shrinking'.[46]

* * *

Epilepsy, in combination with manic-depressive symptoms, played a decisive role in the life and art of a great painter, too. During Vincent van Gogh's last and most productive years, his creative ability – also sometimes influenced by absinthe – was affected by a rare variant of the disease. The toxic effect of this beverage and some medicines (for instance bromides), which he took in increasing amounts, may have exacerbated his condition, bringing on attacks of anguish, confusion, and aggression.

During one of these attacks, Van Gogh first threatened to kill his friend Gauguin, whereupon he cut off the lobe of his ear and made a gift of it to a sex worker. The consequence of this crisis may be seen in one of his self-portraits, with a bandage around the artist's head. Between attacks, Van Gogh was affected by a remarkable and powerful symptom, a compulsively enhanced creative activity called hypergraphia. Since the condition affected a great artist, we owe the existence of an overwhelmingly large number of brilliant paintings – many of them begun and finished on the same day – to a pathological symptom.

Van Gogh himself knew that there was something the matter with him. In letters to his brother Theo, he wrote, 'I am working like one actually possessed, more than ever I am in a dumb fury of work ... I am struggling with all my energy to master my work, thinking that if I succeed, that will be the best lightning-conductor for my illness'. 'And then my brush goes between my fingers as a bow would on the violin.'[47]

One would have thought that Van Gogh's eloquent account of his symptoms would have led to consensus as to the nature of his condition; but no historical personage has been the object of so many shifting suggestions with regard to the nature of his illness – over a hundred diagnoses have been proposed. The latest, advocated in a comprehensive description by

45 Quoted from the second Norton edition of Lewis Carroll, *Alice's Adventures in Wonderland* (New York and London: W. W. Norton, 1992 [1897]), p. 13.

46 Edward Wakeling (1946–2023, a former chairman of the Lewis Carroll Society) in a letter quoted in Morton N. Cohen, *Lewis Carroll: A Biography* (London: Macmillan, 1995), p. 258.

47 Pages 203–204 and 216 in Vincent van Gogh, *Complete Letters of Vincent van Gogh*, Vol. 3, 3rd edn (Boston: Bulfinch Press, 2000).

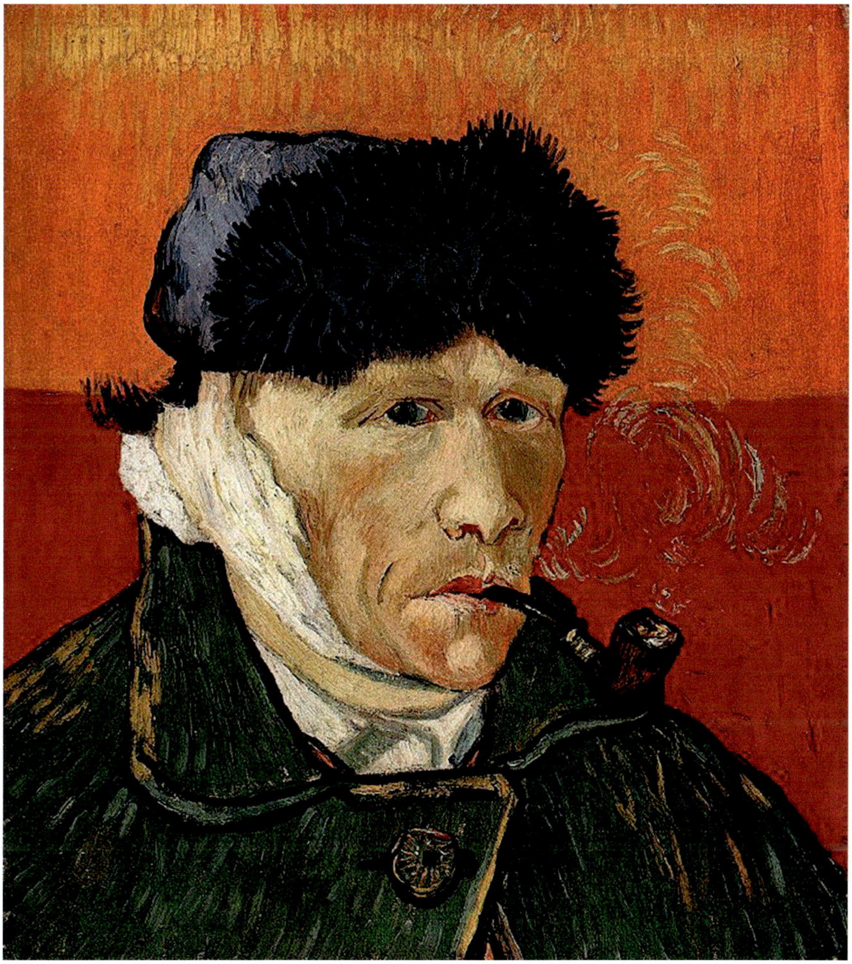

Figure 41 Vincent van Gogh, 'Self-portrait with bandage and pipe', 1889. The artist has cut off the lobe of his ear.

the English physician Wilfred Arnold, is acute intermittent porphyria – a hereditary metabolic disorder in which the body produces poisonous matter that brings on attacks of an epileptic nature.[48] The diagnosis was suggested by Arnold's co-worker Loretta Loftus; and, in a thorough analysis based on Van Gogh's letters, Arnold and Loftus have investigated the extent to which the studied pathology agrees with the hypotheses that have been put forward. They found that about a dozen of these hypotheses – mainly manic-depressive psychosis, alcoholism, syphilis, and lead poisoning – were worth serious consideration. The idea that Van Gogh suffered from Ménière's

48 Wilfred Arnold, *Vincent van Gogh: Chemicals, Crises, and Creativity* (Boston: Birkhäuser, 1992), pp. 141–164.

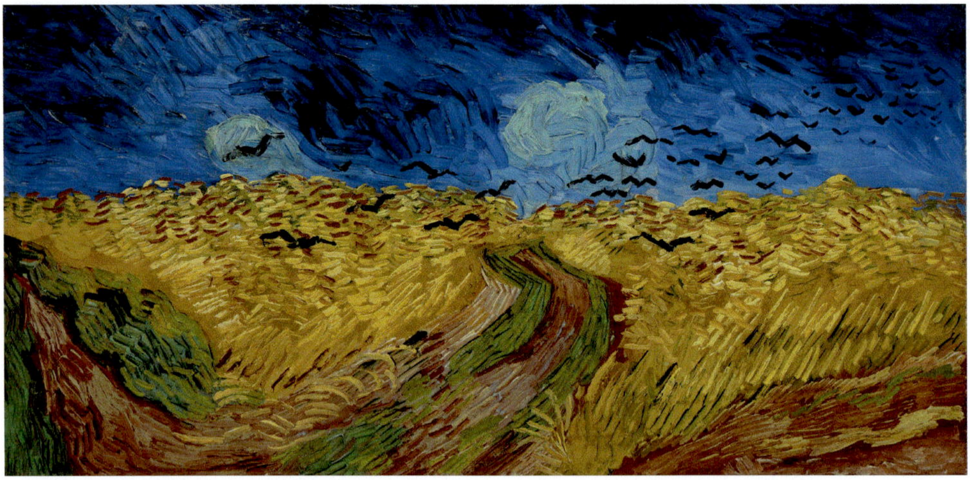

Figure 42 Vincent van Gogh, 'Wheat field with crows', 1890. The same painting comprises both manic manifestations, seen in the bold brush-strokes, and depressive features with a menacing sky and ominous black birds.

ear disease is subjected to a particularly gruff dismissal: 'The presentation exemplifies all of the worst aspects of selective embrace of symptoms ... and misconstruing of quotations in order to shore up an idea.'[49]

Arnold concludes that the acute-intermittent-porphyria diagnosis is the best fit; it encompasses all the symptoms that characterise Van Gogh's illness as recorded, especially regarded against the background of his manic-depressive disposition and his abuse of absinthe. Jan Waldenström, who has conducted fundamental research in the field, has his doubts as a significant symptom, red colouring of the urine, is not mentioned in the correspondence. Kay Jamison, who of course had personal experience of manic-depressive illness which is far more common, supplies strong indications that this was in fact the disease from which van Gogh suffered, adding ironically, 'when one hears hoofbeats it is unlikely to be a zebra'.[50]

In a letter from his last summer, Van Gogh wrote: 'I have painted three more big canvases since. They are vast fields of wheat under troubled skies, and I did not need to go out of my way to try to express sadness and extreme loneliness.'[51] In his final landscape painting, 'Wheat field with crows', the contradictory features of his personality coalesce and attain a tragic climax:

49 Ibid., p. 185.

50 Jamison, *Touched with Fire*, mentioned above in Chapter 2 (note 9). A possible source for Waldenström, an article in *Acta physiat. et neurol.* 14.375 (1939), was unavailable. However, Waldenström was a colleague of Sandblom's, and there may have been direct communication between them on this point.

51 Vincent van Gogh, letter to his siblings, p. 295 in the edition of his letters mentioned in note 47.

the manic dimension is present in the agitated, whirling brush-strokes depicting the waving corn, while anguish is conveyed by the menacing clouds and the flock of black birds. The latter embody the dismal thoughts which would soon drive him to suicide.

* * *

It is difficult to establish the type of mental affliction that destroyed the life but promoted the art of the Italian Renaissance composer Gesualdo, 'the mad Prince of Venosa'.[52] The fact that he ordered the fatal knifing of his wife and her lover in front of him, adding some extra stab wounds himself just for pleasure, was perhaps not so remarkable during this violent period, especially as the couple had been surprised *in flagrante*. But when, uncertain that he was the child's father, he had his own son put to death by having him so vehemently rocked that suffocation ensued, Gesualdo really transgressed the bounds of normal behaviour. He has been described as an eccentric, hardened, and cruel lunatic.

During his final years, after he had ceased composing, Gesualdo was in a state of despondency bordering on insanity, overwhelmed by his guilty conscience over his threefold crime. He is said to have been haunted and tormented by a flock of demons who left him alone only when ten or twelve young men, whom he employed for this express purpose, whipped him three times a day – a masochistic shock treatment if ever there was one.

Gesualdo's highly strung personality is reflected in his compositions which were audacious and fantastic, with dissonances far ahead of his time. With the same violence that characterised his personal life, he broke all the rules; anxious to achieve more powerful expression and find a vent for his inner tempests, he did not shrink from peculiarities in the harmony or from drastic rhythmic interruptions.

Obsessed with the dark aspects of human life, the tragic and the bizarre, Gesualdo wrote the poems for his profane madrigals himself, and they are full of pain and thoughts of death. Slow sequences with rare harmonies and heart-rending as well as melodious exclamations express grief and suffering.

As is the case with so many innovative artists, Gesualdo was misunderstood for a long time – several centuries, in fact. His music was said to evince irregularities that resulted from the confusion and embarrassment of the ignoramus. One of the most beautiful examples of his mature style, the madrigal 'Moro Lasso' (Figure 43), was described as deeply offensive to the ear. The nineteenth century brought a radical change, and these days this madrigal is regarded not as 'stammering and experimental utterances in a new idiom, but as miracles of perfected craft ... one of the crowning glories of the old order of polyphony'. '[Gesualdo] is a perfect master of the short, poignant phrase – precursor of the *leit-motif* – whether it be an expressive

52 See Elena Ferrari-Barasse, 'Gesualdo', in Marc Honegger (ed.), *Dictionnaire de la musique* (Paris: Bordas, 1970), Vol. 1, p. 403.

melodic fall or a striking harmonic progression.'[53] Gesualdo has become recognised as a composer of outstanding genius whose works live on as passionate expressions of a most unusual personality.

***

Handel and Schumann were two composers who alternated between joy in the manic phase and suffering in the depressive one. Like Van Gogh, they created with astonishing ease and swiftness when in a manic state, but slowly and with difficulty after the onset of depression. Schumann conceived

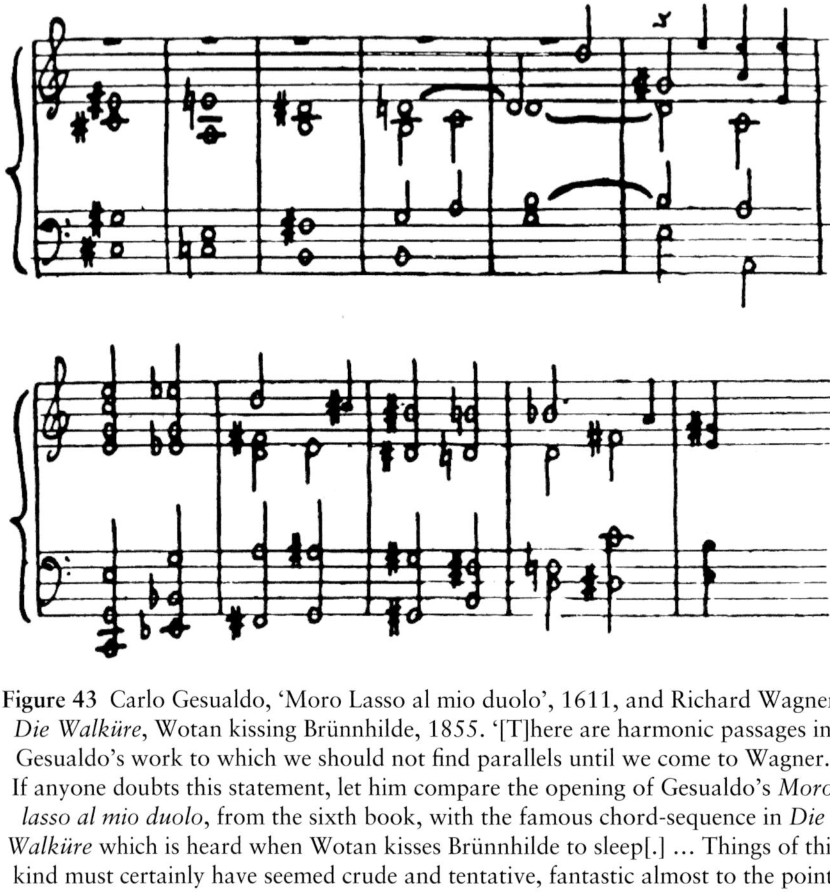

Figure 43 Carlo Gesualdo, 'Moro Lasso al mio duolo', 1611, and Richard Wagner, *Die Walküre*, Wotan kissing Brünnhilde, 1855. '[T]here are harmonic passages in Gesualdo's work to which we should not find parallels until we come to Wagner. If anyone doubts this statement, let him compare the opening of Gesualdo's *Moro lasso al mio duolo*, from the sixth book, with the famous chord-sequence in *Die Walküre* which is heard when Wotan kisses Brünnhilde to sleep[.] ... Things of this kind must certainly have seemed crude and tentative, fantastic almost to the point of insanity, to the historians of the eighteenth and nineteenth centuries.'[54]

53 Philip Heseltine, 'Gesualdo the Musician' in Cecil Gray and Philip Heseltine, *Don Carlo Gesualdo, Prince of Ventosa* (London: Kegan Paul, Trench, Trübner & Co., 1926), pp. 77–130 (the relevant quotations are on pp. 90–91 and 121–123).

54 Ibid., pp. 120–121.

and completed the piano cycle *Kreisleriana*, his most personal work and a highlight of musical Romanticism, in a mere six days. In a letter to his beloved Clara Wieck, Schumann commented: 'I'm overflowing with music and beautiful melodies now – imagine, since my last letter I've finished another whole notebook of new pieces. I intend to call it *Kreisleriana*. You and one of your ideas play the main role in it, and I want to dedicate it to you[55] – yes, to you and nobody else – and then you will smile so sweetly when you discover yourself in it – my music now seems to be so simply and wonderfully intricate in spite of all the simplicity, all the complications, so eloquent and from the heart; that's the way it affects everyone for whom I play it, which I enjoy doing ... When will you be standing at my side when I'm playing the piano? – Oh, we will both cry like children!'[56]

Even if Clara recognised the tonal character of the work, she is sure to have been surprised at how agitated and partly disharmonious it was, and concerned that it might not be appreciated. Like Van Gogh, Schumann had expressed the widely divergent aspects of his own nature in one and the same work, in which he alternately lets us listen to the dreamer Eusebius and the flamboyant Florestan. In the bold composition, gentle pieces succeed wild and demonic ones with a sudden vehemence that astonished the composer himself, driven as he was by unfettered inspiration. The premonition that Schumann had suggested in his letter to Clara was confirmed in due course, and *Kreisleriana* constituted a harbinger of subsequent developments.

Schumann suffered repeated attacks of severe depression: 'on the night of October 17th, 1833, I was suddenly struck by the most horrible thought which anyone can have – the most horrible with which heaven can punish us – that of losing one's mind – it took hold of me with such intensity that all solace, all my prayers were like scorn and derision. This fear drove me from one place to another; I couldn't breathe when I asked myself, "What would happen if you could no longer think," – Clara, if you're shattered like that you're not aware of suffering, sickness, despair – then I ran to a doctor in a state of continual and terrible agitation – told him everything, that I often fainted, that I was so afraid I didn't know what to do, that I couldn't guarantee that in a state of extreme helplessness I wouldn't take my life. Don't be shocked, my angel from heaven; just listen. The doctor kindly consoled me and finally said with a smile, "Medicine won't help at all; find a woman; she will cure you at once." I felt relieved; I thought that would be possible' – and he sang hopefully, using Heine's words in 'Poet's Love':

55 In the end, he dedicated it to Chopin.

56 Letter from Robert Schumann to Clara Wieck, dated 'Saturday before Easter' 1838, in *The Complete Correspondence of Clara and Robert Schumann*, ed. by Eva Weissweiler, trans. by Hildegard Fritsch and Ronald L. Crawford, 3 vols (New York: Peter Lang, 1994), Vol. 1, pp. 141–142.

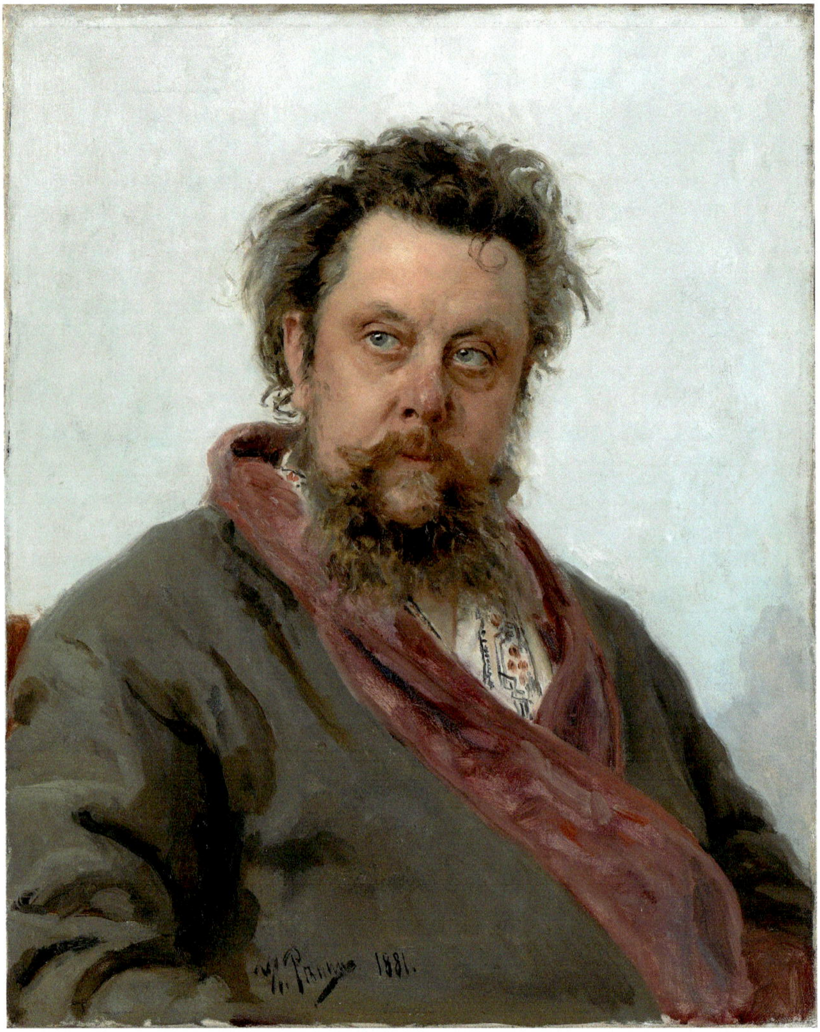

Figure 44 Ilja Repin, 'Portrait of Mussorgsky', 1881.

When I look into your eyes,
All my pain and sorrow vanish;
But when I kiss your lips,
Then I am wholly healed.[57]

57 'Dichterliebe': 'Wenn ich in deine Augen seh / So schwindet all meine Leid und Weh / Doch wenn ich küsse deinen Mund / So werd ich ganz und gar gesund'. English translation by Richard Stokes, from *The Book of Lieder* (London: Faber and Faber, 2005). The letter is dated 11 February 1838, p. 97 in the edition of the Schumann correspondence mentioned in the preceding note (Vol. 1).

Schumann followed the friendly advice, but the cure did not last, and he was afflicted by a delirium with auditory hallucinations.[58] He told Clara how angels sang a wonderful melody which he attempted to write down. However, his creative capability ultimately ended in a state of severe depression. Having attempted suicide in the waters of the Rhine, he was isolated in an asylum whose inhumane directives cut him off from every connection with his wife and his friends. His mental state deteriorated as a result, and he starved himself to death.

Modest Mussorgsky drank himself to death, alcohol being the commonest means of assuaging anxiety and relieving depression.[59] His creative ability was closely bound up with the shifts in his moods, as his letters show. When he was feeling cheerful, plenty of merry notes came into existence; 'the sounds and ideas hung in the air, and now I am gulping and overeating. I can hardly manage to scribble it down on paper.'[60] Light of heart, he composed cheerful pieces almost as if in a delirium, *Pictures from an Exhibition* among them. When he was despondent, feeling that life was meaningless, he was either quiet or engaged on writing sad songs full of despair, like the ones he collected under the title *Sunless* (compare Nietzsche below) or *Songs and Dances of Death*. Mussorgsky spent his last few years in the misery of chronic alcoholism and its complications, *delirium tremens* and epileptic seizures. A late portrait painted by Ilja Repin has left us a harrowing picture of his mental and physical decline.

Even so, symptoms of manifest mental illness are more seldom seen in music than in literature and pictorial arts; at any rate, they are harder to trace in music. An accelerated inner pace during Schumann's manic periods may account for the extremely rapid tempi he occasionally prescribed in his compositions; they made his contemporaries suspect that there was something wrong with his metronome. As the conductor von Karajan has pointed out, however, there is a more convincing example in Schumann's Fourth Symphony, a musical phrase that is repeated excessively.[61] This is a schizophrenic symptom to which psychiatrists refer as 'fil circulaire' or verbigeration and which has a counterpart in the pictorial arts in the phenomenon called perseveration, endlessly repeated signs (cf. Figure 29). The same symptom, albeit more pronounced, is seen in an even more advanced case of mental illness, the final stage of Hölderlin's schizophrenia. One of his friends was most concerned and observed that Hölderlin still played the piano correctly, though in a highly singular fashion. Once started, he would

58 John O'Shea, *Music and Medicine: Medical Profiles of the Great Composers* (London: Dent, 1990), p. 130.

59 See Vladimir Lerner, 'The Pathography of Composers: Modest Mussorgsky', *Journal of Medical Biography* 6.3 (1998), 175–181.

60 Quoted from a letter to Vladimir Stasov, [12?] June 1874, in *The Musorgsky Reader: A Life of Modeste Musorgsky in Letters and Documents*, ed. and trans. by Jay Leyda and Sergei Bertensson (New York: W. W. Norton, 1947), p. 271.

61 Sandblom refers to Richard Osborne, *Conversations with Karajan* (Oxford: Oxford University Press, 1989); however, it was not possible to locate a page reference for this claim.

go on for days, pursuing one childishly simple idea and playing it over hundreds and hundreds of times, to such an extent that no one could endure it.[62]

Friedrich Nietzsche is an example of how severe mental symptoms in life and work may be caused by organic changes in the brain. His derangement, caused by tertiary syphilis, led to a mental breakdown and *paralysie générale*.[63] Symptoms of his illness are increasingly evident in his late works, and it can be difficult to decide where normality leaves off and pathology comes in; for instance, what role did his syphilis play when he conceived his notion of 'der Übermensch'?

The triumphant self-assertion that is the first sign of this mental disorder comes out in the following quotation from the somewhat bizarre *Ecce Homo*: '[G]enius is conditioned by dry air, clear sky – that is to say by rapid metabolism, by the possibility of again and again supplying oneself with great, even tremendous quantities of energy.'[64] This self-assurance becomes moving when viewed against the background of Nietzsche's feeble health. He suffered from severe attacks of migraine, frequent stomach pains, and, above all, a tormenting insomnia which caused him to take vast quantities of chloral and veronal. No wonder he made Zarathustra praise sleep: 'Still! Still! Did not the world just become perfect? But what is happening to me? Just as a delicate breeze, unseen, dances upon an inlaid sea, lightly, featherlightly: so – sleep dances upon me.'[65] Nietzsche was a musician, too. The poem by Byron which he selected for setting to music dealt with the moon, 'Sun of the Sleepless'.

* * *

Alzheimer's disease entails a gradual destruction of nerve cells in the cerebral cortex; growing numbers of these cells seemingly die by suicide through an enzymatic process.

The famous author Iris Murdoch was affected. The loss of mental capacity that attends this illness unfortunately meant that she was unable to describe the symptoms of which she grew less and less aware. Her husband of 40 years, John Bayley, did so, however, in his book *Elegy for Iris* (1999), with such profound insight and compassion that I quote him fairly liberally in these pages.

62 Wilhelm Waiblinger, 'Friedrich Hölderlins Leben, Dichtung und Wahnsinn', in *Wilh. Waiblingers gesammelte Werke: mit des Dichters Leben*, 9 vols, Vol. 3 (Hamburg: Georg Heubel, 1839), pp. 219–261, p. 248.

63 Frederick Copleston, *Friedrich Nietzsche: Philosopher of Culture* (London and New York: Search Press and Harper & Row, 1975), p. 27.

64 Friedrich Nietzsche, *Ecce Homo: How One Becomes What One Is*, trans. R. J. Hollingdale (London: Penguin, 1979), p. 55.

65 Friedrich Nietzsche, *Thus Spoke Zarathustra: A Book for Everyone and Nobody*, trans. Graham Parkes (Oxford: Oxford University Press, 2005), p. 241. (The passage occurs in the fourth and last part, section 10.)

Alzheimer's disease resembles a creeping fog which the sick person hardly notices until everything around him or her has vanished. At that stage, it becomes difficult to even imagine that there is a world outside.

Competent nursing remains the only therapy. Medicinal treatments have been disappointing. Medicines that bring some improvement are effective for too short a period; and they threaten to confuse, even terrify patients during brief lucid spells when the mercifully concealing fog is dispersed and sufferers suddenly see an abyss opening before their feet.

As the illness progresses, both speech and writing are affected. Murdoch's husband records the following experience at an early stage, in connection with her addressing an audience: 'The chairman was sympathetic, but he soon became baffled and uncomfortable by Iris's inability to summon the words she seemed to want. Her delivery had always been slow and thoughtful and a little hesitant, and at first I was not perturbed, sure that she would recover in a few minutes, when she got the feel of the gathering. It was hard to say how conscious she was of her own difficulty, but the effect soon became paralysing, for the listener as well as for her.'[66]

A greater disaster ensued when the author lost her ability to write. She would, for instance, complain that she was stuck, that she could not continue with the novel on which she was engaged. '"It's this man Jackson," she said to me one day with a sort of worried detachment. "I can't make out who he is, or what he is doing"' (p. 213) – a welcome sidelight on her close relationships with the characters in her fiction. Bayley continues: 'I had known before that the mood would pass, and this one, though much odder, would, too – I could not imagine anything else. But suddenly, standing blinking in the dry, dusty sunlight of the Negev, I realised for the first time that something might be seriously wrong. ... For the first time, I took to enquiring about her ideas for a next novel. She had ideas, she said, but they wouldn't come together. She was trying to catch something by its tail, and it always eluded her' (pp. 213–214 and 217). Murdoch's ability to concentrate was lost, as was her ability to form coherent sentences. She no longer knew that she had written twenty-six remarkable novels: 'We had ... told and listened and communed together, until communication had dwindled and faltered and all but ceased. No more letters, no more words. ... The face of the Alzheimer's sufferer indicates only an absence: It is a mask in the most literal sense' (pp. 50 and 53).

One of the dominant symptoms of Alzheimer's, anxiety, left its mark on much of what Murdoch said. The constantly repeated question 'When are we leaving?' is an example, and another is the most pathetic question of all, as if she was thinking of what the blinded airman says in Faulkner's *Soldier's Pay*: 'When are they going to let me out?' (pp. 63–64).

Bayley described Murdoch's fear of being alone, of being cut off from familiar surroundings, as a feature of Alzheimer's, observing that '[i]f Iris

---

66 John Bayley, *Elegy for Iris* (New York: St Martin's Press, 1999), p. 212. Subsequent page references in parentheses in the running text.

could climb inside my skin now, or enter me as if I had a pouch like a kangaroo, she would do so' (p. 127).

As Alzheimer's disease progresses, it torments the partner more than the sick person, and the sufferer's spouse may develop what Bayley refers to as the terrible need to point out how difficult everything has become and compel the sick person to share in that experience. He loses his patience occasionally, sometimes intentionally. A fit of rage affords him relief and may even be therapeutic for the patient thanks to the sudden break in the routine (p. 233).

The sole thing that finds its way into the sufferer's consciousness is a joke: 'Humour seems to survive anything. ... Teasing nonsense rituals once lovingly exchanged awake an abruptly happy response, and a sudden beaming smile ... That is something to be tried for all the time. It transforms her face, bringing it back to what it was, and with an added glow that can seem almost supernatural' (pp. 54, 51, and 53). Iris's reactions become increasingly pointless, however, and daily habits replace what used to be her memory. Since her husband is fully aware of the erasure of her brain, he realises that her statement about how she feels that she is sailing into the darkness does not amount to a cruelly clear-sighted account of what is happening; she must have assimilated a suggestion from the couple's friends without being aware of doing so (p. 259). Bayley comments, '[t]he wish to be back beside me ... seems less and less forlorn, more simple, more natural. She is not sailing into the dark: The voyage is over, and under the dark escort of Alzheimer's, she has arrived somewhere. So have I' (p. 266).

* * *

The Swedish author Ulla Isaksson has written a memoir resembling that of John Bayley, *Boken om E* ('The book about E', 1994), which describes how her husband, the brilliant essayist Erik Hjalmar Linder, passed through the stages of increasing dementia up to the total annihilation of the life of his mind. 'What I have not yet said, hardly even thought: it seems a universe is going to pieces. I could not say more; I was trembling all over.' Like Bayley's, her book is characterised by profound insight and loving observation; 'blindly and childishly, I struggled against this strange thing that I felt had come between us'.[67]

Linder found it increasingly hard to concentrate in his writing, but his wife assisted him. A couple of knowledgeable friends had read part of his memoirs but found them disappointing. Isaksson describes how the couple had spent an evening with their friends, talking about their memories. Her husband had participated with alacrity, but the next day it was as if everything that had been called to life during the preceding evening had

67 Ulla Isaksson, *Boken om E* (Stockholm: Albert Bonniers förlag, 1994). Unfortunately it was not possible to identify the pages in this Swedish original version.

disappeared down a black hole. At that point, she offered to take the chapter in hand; it turned out quite well, and E was very pleased.

When Linder attempted to write a study of the style of a novel, the finished text consisted of 22 quotations introduced by a single sentence – the title of the novel was not even mentioned. Several of the quotations were faulty, and some appeared in more than one place; E had not drawn a single conclusion, nor had he made the slightest attempt at formulating a characterisation.

Isaksson found it hard to accustom herself to, and live with, the waning sense of togetherness and love. There was a widening gulf between the spouses, and vehement outbursts became more frequent: 'But the appalling Wrath that persecuted me like a shameful disease during the first "sick" years was certainly no laughing matter. I can feel it, though my pen is trembling. Three years of our life together have been lost to me. I was and was not there, I saw and heard, but understood nothing ... And yet, its hands tied behind its back, wretched love was constantly struggling to break free. We saw and heard it, we stretched out our arms towards it, and time and again it blessed us as we were on the brink of utter ruin. Now, too, it is love that drives me. I have to recover what I lost in order to be able to surmount that which drove us apart. In order to understand.'

* * *

Maurice Ravel, who fell silent during his last few years, was also obliged to experience how Alzheimer's disease destroys creative ability. The first sign of the loss of his powers was a difficulty in expressing himself. Finding that he was no longer able to write his music down, the desperate musician described the 'terrifying shadow' that extinguished his ideas.[68]

68 Valentine Hugo, 'Trois souvenirs sur Ravel', *La Revue musicale* 210 (January 1952), 137–146 (p. 145).

Chapter 6
Congenital malformations

Turning to purely physical illnesses, it is natural to begin with inherited disorders, as congenital malformations are. Humanity harbours an instinctive loathing of these defects; for that reason they often engender irrational feelings of shame in those affected, as well as a sense of repulsion in their fellow human beings. The unfortunate victims sometimes react with quiet resignation, but more often with revolt and attempts to gain compensation for themselves, in some cases by means of artistic activity.

This is how Sir Francis Bacon expresses their plight: 'Whosoever hath any thing fixed in his person that doth induce contempt, hath also a perpetual spur in himself to rescue and deliver himself from scorn. Therefore all deformed persons are extreme bold.'[1] Charles Lamb observed the same characteristic in Daniel Defoe, who lacked external ears: 'Neither have I incurred, nor done any thing to incur, with Defoe, that hideous disfigurement, which constrained him to draw upon assurance – to feel "quite unabashed," and at ease upon that article.'[2] Extremely developed facial features may be equally disfiguring. Nicolai Gogol was endowed with a huge, mobile nose which made him an object of ridicule. He compensated himself by making fun of his hideous appearance. In one of his short stories, he lets the nose of a conceited bureaucrat disappear, only to be subsequently discovered strutting down the street.

However, nobody has succeeded in compensating himself in a more sublime manner than Michelangelo, who had a melancholy disposition. Distressed and embarrassed by his malformed nose, broken during a fist-fight in his childhood, the vain artist proved that such a feature could coexist with great beauty by equipping one of his Holy Virgins with a comparable feature.

In the early eighteenth century, 'The Hunchback Song', a mock-celebration of that deformity, was very popular. The author himself had a huge hump

1 Francis Bacon, *The Essays or Counsels Civil and Moral*, ed. by Brian Vickers (Oxford: Oxford University Press, 1999), p. 99.

2 Charles Lamb, 'A Chapter on Ears', from *Quotidiana* (1823); quoted from Patrick Madden's edition, http://essays.quotidiana.org/lamb/chapter_on_ears.

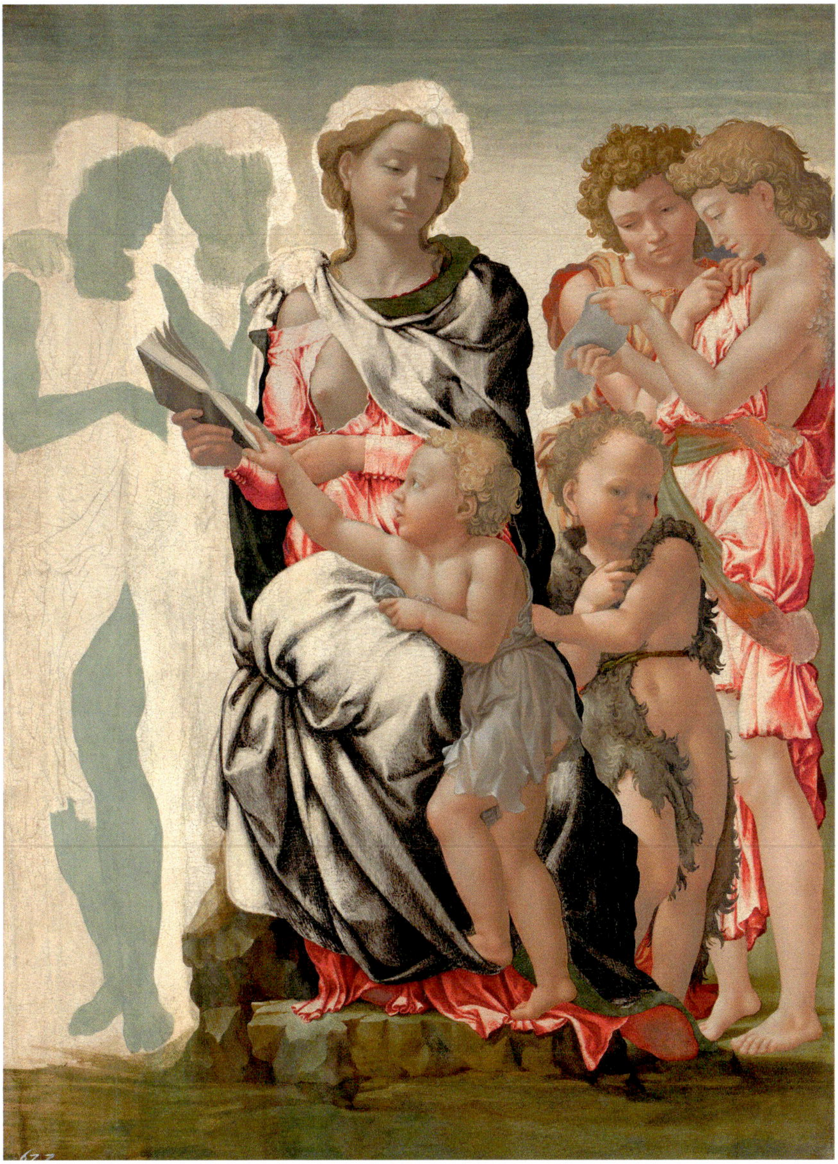

Figure 45 'The Manchester Madonna', ascribed to Michelangelo. The fact that the artist painted the Madonna with a somewhat irregular nose, which bears comparison to Michelangelo's own, supports the attribution to this master.

but was the first to mock it. In the course of history, hunchbacked persons have frequently been described as entertaining, and they would often play the part of jesters. When the song was performed for the first time, the poet gave a great dinner; but only hunchbacks were invited to it.

* * *

One of the best examples of the profound effect that a malformation may have on a person's life and personality, and hence also on any creative activity he or she may have pursued, is found in Lord Byron, whose club foot was, as his biographer-editor Thomas Moore put it, the 'curse' of his life.[3] Byron was intensely conscious of his deformity and went to great lengths to conceal it; any allusion to it would make him furious, especially if uttered by a woman. He happened to hear a young woman he loved say to her maid, 'Do you think I could care any thing for that lame boy?'[4] His own mother did not conceal her disgust with the child, to whom she once referred as a horrid 'abortion', and she had him exposed to extremely painful treatment by a quack. Byron took his revenge on her by means of a scene in his play *The Deformed Transformed*:

> *Enter* Arnold *and his mother* Bertha.
> Bertha: Out, hunchback!
> Arnold: I was born so, mother!
> Bertha: Out,
> Thou incubus! Thou nightmare! Of seven sons,
> The sole abortion!
> Arnold: Would that I had been so,
> And never seen the light!
> Bertha: I would so too![5]

Byron's wounded pride was decisive in forming the arrogant independence in his personality, and it stimulated his youthful genius in the creation of his early masterpieces. Any doubts about the connection are dispelled by his own words:

> ... deformity is daring.
> It is its essence to o'ertake mankind
> By heart and soul, and make itself the equal –
> Ay, the superior of the rest. There is
> A spur in its halt movements, to become
> All that the others cannot, in such things
> As still are free to both, to compensate
> For stepdame Nature's avarice at first.[6]

---

3 *Life, Letters, and Journals of Lord Byron: Complete in One Volume, with Notes* (London: J. Murray, 1844), p. 45: 'But the embittering circumstance of his life, – that, which haunted him like a curse, amidst the buoyancy of youth, and the anticipations of fame and pleasure, was, strange to say, the trifling deformity of his foot.' Byron called it the 'bane' of his life; Leslie A. Marchand, *Byron: A Biography*, 3 vols (New York: Alfred A. Knopf, 1957), Vol. 3, p. 1052.

4 Page 28 in Moore's volume; the woman was one Miss Chaworth. All these passages are also quoted in J. V. Hirschmann, 'Lord Byron's Deformed Foot: A Medical and Biographical Assessment', *Byron Journal* 48.1 (2020), 57–70.

5 Part I, Scene 1; p. 595 in the 1911 Oxford University Press edition of *The Poetical Works of Lord Byron.*

6 Ibid., p. 599.

All his life, Byron pursued strife and difficulty. His works reveal a predilection for rebels such as Don Juan and Cain, solitary outsiders. Cain's development adheres to a Byronic pattern: a stranger to his fellow men, he rose up against all authority and became an outcast.

In his contempt for humankind, Byron only finds a single person for whom he feels unrestricted love and respect – his half-sister (and half-bride?) Augusta Leigh:

> Though I feel that my soul is deliver'd
> To pain – it shall not be its slave.
> There is many a pang to pursue me:
> They may crush, but they shall not contemn;
> They may torture, but shall not subdue me –
> 'Tis of *thee* that I think – not of them.
>
> Though human, thou didst not deceive me,
> Though woman, thou didst not forsake[.][7]

***

For Henri Toulouse-Lautrec, who was far worse deformed than Byron, there were hardly any options except resignation and withdrawal from the world. Belonging to the aristocracy, he would surely have had a military career if it had not been for his malformed body with very short legs and a misshapen head, evident in numerous self-portraits. Toulouse-Lautrec himself said that, if he had had longer legs, he would never have been an artist. He adapted himself to his situation by associating with sex workers and finding his motifs in brothels, where his social position was of little significance and nobody cared what he looked like.

Defying his disabilities, he adopted the motto 'Paint, drink, and love', ending his days as a great artist, an alcoholic with attacks of *delirium tremens*, and a syphilitic. Jean-Edouard Vuillard was an eye-witness to his decline: 'Lautrec was too proud to submit to his lot, a physical freak, an aristocrat cut off from his kind by [his] grotesque appearance. He found an affinity between his own condition and the moral penury of the prostitute. He may have seemed cynical, but if so it was from an underlying despair ... I was always moved by the way in which Lautrec changed his tone when art was discussed. He who was so cynical and so foul-mouthed on all other occasions became completely serious. It was a matter of faith with him. ... Poor Lautrec! I went to see him one day, just after he had been put in a home in Neuilly. He hadn't long to live. He was a dying man, a wreck. His doctor had told him to "take exercise", so he had bought a gymnasium horse, Lautrec, who couldn't even get his foot on the pedals! A cruel irony – and yet it symbolized his whole life!'[8]

7 From 'Stanzas to Augusta', stanzas III and IV; p. 88 in the 1911 Oxford edition.

8 This passage appears to be Philip Sandblom's own translation from an article by G[ermain] B[azin], 'Lautrec raconté par Vuillard', *L'Amour de l'art* 12.4 (April 1931), 141–142.

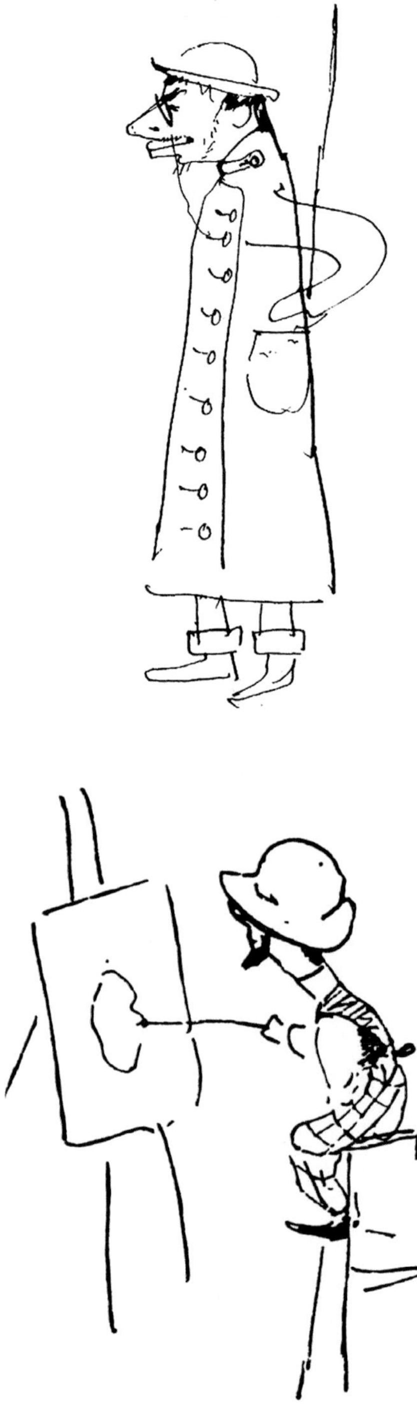

Figure 46 Henri de Toulouse-Lautrec, drawings. In his self-portraits, the artist demonstrates both his short legs and his deformed head.

Another famous painter whose whole life was influenced by a congenital defect was the Mexican artist Frida Kahlo. The reason for the desperation expressed in her works is the perennial pain caused by her *spina bifida*, with progressive ulcerations on the legs; see p. 2.

* * *

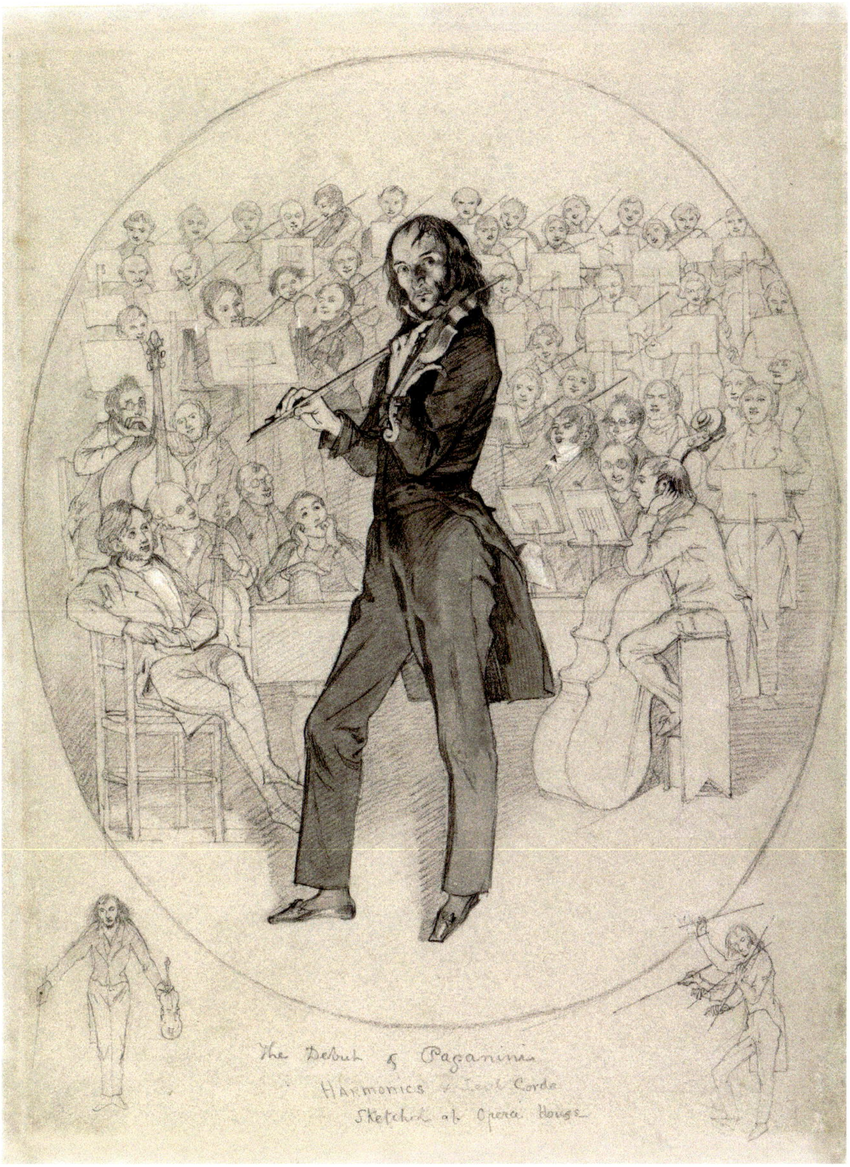

Figure 47 Daniel Maclise, 'Nicolò Paganini', 1831. In this drawing of the violin virtuoso, the abnormally flexible joints that are characteristic of his congenital disorder are clearly visible – note the backwards-bending thumb.

There is a peculiar case of a congenital physical disorder that actually promoted artistic activity. One of the greatest violinists of all time, the demonic Paganini, was marked by disease. Rarely has a great artist worked under more pitiful conditions. There was no end to his illnesses – he suffered from tuberculosis and syphilis, osteomyelitis of the jaw, diarrhoea, haemorrhoids, urinary retention, and sundry infections. His ill health, and not least the therapies he underwent, gave him an emaciated and increasingly odd appearance; the mercury cures prescribed for his syphilis caused his teeth to fall out and discoloured his skin. Evidently, chemotherapy was attended by distressing complications from the very beginning.

Even so, the most remarkable feature in his state of ill health was a congenital disorder, the Ehlers-Danlos syndrome, which formed the basis for his virtuosity as a violinist. This condition is characterised by an excessive flexibility of the joints. That made it possible for Paganini to perform the astonishing double-stoppings and roulades for which he was famous. His wrist was so loose that he could move and twist his hand in all directions, and his thumb could be bent backwards so that it reached his forearm. Although his hand was not malformed in itself, its reach was doubled: with his left thumb placed across the middle of the fingerboard, he was able to play in the first three positions without shifting.

This disorder, which is usually troublesome for the sufferer, became an artistic boon in Paganini's case – it was, indeed, a blessing in disguise. And what a disguise that was! Contemporaneous accounts describe how his strange appearance, his odd movements like those of a puppet, and the deathly pallor of his skin made him look almost ridiculous. However, this impression was dispelled the moment the master placed his violin beneath his chin and began to play: the first strokes of his bow were like an electric shock that gave him new life. 'He *throws* the bow on the strings and runs up and down the scales with marvellous rapidity, the cadences rippling out from beneath his fingers like so many strings of pearls.'[9]

Paganini's trills of ease were trills of disease. Liszt wrote in his obituary that 'the wonderful meeting of such a mighty talent with circumstances so adaptable to an apotheosis will remain a singularity in the history of art'.[10]

9 This is an English translation of a passage from Carl Guhr, *Über Paganinis Kunst die Violine zu spielen* (Mainz: B. Schotts Söhne, ?1830), p. 9. The translation is found in J. G. Prod'homme, *Nicolo Paganini: A Biography*, trans. Alice Mattullath (New York: Fischer, 1911), p. 24. (Guhr's book has been translated into English in its entirety.)

10 Franz Liszt, 'Sur Paganini: à propos de sa mort', *La Revue et Gazette Musicale* 7.50 (1840), 431–432 ('La combinaison singulière d'un talent colossal avec toutes les circonstances les plus propres à l'entourer de prestige, restera comme un fait isolé dans histoire de l'art'). The translation seems to have been Sandblom's own.

Chapter 7
Old age, debility, and death

As we approach the end of life, we encounter the condition that becomes the fate of everyone who lives long enough, namely old age. While old age is not always associated with retrogression, creative ability usually declines with advancing years. A few individuals, including Milton and Goethe as well as Titian and Verdi, continued to do powerful creative work well into senescence; but such endeavour is made increasingly difficult as one's powers decrease and infirmity comes into one's life.

Pictorial artists and sculptors tend to retain their creative ability longer than authors and composers; in addition, they often succeed in renewing their modes of expression as they near the end. Such a development may be seen in Titian, Rembrandt, Cézanne, and Klee.[1] Simone de Beauvoir observed that old artists were fortunate in comparison with writers; according to her, artists are not obliged to draw on their own experiences. Living not in the past but in the present, they are receptive to the colours, shapes, and flashes of inspiration that are still offered by the world.[2]

As darkness falls across one's path, one's thoughts – and consequently creative pursuits – turn increasingly to the brevity of life and its essential vanity. Unexpectedly early, there is sorrow over the loss of the bloom and attractiveness of youth. The ageing Montaigne provided an apt metaphor when he said that youth looks forward whereas age looks back; this, he said, was the essential meaning of the double face of Janus. If the years were to drag him along, he asked that they would do so backwards, affording him glimpses of the sweetness of the stage of life which was now over. Memories of youth would stay with him, and he quoted Martial saying that those who can remember the past live twice.[3]

* * *

1 See E. Andersson, S. Berg, M. Lawenius, and J.-E. Ruth, 'Creativity in Old Age: A Longitudinal Study', *Aging Clinical and Experimental Research* 1 (1989).

2 Simone de Beauvoir, *La Vieillesse* (Paris: Gallimard, 1970), p. 429. There is an English translation by Patrick O'Brian; see Simone de Beauvoir, *The Coming of Age* (New York: W. W. Norton, 1996), p. 406.

3 Michel de Montaigne, *The Complete Essays*, ed. and trans. by M. A. Screech (London: Penguin, 1987); Book III, Section 5, p. 949. The reference to Martial is to his *Epigrams*, X.xxiii.

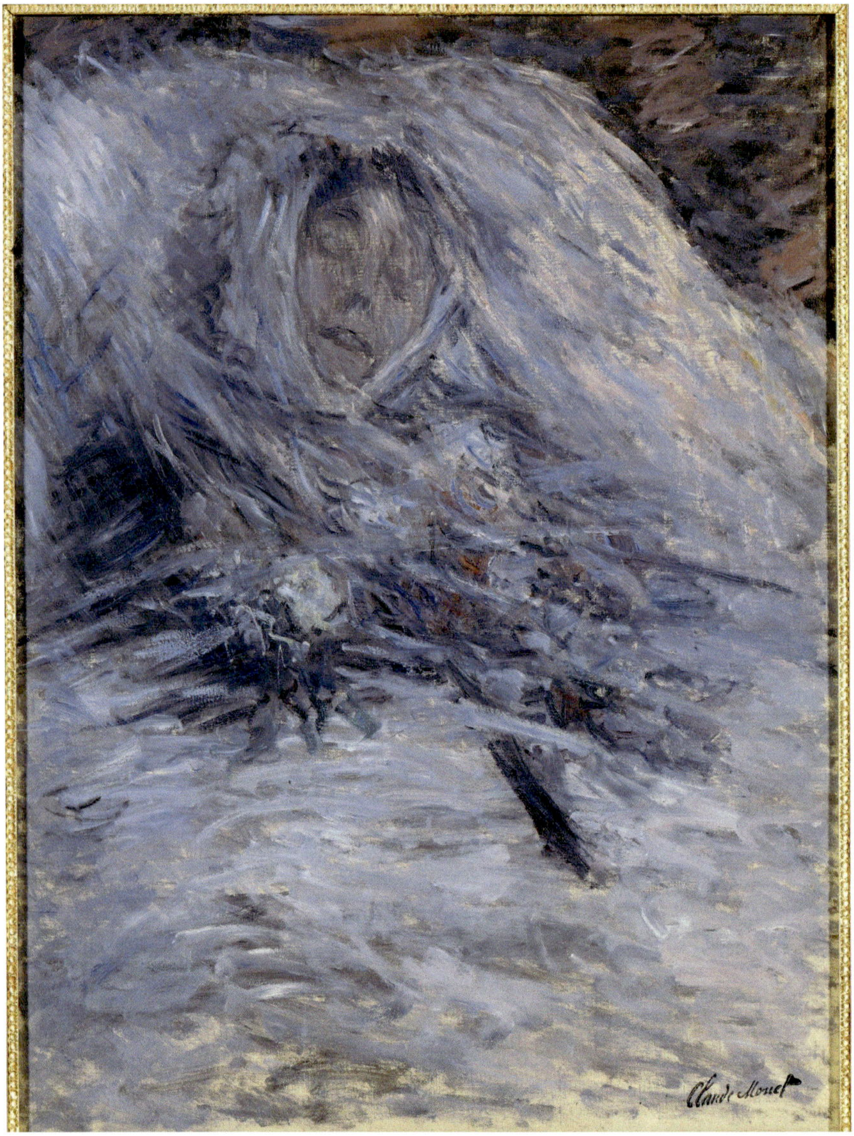

Figure 48 Claude Monet, 'Camille on her deathbed', 1879. Monet painted a portrait of his dying 32-year-old wife. He commented that he had caught himself studying her tragic temples, almost automatically searching for the series of shifting colours – blue, yellow, grey, and others – that death had created on her stiffened face.[4]

4 Georges Clemenceau, *Claude Monet: les nymphéas* (Paris: Plon et Nourrit, 1928), p. 19.

A mere fifty years old, Pierre de Ronsard was obliged to endure the bitterness of being rejected on account of his age, no longer being welcome to take part in the games and pleasures of love. He saw his beloved sitting, bored and uninterested without deigning to afford him so much as a look, whereas her cousin at least threw him a passing glance:

> Viste comme un esclair sur moy jetta son oeil.
> Toy, comme paresseuse et pleine de sommeil,
> D'un seul petit regard tu ne m'estimas digne[.][5]

Frightened by her silence, the poet slipped away, afraid that his greeting would displease her.

Voltaire was also sadly conscious of the fact that the time for love had expired and was in despair over the loss of its pleasures. To his friend Mme du Châtelet he addressed the following lines:

> One dies twice, I see that now:
> To cease to please and be worth loving
> Is an unbearable death;
> To cease living is nothing.[6]

In exchange for love, he received friendship that was sweeter and more gentle, but far less vivid. Captivated by this new beauty with an enlightened soul, he followed her willingly, but wept at his inability to follow anybody else but her.[7]

The Swedish poet Esaias Tegnér (1782–1846) expressed himself with great pathos: for 'an eternal youth with an eternal desire', growing old and falling ill was particularly bitter. 'The older, the more infirm, and the more dejected we become, the more we treasure our youthful memories. If trees were capable of longing, I am convinced that their thoughts would be of spring as their leaves fell.'[8] At the same age, and maybe in a similar mood, Richard Strauss composed *Der Rosenkavalier*. In this autumnal opera, attention is focused not on a bold Salome discarding her seven veils but on

---

5 Poem number XVI in Book I of the sequence 'Des sonnets pour Hélène'. Page 222 in the first volume of Pierre de Ronsard, *Œuvres complètes*, ed. by Gustave Cohen (Paris: Gallimard, 1950), two vols.

6 'On meurt deux fois, je le vois bien: / Cesser d'aimer et d'être aimable / C'est une mort insupportable, / Cesser de vivre ce n'est rien.' From 'Stances X [the number varies in different editions]: A Madame du Chatelet' (1741). In *Epitres, stances, et odes par Voltaire*, Vol. 2 (Paris: L. de Bure, 1823), 100–102 (p. 101).

7 'Du ciel alors daignant descendre, / L'Amitié vint à mon secours; / Elle est plus égale, aussi tendre, / Et moins vive que les Amours. // Touché de sa beauté nouvelle, / Et de sa lumière éclairé, / Je la suivis, mais je pleurai / De ne pouvoir plus suivre qu'elle.' Pages 101–102 in the edition mentioned in the previous note (Vol. 2).

8 The designation 'an eternal youth' etc. comes from Fredrik Böök, *Esaias Tegnér: Senare delen* (i.e., Part 2) (Stockholm: Bonniers, 1946), p. 219. The words about treasuring youthful memories, translated by Sandblom, come from a letter of Tegnér's to M. Lagerlöf, of 23 December 1833; *Esaias Tegnérs brev*, ed. by Nils Palmborg, Vol. VII: 1833–1835 (Malmö: Allhems förlag), p. 120.

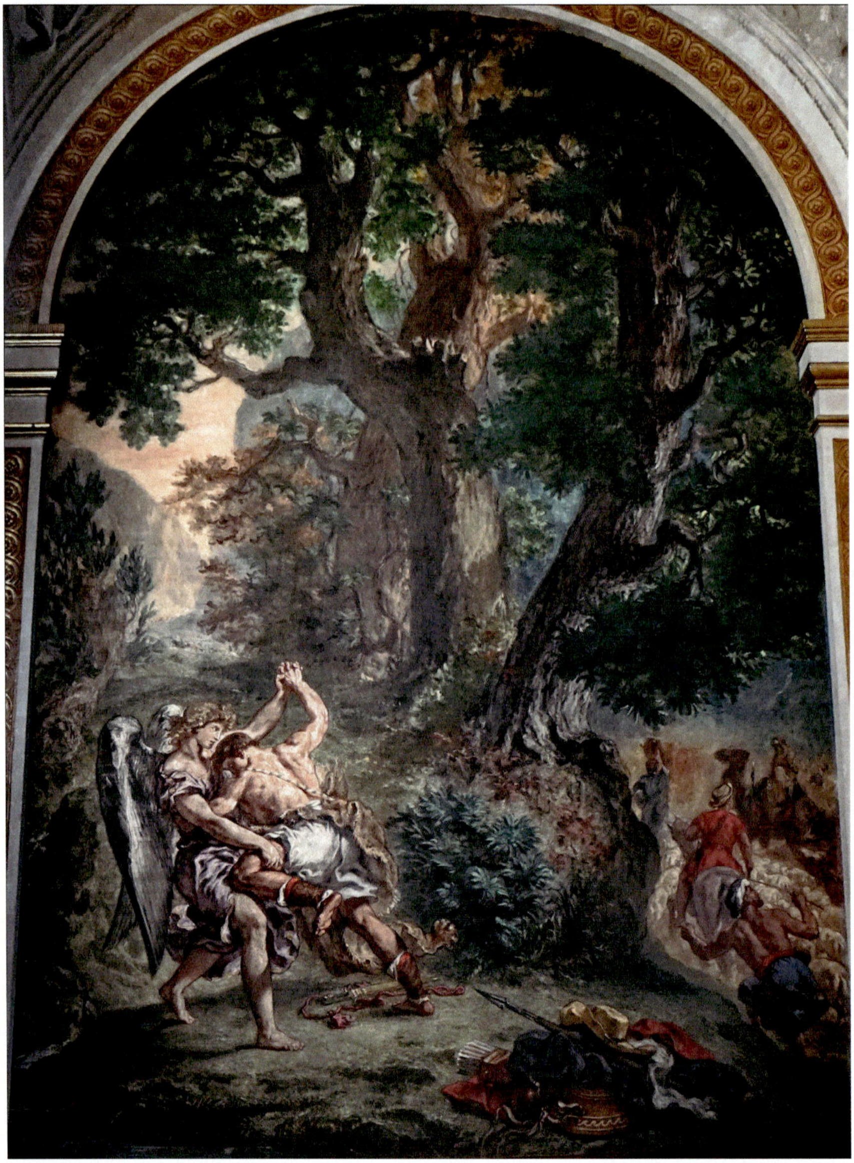

Figure 49 Eugène Delacroix, 'Jacob wrestling with the angel', 1850–61 (cropped). A human being struggles against his destiny, a struggle he cannot but lose.

an ageing Marschallin who laments the loss of her youthful allure, and with it her beloved Rosenkavalier, in wistful melodies.

* * *

During the last years of his life, Eugène Delacroix struggled against fatigue, weakness, and a feeling of helplessness while endeavouring to finish the

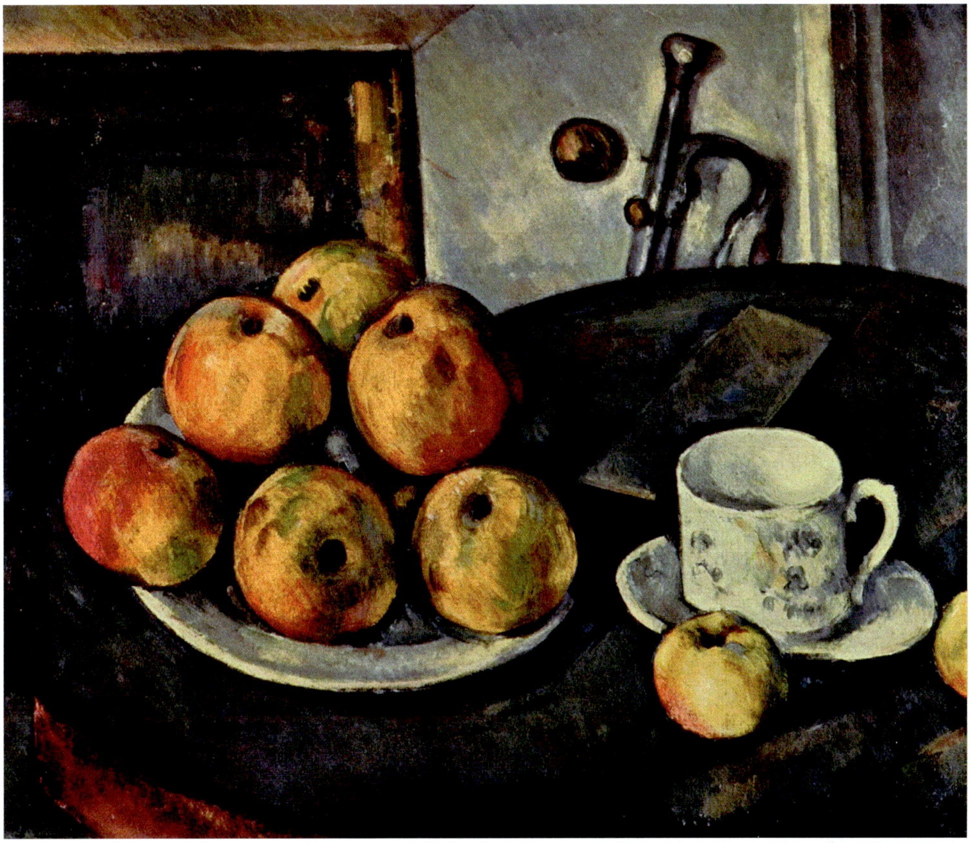

Figure 50 Paul Cézanne, 'Still life with apples and a cup', 1890. The artist's apples form a harmony of the spheres.

most demanding of his works, the paintings in Saint-Sulpice. In the picture of Jacob wrestling with the angel, he reproduces his own plight as a human being struggling with his destiny. The struggle itself is what matters, since the final outcome – defeat and annihilation – is settled in advance.

Paul Cézanne, solitary pioneer in art, became increasingly frail towards the end of his life and realised that his days were numbered; he said that he could see the promised land but feared that he would not be allowed to enter it, thus sharing the fate of Moses.[9] A few days before his death, he wrote to his son that he laboured on, hoping that his efforts would lead to something, and that that was what mattered in the end.[10] In late paintings, his beloved apples, arranged in a harmony of spheres, are replaced by human skulls, the

9 Remarks addressed to Ambroise Vollard on 9 January 1903, quoted in Ambroise Vollard, *En écoutant Cézanne, Degas, Renoir* (Paris: Bernard Grasset, 1938), p. 80.

10 Letter to Cézanne's son of 15 October 1906; Paul Cézanne, *Correspondance*, ed. by John Rewald (Paris: Bernard Grasset, 1937), p. 297.

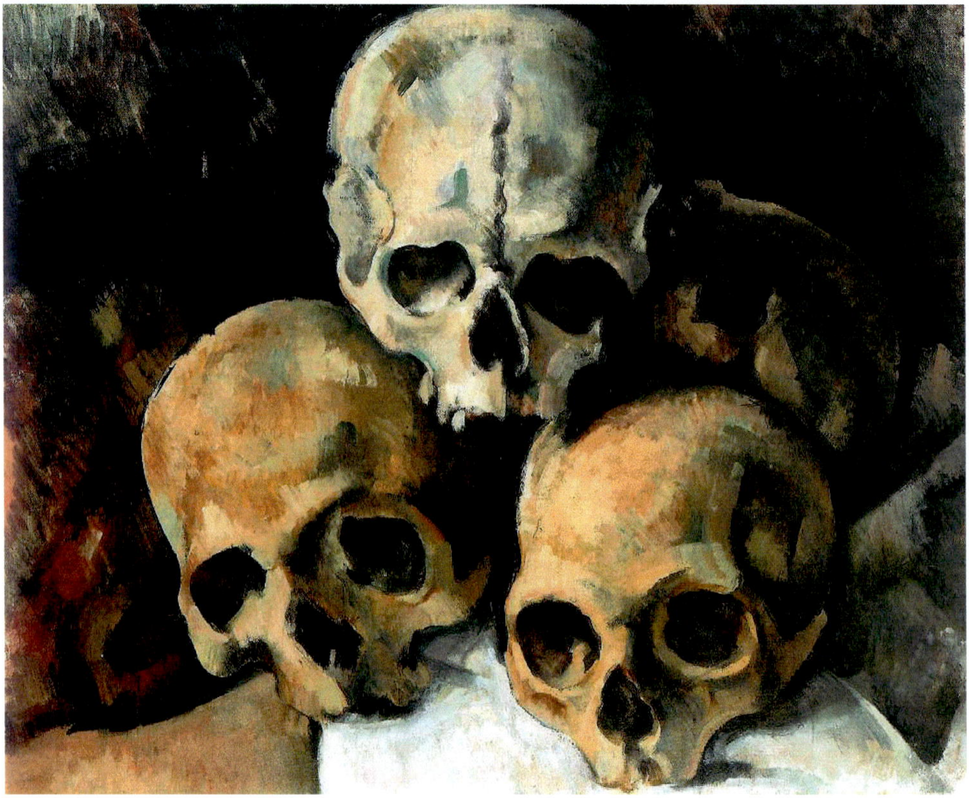

Figure 51 Paul Cézanne, 'Pyramid of skulls', 1901. The artist in his old age exchanges his apples for skulls, the symbol of mortality.

very emblems of vanity. In comparison with the luminous paintings from the 1890s, where joy shines through as well as the white background, the colours are increasingly sombre; the harmony adopts a minor key, and the impression is deeply tragic. An even more pronounced development of this type is seen in Mark Rothko. As his health failed, death itself became an obsession; it is the principal theme in the Rothko chapel in Houston, where light and life fade into an almost black purple.

Other artists form examples of mental depletion accompanying the degeneration of the body. For each year that passes, one or more strings of the soul snap; its chords sound increasingly thin, and a lingering note that used to enrich the harmony may cause a shrill dissonance.

The erotic tone, often merely hinted at by a wavy line or by a complete omission of intimate details, that invested the works of the young Picasso with abundant humanity, could sometimes come across as boyishly mischievous; it is only much later, when this tone is sounded in monotonous isolation by the ageing man, that it degenerates into pornography. On his artistic exploration past the curves and crannies of the female body, he neglects to have himself tied to the mast like Odysseus and is seduced by the

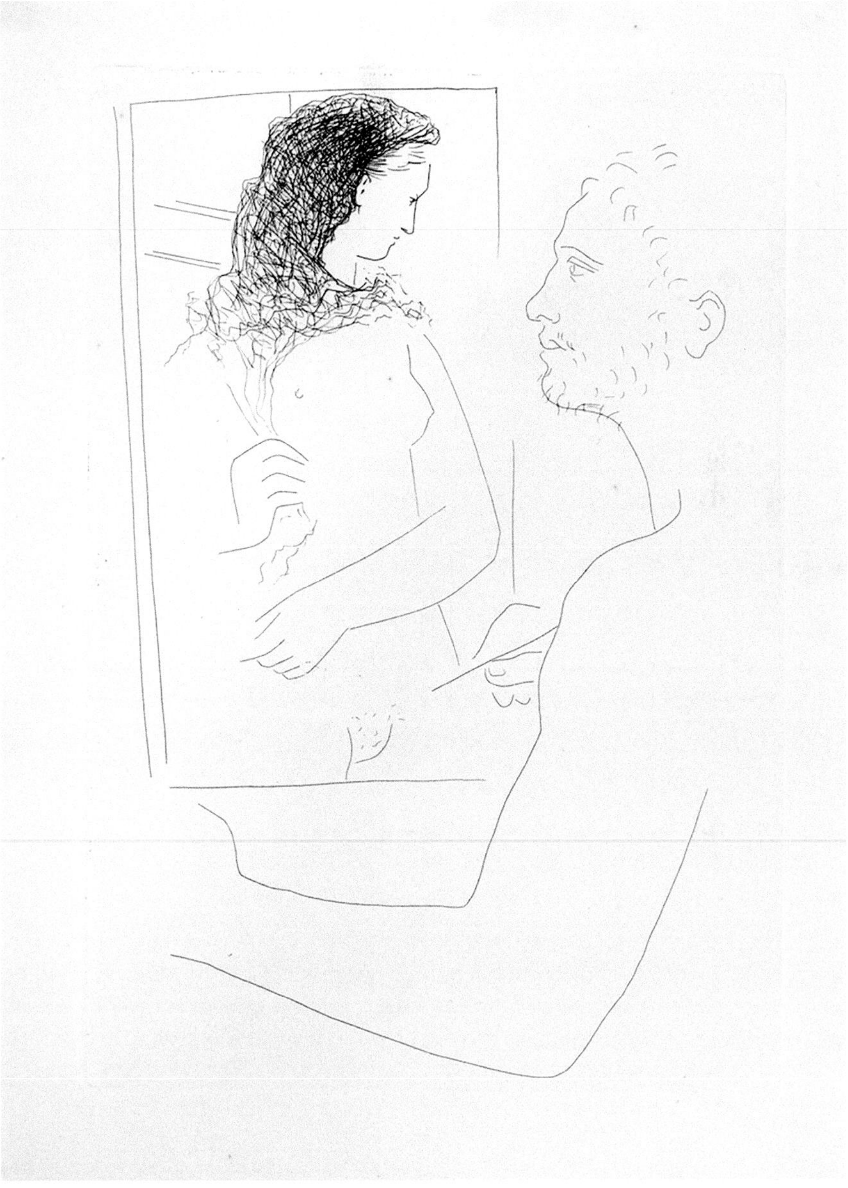

Figure 52 Pablo Picasso, 'Painter in front of his painting'. The young artist studies his model with tenderness and discretion. From Honoré de Balzac, 'The unknown masterpiece' (1831), in an edition from 1927.

sirens he has himself created. The artistic vision becomes an obscene viewing with the artist himself as a Peeping Tom.

Even so, Picasso retained a vigorous power of expression into his old age, a quality which makes many of his pictures veritable apogees of erotic art. It would be more natural to ascribe the phrase that he painted

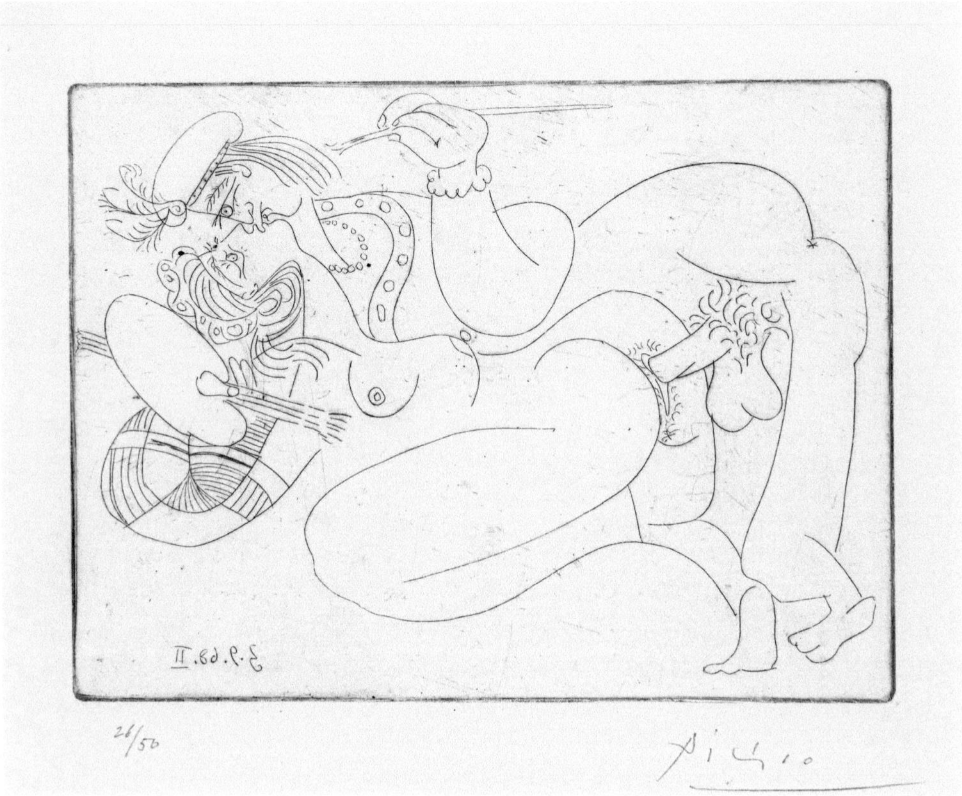

Figure 53 Pablo Picasso, 'Raphael et la Fornarina XIV: le Pape s'est éclipsé', 1968. With increasing senile eroticism, the ageing master is seduced by his own art and makes shameless use of the fact. From the 'Suite 347'.

'with [his] prick' to him rather than to Auguste Renoir, who is said to have uttered it.[11] With regard to the latter, such a choice of words seems far too coarse as a designation for the elementary eroticism that formed an undercurrent in his work as a painter.

* * *

Renoir was one of those fortunate artists whose mental powers last well into old age, even when it comes with pronounced ill health. In these artists, we often observe a yearning for the joy of youth. In middle age, Renoir was for a time the victim of an ambition one sometimes finds among artists, namely that of reaching beyond their ability. In his efforts to adapt to Classical

11 Jean Renoir, *Renoir, My Father*, trans. Randolph and Dorothy Weaver (Boston: Little, Brown and Company, 1958), p. 205. For a discussion as to whether or not this quotation is apocryphal, see https://quoteinvestigator.com/2012/05/28/renoir-paint/.

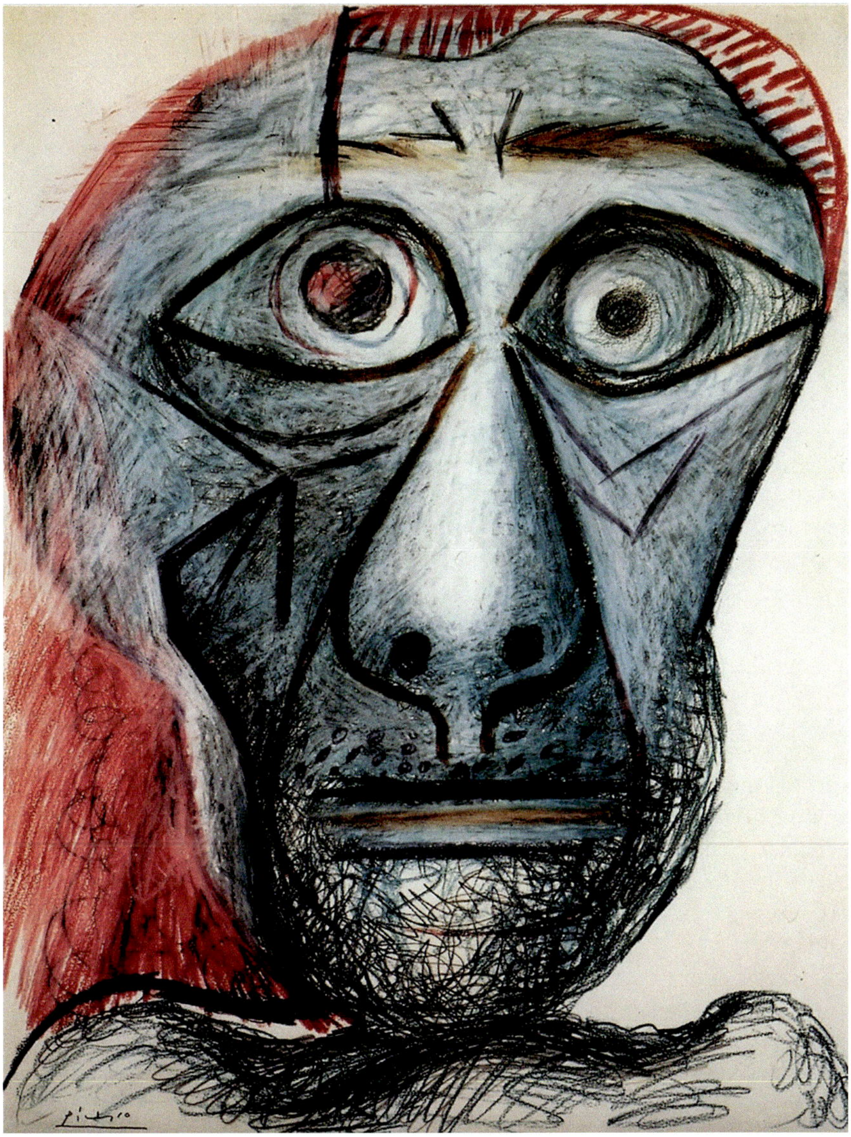

Figure 54 Pablo Picasso, 'Self-portrait facing death', 1972. As Picasso approached 90 years of age, he sometimes turned his gaze away from erotic scenes to the final annihilation, as in this self-portrait from the year he died – a picture of the undisguised agony of death.

ideals, he could be dry and cold. In the course of the years, however, he regained his powerful artistic individuality. Although he suffered from painful old-age arthritis, which forced him to attach cotton wool to the palm of his hand so he could hold the brush, he painted pictures radiating youthful delight and loved representing children, young girls, and the flowers of spring (see Figures 8 and 9).

One has a feeling that Renoir also treasured the memories of his early years, but in a healthy, vigorous manner; and we can see how naturally and freely he adapted his landscapes to the rules of Classical composition. At this stage of his life, his colours turned brighter and moved towards red on the spectrum, possibly owing to cataracts but surely also quite deliberately, as part of an endeavour to attain a warmer overall tone.

It should be pointed out in this context that there is a hypothesis according to which Renoir's arthritis was an occupational illness, caused by poisoning through his paint. As his light colours called for heavy lead, he might have had to pay with his own health for the radiance that captivates us in his art.

The same explanation has been offered with regard to Raoul Dufy's rheumatoid arthritis, but this artist's medical history differs from that of Renoir in two essential respects: his illness had begun earlier and was even more disabling, and furthermore he had medical treatment which improved his health significantly. In the words of his physician: 'The medical story of Raoul Dufy represents one of those rare instances in which a medical advance is made at exactly the right time to salvage creative functioning in an important person and thereby enrich our heritage.'[12]

This singular circumstance makes it possible for us to study not only how Dufy's art was, like his body, crippled by his illness, but also how it reverted to its original greatness and perhaps even progressed further thanks to medical treatment. It happened when Dufy was 73, frail and completely immobile after 15 years of illness. His drawing had become laboured and his lines as rigid as his joints. The physician Dr Homburger, who had always taken a keen interest in art, heard of his plight; and as Homburger had just received a batch of drugs for preliminary trials with ACTH and cortisone (then newly discovered hormones that counteract inflammatory processes), he wrote to Dufy and invited him to Boston in order to become one of the first patients to be treated with the new medicinal substances. The result was dramatic: within a few days, mobility increased in Dufy's joints. For the first time in many years, he was able to squeeze the paint out of his tubes unaided. After another six weeks he was on his legs again, alert and active and enjoying life. The effect on his work is evident when one compares his handwriting as well as his pictures painted before and after treatment. His art flourished, and once more he found himself in complete control of his means of expression. These drugs frequently induce euphoria, and Dufy sensed it, naming one of his marvellous still-life pictures with flowers 'La Cortisone'.

Did Dufy's recovery also entail further development in his artistry? Maybe the artist himself has the best answer to that question. He said that things continued to go well for him and that irrespective of whether it was the cortisone or the hormones that he had to thank for it, he was now

12 F. Homburger and D. D. Bonner, 'The Treatment of Raoul Dufy's Arthritis', *New England Journal of Medicine* 301.12 (1979), 669.

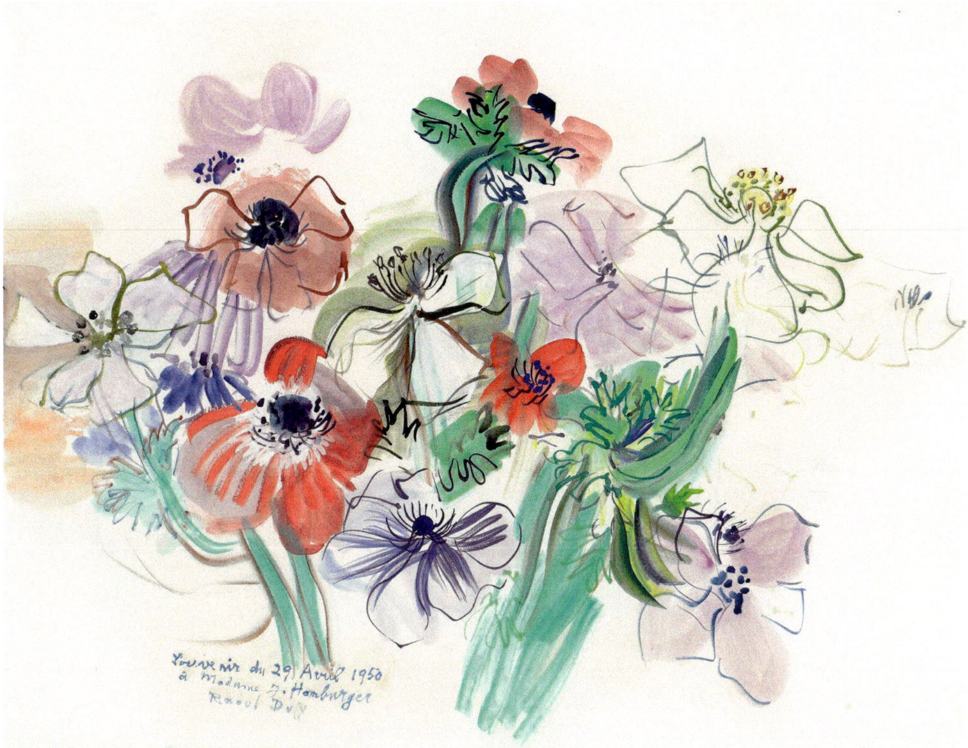

Figure 55 Raoul Dufy, 'Souvenir du 29 Avril 1950 à Madame F. Homburger', 1950. Rigid and jerky lines in artwork and handwriting at the peak of the illness.

painting things he had studied in his youth and not then managed to perform to his satisfaction. For works composed in the spirit of Cézanne, he said, he had used pure and uncommon colour compositions in a manner he had not managed to accomplish over the past 30 years. He posed the question whether that signified a rebirth or a swan song for Fauvism, mentioning the possibility that his happiness in achieving success in his work might have led his senses astray.[13]

* * *

When the ageing Joseph Haydn did not manage to finish his last string quartet, he published the two completed movements along with a comment to the effect that he had no strength left, being old and feeble – words he also had put on his calling cards, so as to be spared continued demands on his capabilities.

13 Ibid., 671.

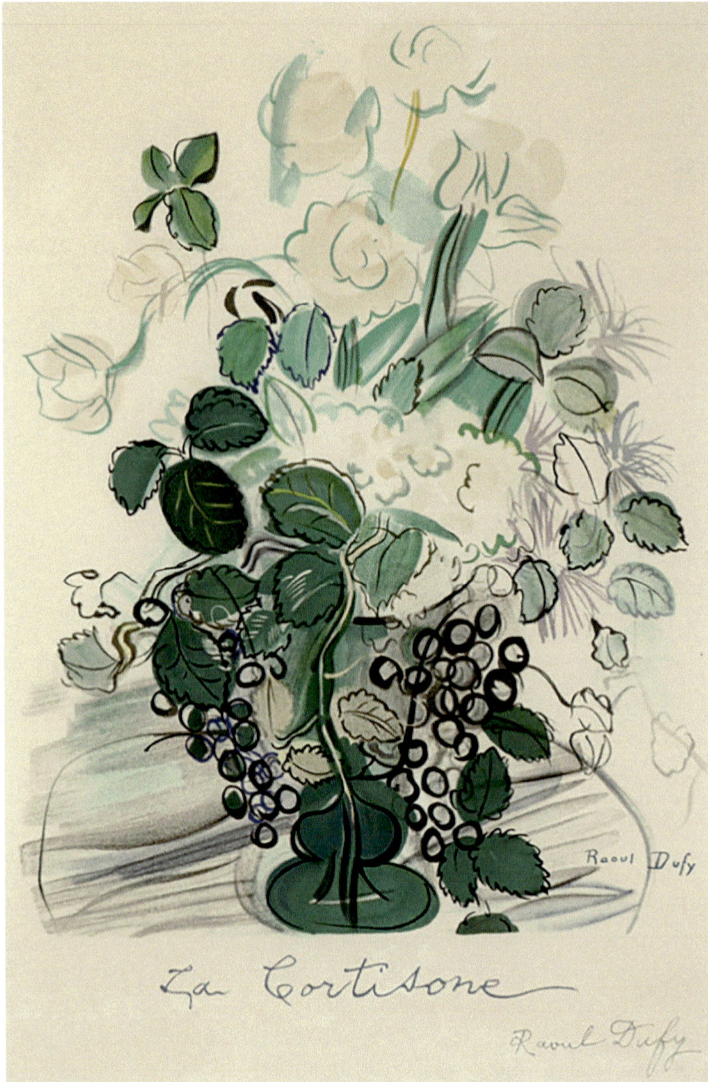

Figure 56 Raoul Dufy, 'La Cortisone', 1951. After recovery, the lines are softer and the whole image flourishes.

Giuseppe Verdi had less reason to worry about his ageing having a deleterious effect on his abilities. At the age of 60 he regarded his life's work, the composing of operas, as concluded. Every proposal that he continue to compose was rejected with irritation; he did not feel obliged to go on working, suggesting that those who tried to make him knew as well as he that he was finished. His wife had to enter into a conspiracy with four of his friends in order to persuade the obstinate composer to resume collaboration with his librettist. After a long period of preparation, his late masterpiece *Otello* came into being – an unsettling drama in which music, words, and actions come together in demonstrating how evil assumes control by cruelly and cunningly exploiting jealousy.

In his final years, Franz Liszt endeavoured to capture his melancholia and insomnia in a nocturne. 'Schlaflos, Frage und Antwort' ('Sleepless, Question and Answer') is a piece of programmatic music in which he expressed the feelings of many an ageing person. In *Valses oubliées* ('Forgotten waltzes), he glumly recollected the pleasures of his distant youth.[14]

* * *

When the body loses its final battle for life, we leave things temporal for eternity. Since death is always ahead of us, we can only have faint ideas about how we will experience it. In some creative people, for instance Paul Klee, its imminence may produce a final blazing-up of creative power; for others, it extinguishes that flame for good. The latter happened to Theodor Storm.

This German author, who developed stomach cancer, requested that his doctor tell him the whole truth, 'between men'. However, the somewhat naive writer had overestimated his own resilience and broke down on hearing his diagnosis. To help him, his brother summoned another physician who mendaciously told Storm that his illness was not fatal. Storm believed him implicitly and experienced a trouble-free summer during which he crowned his literary career with a classic masterpiece, *Der Schimmelreiter* (*The Rider on the White Horse*). Consequently, we owe the existence of this great work to a merciful fraud. But the period of grace turned out to be a brief one, and the vision he had once described in a poem became reality:

> So strangely alien the world becomes,
> And quietly you're abandoned by all hope,
> Until you know at last, at last,
> That the arrow of Death has struck you.[15]

* * *

The dying Ivan Ilyich in Tolstoy's novella ('The Death of Ivan Ilyich') felt humiliated and abandoned when his friends persisted in lying to him about his condition and began to avoid his company, much in the same way as when someone enters the drawing-room smelling bad.

There was a real-life counterpart to Tolstoy's invented drastic situation when Franz Kafka found himself in the same predicament. Kafka makes us

---

14 John O'Shea, *Music and Medicine: Medical Profiles of the Great Composers* (London: J. M. Dent, 1990), pp. 167–168. With regard to Haydn, see Rosemary Hughes, *Haydn* (London: J. M. Dent & Sons, 1974), p. 105; for Verdi, see James A. Hepokoski, *Giuseppe Verdi: Otello* (Cambridge: Cambridge University Press, 1987), pp. 21–29.

15 'So seltsam fremd wird dir die Welt / Und leis verlässt dich alles Hoffen, / Bis du es endlich, endlich weisst, / Dass dich des Todes Pfeil getroffen'.

understand how abandoned and uncertain patients may feel when they are being deceived and left in a state of ignorance. From the sanatorium where he was to die two months later, he wrote to a friend that he learnt nothing definite from anything anyone said to him, for, as soon as the disease was the topic of conversation, everybody would adopt an evasive, embarrassed, or non-committal way of expressing themselves.[16] I have reason to believe that both Storm and Kafka could have coped with learning the truth if they had had adequate compassionate support.

Few of us attain the stoic frame of mind at which Samuel Johnson hinted when he said that knowledge of being due to be hanged in a fortnight concentrates a man's mind wonderfully.[17] Nor are we likely to emulate François Villon, who had good reason to fear this particular fate and therefore expected the executioner's noose soon to inform his neck of the weight of his bottom.[18]

Sick of life, the melancholy Swedish Romantic poet Stagnelius summons putrefaction and combustion, the final indignities visited on the human body:

> Decay! Make haste, beloved Bride!
> to make our lonely bed!
> Rejected by man and rejected by God,
> I have no hope but in you.
> ...
> Fold my yearning body into thy bosom,
> Stifle my pain in thy embrace,
> In worms let my thoughts and feelings dissolve,
> In ashes my burning heart ...

However, knowledge that you did credit to your talents and left a lasting impression of your personality in art or science may help you face the end with equanimity. In his *Menschliches Allzumenschliches* (*Human, All Too Human*), Nietzsche did so, finding comfort in a grimly humorous imagined scene: the thinker, he says, like the artist who has given the best of himself in his work, watches the gradual destruction of his body and mind with malicious joy; it is as if, hidden in a corner, he sees how a thief is opening a safe which he knows is empty, the treasure being in safe keeping somewhere else.[19]

* * *

16 Franz Kafka, *Letters to Friends, Family and Editors*, trans. by Richard and Clara Winston (New York: Schocken Books, 1977), p. 411.

17 *Boswell's Life of Johnson*, ed. R. W. Chapman (London: Oxford University Press, 1953 edition), p. 849 (Friday 19 September, 1777).

18 'Et de la corde d'une toise / Scaura mon col que mon cul poise' (from an epigram beginning 'Je suis Françoys, dont il me poise').

19 Friedrich Nietzsche, *Menschliches Allzumenschliches: Ein Buch für freie Geister* (Cologne: Anaconda Verlag, 2006), p. 157. For an English translation, see Friedrich Nietzsche, *Human, All Too Human: A Book for Free Spirits*, trans. R. J. Hollingdale (Cambridge: Cambridge University Press, 1996), p. 97.

For those who never give a thought to death, ignorance is bliss; but to most of us death retains its sting, and we tend to share La Rochefoucauld's opinion that there are two things we cannot look upon with a steady gaze, namely the sun and death. Even Dr Johnson's stoicism was artificial; he is on record as saying that '[n]o rational man can die without uneasy apprehension'.[20] It is small comfort to know that we share our ultimate destiny with every other human being, for, as Pascal realized, 'we shall die alone'.[21]

Though medical care makes death increasingly easy nowadays, not many of us will be entirely spared its agony. In the end, it will destroy us in the same way as a savage beast rends its prey; but it is the sensitive artist who most vividly imagines the hot and stinking breath of the beast as it overpowers us (Figure 70). This feeling of horror and disgust has found searing expressions in the works of artists and writers. Baudelaire's description of the dead human body, coloured by his syphilitic state of mind, is as cynical as Flaubert's account of the living human frame (see p. 21) and Théodore Géricault's of the decapitated (Figure 57). Accompanied by his mistress, the poet finds 'A corpse' ('Une charogne') rotting on the pebbled road,

> Its legs raised in the air, like a lewd woman,
> Burning and dripping with poisons,
> Displayed in a shameless, nonchalant way
> Its belly, swollen with gases.[22]

However, even such loathsome matter may be spiritualised by art. When the stench makes his beloved stagger, Baudelaire consoles her by saying that, when her beauty has been ravaged by worms, he will have preserved the form and the divine essence of her body. Rarely has a thought been given such dissimilar expression as this one – drastic by Baudelaire, and with exquisite grace in a sonnet by Shakespeare:

> But thy eternal summer shall not fade,
> Nor lose possession of that fair thou ow'st,
> Nor shall Death brag thou wander'st in his shade,
> When in eternal lines to time thou grow'st;
>
> So long as men can breathe or eyes can see,
> So long lives this, and this gives life to thee.[23]

---

20 Page 949 in the 1953 Oxford University Press edition quoted above; Wednesday 15 April 1778. (Johnson's biographer James Boswell often refers to his fear of death.)

21 Blaise Pascal, *Pensées and Other Writings*, trans. Honor Levi (Oxford: Oxford University Press, 1995), p. 58.

22 *Les Fleurs du mal*, 'Spleen et idéal', XXIX: 'Les jambes en l'air, comme une femme lubrique, / Brûlante et suant les poisons, / Ouvrait d'une facon nonchalante et cynique / Son ventre plein d'exhalations'.

23 Sonnet 18.

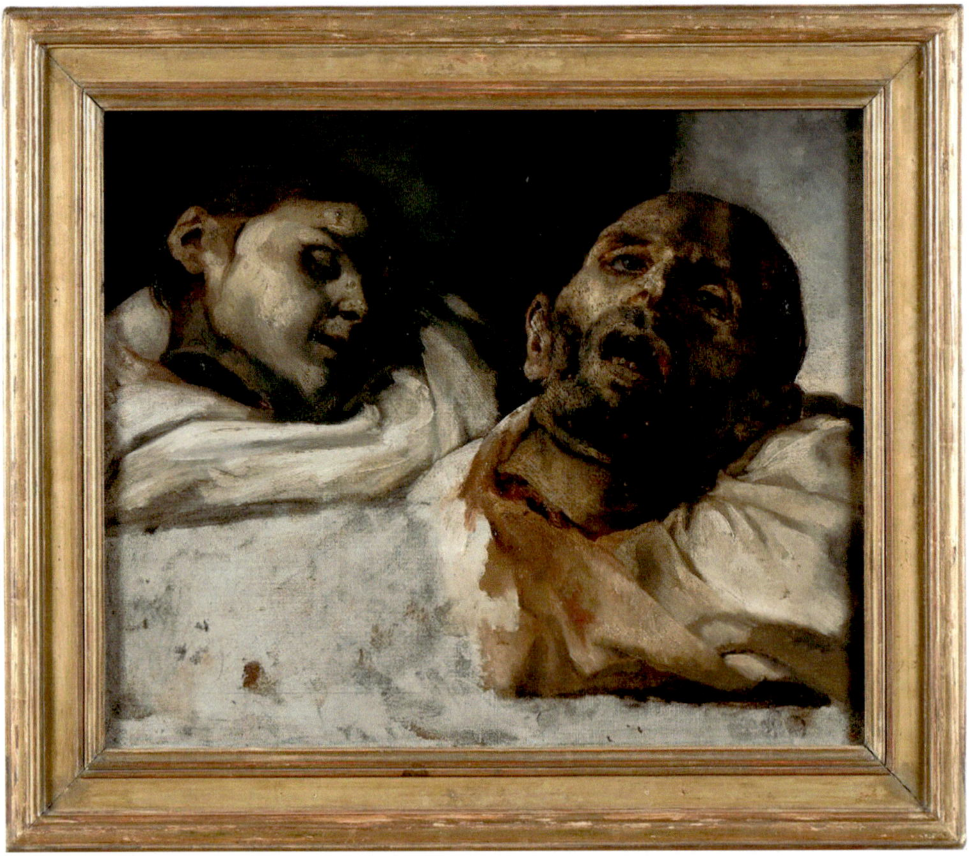

Figure 57 Théodore Géricault, 'The severed heads', 1818. The artist was greatly interested in all kinds of human degradation, physical as well as mental, and studied it in prisons, asylums, and mortuaries. The female head belonged to a sex worker, the male to a beheaded thief.

Despite the horrors in store for him, Baudelaire was longing to become 'Le Mort joyeux', 'the happy dead man'; but, as he detested grieving people, he instead invited the ravens to feast on his dead body and the worms to explore whatever torture might have left of his aged body.[24]

Similar contrasts between the horrific and the pleasing may be found in art and music alike. Géricault paints pictures of the cut-off heads of a thief and a sex worker with the same directness and hardened cynicism that Baudelaire expresses in his poetry. Conversely, nothing could be more intense and moving than Monet's portrait of his young wife on her death-bed (Figure 48). A tender love is revealed in the brush-strokes caressing her features, bringing out the spiritualised beauty that he wishes to preserve for ever, as Shakespeare did in his sonnet. At the same time, though, Monet's

24 Poem No. LXXII in 'Spleen et idéal', *Les Fleurs du mal.*

artistic dedication to the truth compelled him to reproduce the *livor mortis* with the same cynical candour that Géricault displays in his severed heads.

In the realm of music, corresponding contrasts may be seen in the difference between Shostakovich and Mozart. In words as well as tones, the former renounces all hope that death will be followed by new life; death, to Shostakovich, is not a beginning but an end, the end of everything.[25] The melancholy songs in his Fourteenth Symphony, where a horror of death forms a theme, range from infinite sadness, 'De profundis', by Federico García Lorca, to the fury of Rainer Maria Rilke's 'Schluss-Stück':

> Death is huge
> We are his
> Even as our mouths are laughing.[26]

We hear death banging on the door with a gnarled fist, answered by screams of horror, in a sense of despair totally unlike Mozart's composure and gravity in the unfinished *Requiem* in D Minor. In an earlier letter to his dying father, he had called death the best and truest friend of humankind, declaring that the idea of death is not just less frightening to him now but actually soothing and consoling.[27] The last notes he recorded on his deathbed were eight bars from 'Lacrimosa', bars which were also his own tears of regret as he bid life farewell.

***

When George Orwell was once hospitalised with pneumonia in a general ward, he watched with disgust 'How the Poor Die', helpless and abandoned, and lamented: 'People talk about the horrors of war, but what weapon has man invented that even approaches in cruelty some of the commoner diseases? "Natural" death, almost by definition, means something slow, smelly and painful.'[28]

In employing the expression 'A very easy death' about her mother's demise, the coldly furious Simone de Beauvoir is mordantly sarcastic when she describes the actual process: 'Then suddenly she cried out, a burning pain in her left buttock. It was not at all surprising. Her flayed body was bathing in the uric acid that oozed from her skin ... [O]n the edge of shrieking, she moaned, "It burns, it's awful; I can't stand it. I can't bear it any longer." ... She suddenly cried, "I can't breathe!" Her mouth opened, her eyes stared wide, huge in that wasted, ravaged face: with a spasm she entered

25 It was not possible to find a source for this observation.

26 'Der Tod ist gross / Wir sind die Seinen / lachenden Munds.'

27 Letter written on 4 April 1787; quoted in William Stafford, *The Mozart Myths: A Critical Reassessment* (Stanford: Stanford University Press, 1991), p. 209.

28 George Orwell, 'How the Poor Die', in *Shooting an Elephant and Other Essays* (London: Secker and Warburg, 1950), p. 25.

into coma. ... "But, Madame", replied the nurse, "I assure you it was a very easy death."'[29]

A forthright and unrestrained anger against death was voiced by Dylan Thomas witnessing the end of his father's life:

Do not go gentle into that good night.
Old age should burn and rave at close of day;
Rage, rage against the dying of the light.[30]

* * *

Humankind's fear of death and annihilation gave birth to the idea of an eternal life, faith in which has brought comfort to many throughout the millennia. Alongside the conception of celestial powers, it has inspired the creation of magnificent architecture, art, and music in praise of the Divine. These riches bring bliss and delight to everybody, irrespective of religion.

The secularised human being who prefers to stay within the boundaries of reason and doubts the possibility of eternal life resigns willingly, indifferently, or like Philip Larkin in the poem 'Aubade' bitterly, in anticipation of

The sure extinction that we travel to
And shall be lost in always.

This misery is brought out with beautiful sharpness:

This is a special way of being afraid
No trick dispels. Religion used to try,
That vast moth-eaten musical brocade
Created to pretend we never die,
And specious stuff that says *No rational being*
Can fear a thing it will not feel, not seeing
That this is what we fear – no sight, no sound,
No touch or taste or smell, nothing to think with,
Nothing to love or link with,
The anaesthetic from which none come round.[31]

We might dispel our fears and gain wisdom by means of a 'trick' provided by Tacitus, who declared that the inmost essence of philosophy is to prepare for death. Anyone who reflects deeply on the subject may be rewarded by the thought that even if death robs us of our one and only life, 'not to be' might still become a longed-for, peaceful rest.

---

29 Simone de Beauvoir, *A Very Easy Death*, trans. Patrick O'Brian (New York: Pantheon, 1985), pp. 80–81 and 88. The French original, *Une mort très douce*, appeared from Gallimard, Paris, in 1964; see pp. 115 and 126–127.

30 'Do not go gentle into that good night', p. 116 in Dylan Thomas, *Collected Poems 1934–1952* (London: J. M. Dent & Sons, 1952).

31 According to Anthony Thwaite's 1988 edition of Larkin's *Collected Poems* (The Marvell Press and Faber and Faber, London), p. 209, the poem was first published in 1977.

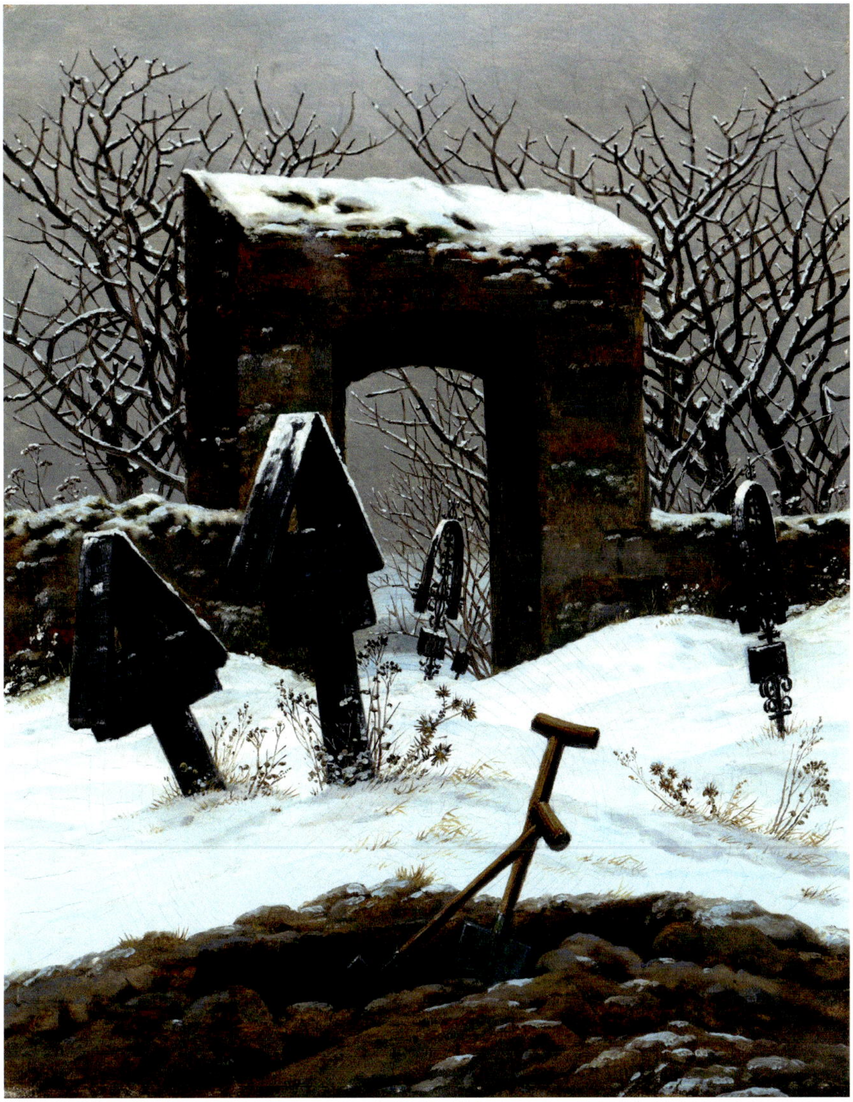

Figure 58 Caspar David Friedrich, 'Graveyard under snow', 1826/1827.

Friedrich Schlegel had an ecstatic premonition that death might actually be welcome, a joy and a haven; he said that he understood how human beings might yearn for annihilation and liberation even when at the peak of their powers, and look forward to resurrection as a morning ray of hope.[32]

Among those who shared that thought we find, among others, Ronsard (p. 156), Keats (pp. 178–180), Chekhov (p. 185), the frequently depressed Caspar David Friedrich, who helps us grasp the infinite peace beneath

32 Regrettably, it was not possible to find a source for Schlegel's premonition.

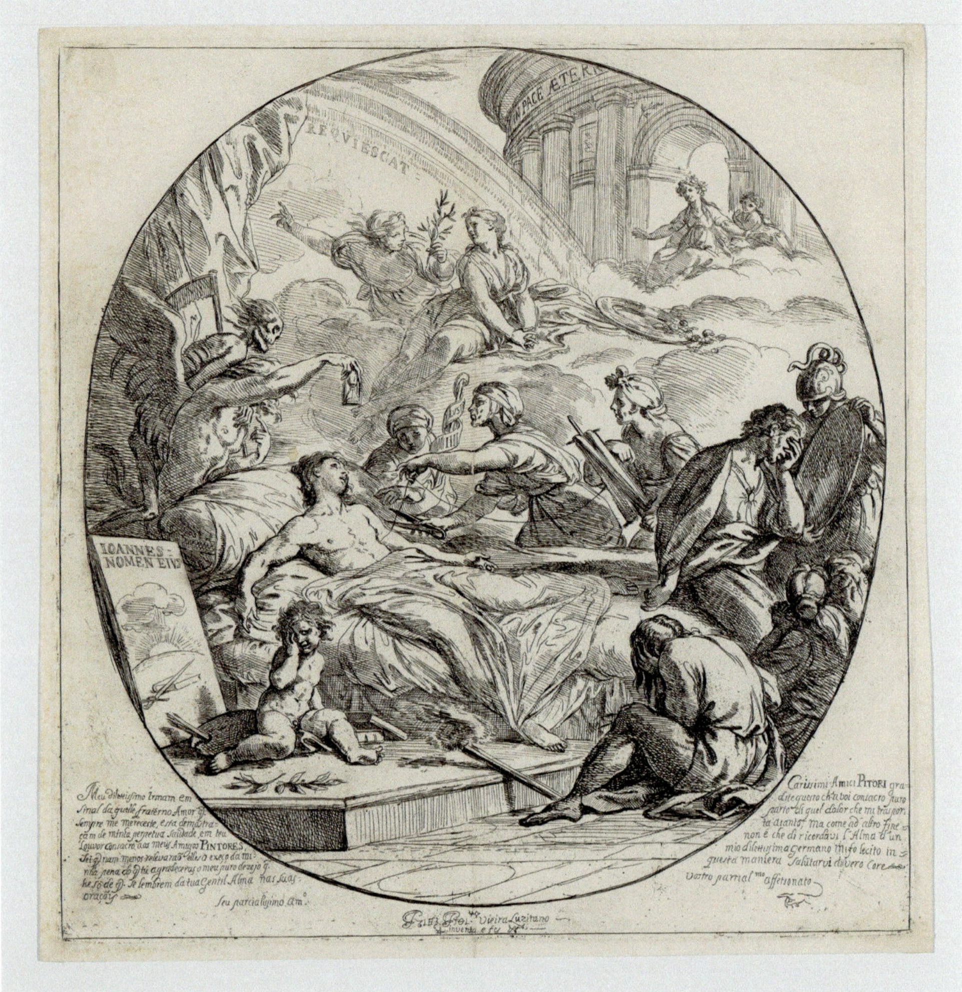

Figure 59 Vieira Lusitano, 'The three Fates' ('As três Parcas'), 1714–20. Anyone who trawls through books on death in the arts, looking for an image where death is represented as a good thing, soon becomes overwhelmed by the sheer number of scary images of the Dance of Death and the Man with the Scythe who rapes a virgin; those pictures probably correspond to the general idea of death as horrible. In this allegory of the death of a young artist, however, all the attributes of death are present, but the scene is flooded with the bright hope of *pax eterna*, everlasting peace.

snowy tombstones, and Gustav Mahler, whose Ninth Symphony extends a tenderly hesitant farewell, a passionate goodnight kiss, to life. As stoics, Arthur Rimbaud is lapidary and Benjamin Britten painfully beautiful in his musical expression when they, prepared to depart, declare that they have seen, had, and felt enough ('Assez vu, assez eu, assez connu').[33]

33 Arthur Rimbaud, *Les Illuminations*, set to music by Benjamin Britten in 1939.

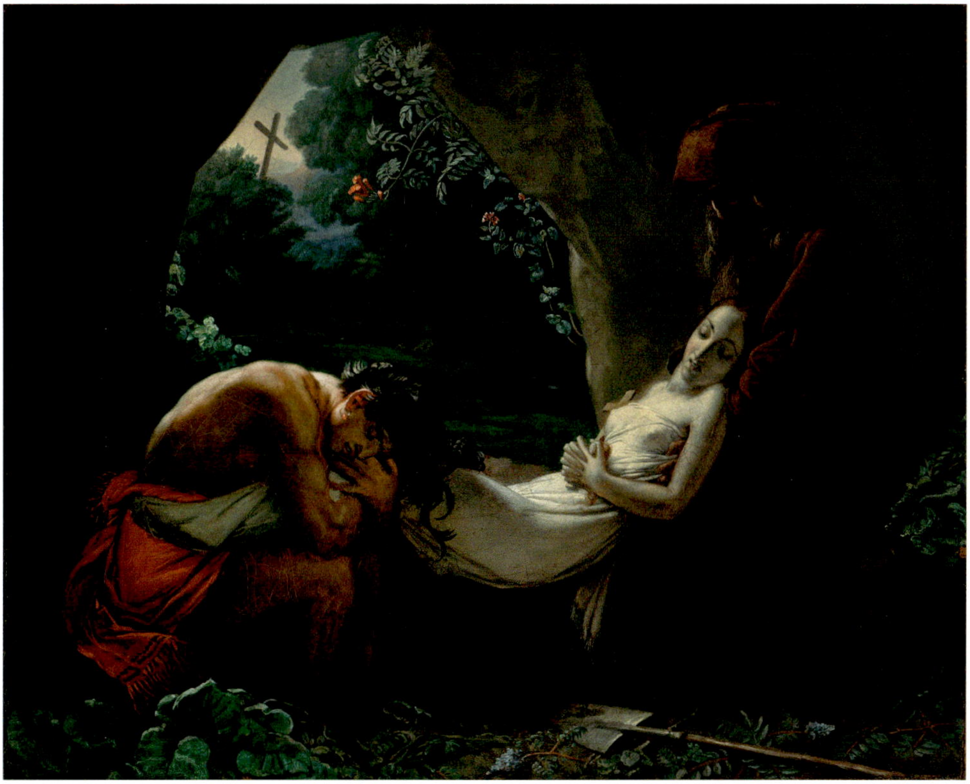

Figure 60 Anne-Louis Girodet-Trioson, 'Atala au tombeau', 1808. The same bright hope for peace suffuses the slightly erotic burial of Atala, who, according to François-René de Chateaubriand (in his novella *Atala*, 1801), lived like a flower and wilted like a herb in the field.

It would be possible to name Edmund Spenser in this company, as his *The Faerie Queene* maintains that ultimate peace is worth dying for, even if the end is painful:

> Sleep after toil, port after stormy seas,
> Ease after war, death after life does greatly please.[34]

However, these lines do not afford much consolation when one remembers that they were uttered by 'Despair', advancing the argument that desolation is the primary feature of life and that the only action worth undertaking is that which hastens our departure from it.

Ahasuerus, the Wandering Jew, provides us with a better argument – a better reason to long for, or at least accept, death. His terrible punishment (for having refused Jesus his aid on the path towards Crucifixion) was to be condemned to live for ever, never attaining an increasingly yearned-for death.

34 From Book I, canto 9, stanza 40 of *The Faerie Queene*.

Shakespeare offers us grave and exquisite comfort in the words (Act III, scene 1) in which he clothes Hamlet's thoughts about life and death:

> To die – to sleep,
> No more; and, by a sleep to say we end
> The heart-ache and the thousand natural shocks
> That flesh is heir to, 'tis a consummation
> Devoutly to be wish'd.

* * *

There is a time for everything, even for eternity – in ways humanity cannot fathom – and for our lives, the strange and wondrous experience of being alive and aware for a time upon this earth, an extraordinary opportunity. It would be presumptuous to demand a meaning to it all beyond this.

Many people have agreed with Marcus Aurelius that there may not be any meaning at all, merely 'a brief sojourning in an alien land; and after repute, oblivion'.[35] As the Swedish poet Erik Blomberg (1894–1965) wrote in a poem repeatedly set to music, 'The earth is humanity's home'.

It remains for us mortals to place our trust in the immortal genome of which we are the temporary, but essential, offshoots, custodians for future generations. But it is small consolation, for the genome dilutes rapidly.

As our last moment draws near, we all hope to 'pass away quietly', 'cease upon the midnight with no pain'.[36] Joseph von Eichendorff almost succeeds in making us long for it in his poem 'Im Abendrot' ('At sunset'), especially if we hear its words set to the beautiful musical language of Richard Strauss, which makes our souls join in the singing. Arrived at a great age, the composer felt 'wandermüde', weary with wandering, after his long and rich musical life; but his son encouraged him to gather his powers for a final farewell. He accomplished it with *Vier letzte Lieder* (*Four Last Songs*), where he finally welcomes death in peace of mind and with gratitude to the woman who had been his companion on his wanderings:

> O vast, tranquil peace!
> So deeply set in the glow of evening.
> How weary we are with wandering –
> Might this be death?[37]

35 Marcus Aurelius, *Meditations*, trans. Maxwell Staniforth (Harmondsworth: Penguin, 1964), p. 51.
36 The last quotation is from John Keats's 'Ode to a Nightingale', line 56.
37 'O weiter, stiller Friede! / So tief im Abendrot. / Wie sind wir wandermüde – / Ist dies etwa der Tod?'

Chapter 8
Disturbances affecting sight and hearing

> What unfortunate condition of humanity, their spirit has hardly matured when their body begins to deteriorate.
>
> Montesquieu

It is natural that artists, who rely so greatly on their sensory perceptions, should be highly dependent on their senses, especially sight and hearing. The senses frequently decline with advancing age, but of course they may also be damaged by illness. One would assume that changes to a person's eyesight would have a particularly marked effect on a pictorial artist and his or her work. That Whistler and Léger were colour-blind is something that specialists have been able to conclude from looking at their paintings. When Degas's eyesight began to diminish, he made the transition from painting to sculpture, where he was better able to rely on his tactile sense. The painter Georgia O'Keeffe, who found herself in the same predicament as she grew older, also attempted sculpture but was disappointed: 'The clay controls me, I can't control it', she lamented, and began to long for the more compliant brush. One day she seized such an object from a young girl who was applying a coat of varnish, exclaiming, 'I just have to hold a brush!' Brush in hand, she defied her diminished eyesight and went on painting animated, sensuous pictures of flowers.[1]

* * *

Even so, the commonest and most explicit manifestation of illness affecting eyesight is that arising from cataracts, an opacity of the lens. Claude Monet, one of the greatest colourists of all time, gave us the most radiant pictures of Impressionism. He loved painting the same motif, for instance 'The Japanese bridge', over and over again at different times of day. The shifting light of Nature generated a change of colours as the day went on, and the delighted master reproduced it with sensitive brush-strokes in subtle and vivid colour harmonies.

---

1 Unfortunately, it was not possible to identify the source of this quotation.

Monet was of course devastated when this disorder impaired his eyesight.[2] Its effect on his painting is tragically obvious; he said that comparisons with his earlier works sent him into an uncontrollable rage and caused him to attack his canvases with a penknife.[3] Outlines dissolved and shapes became indefinite – according to him, he saw everything as in a fog – and his brush-strokes grew rough, occasionally vehement, as if made in a state of despair. His sense of colour changed, the colour scale being pushed in the direction of red as his opaque lenses reduced every other colour; even his blues acquired a touch of purple. The master himself observed that they became abominably false.[4]

Following an operation for his cataracts, Monet's eyesight was much improved, but he was not at all happy when he saw the reddish landscapes from the last few years: 'The distortion and exaggerated colours that I see are quite terrifying ... and if I was condemned to see nature as I see it now, I'd prefer to be blind and keep my memories of the beauties I've always seen.' To his doctor he wrote, 'It makes me sorry that I ever decided to go ahead with that fatal operation. Excuse me for being so frank and allow me to say that I think it's criminal to have placed me in such a predicament.'[5] He corrected the colours on some of his paintings and destroyed others, even kicking them, shattering the canvases. His friends managed to save some of them.

Now that the opaque lenses had been removed, Monet exaggerated the blue tones instead, and he noticed it himself, saying that all he could see was blue and that it was disgusting. Since that is how Monet himself saw his motif, it was his own personal realism; and one can only wonder what 'realism' actually is – reality for whom?

As if Monet wished to help us perceive and comprehend the effects of cataracts, he kept returning to the Japanese bridge, painting yet another series in different colours. This time, though, the variation was involuntary and deceptive, arising from a change of the inner light in the master's eyes – a change caused by the illness and the ensuing operation.

Many art historians have misunderstood or underestimated the powerful influence of Monet's reduced vision on his painting; they have interpreted his difficulties – difficulties which he himself described as distortions and exaggerations – as a conscious ambition in the direction of greater abstraction, Impressionism being replaced by Expressionism,

2 On Monet's cataracts, see P. D. Trevor-Roper, *The World through Blunted Sight* (Indianapolis and New York: Bobbs-Merrill Company, 1970), p. 89.

3 François Thiébalt-Sisson, 'Les Nymphéas de Claude Monet', *La Revue de l'Art Ancien et Moderne* 52 (1927), 41–52 (p. 46).

4 Richard Kendall, *Monet by Himself* (London: Macdonald & Co., 1989), p. 259.

5 The first quotation is from a letter to Georges Clemenceau of 30 August 1923, the second from a letter to Dr Charles Coutela, of 22 June 1923; both references are in Kendall, *Monet by Himself*, pp. 261–262.

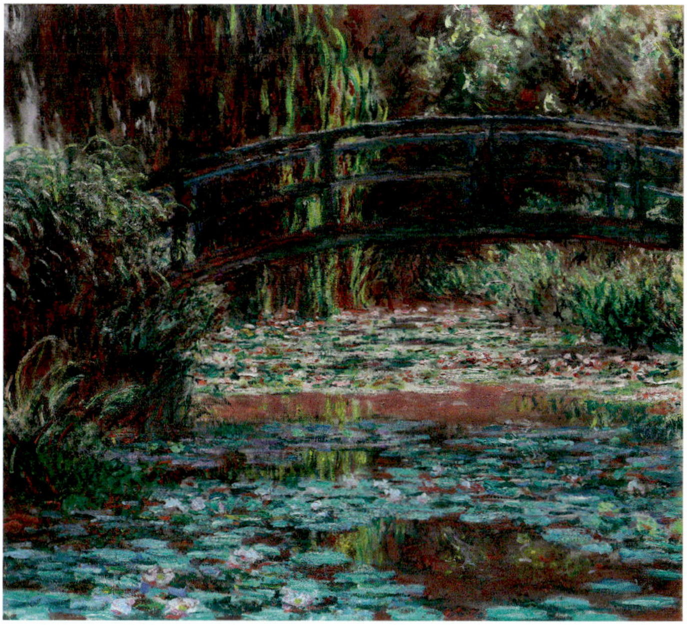

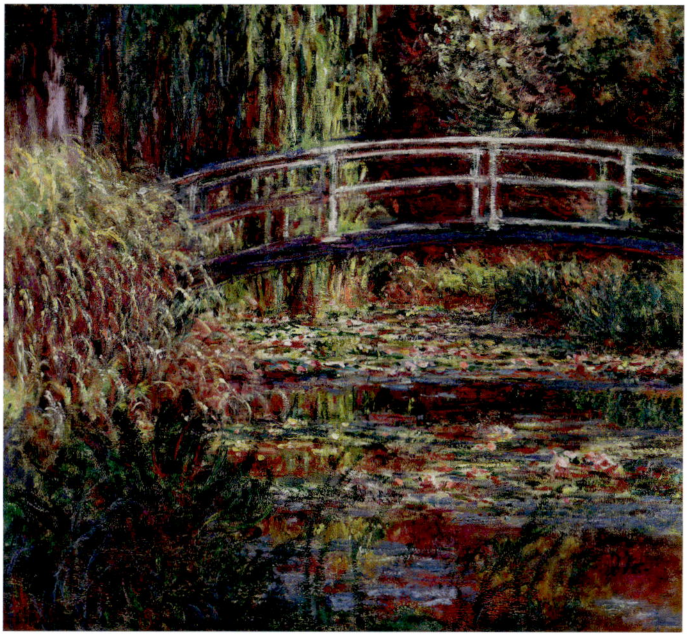

Figures 61 and 62 Claude Monet, 'The water-lily pond', two paintings, 1900. The five Monet reproductions, 61–62 and 63–65, show a corner of Nature, seen through one and the same temperament but looked at with different eyes: in 61–62, the Japanese bridge is seen painted in a state of health, whereas Figures 63–65 are paintings by an artist whose eyes are affected by disease. With healthy eyes, the colour varies according to the time of day – predominantly blue at lunchtime, veering towards red at dusk.

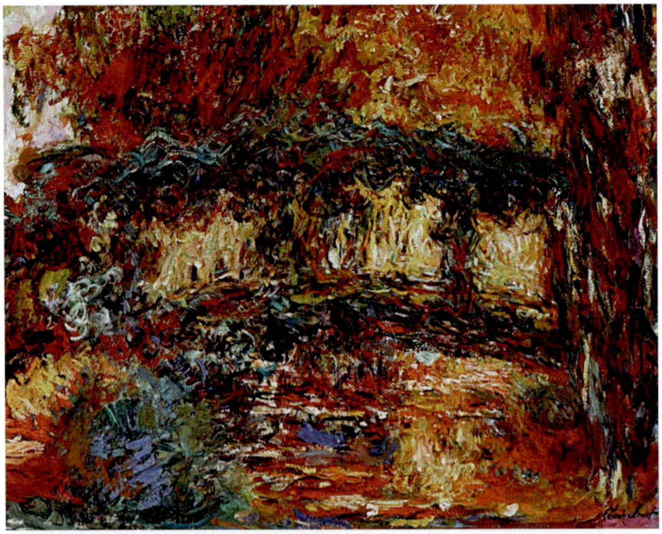

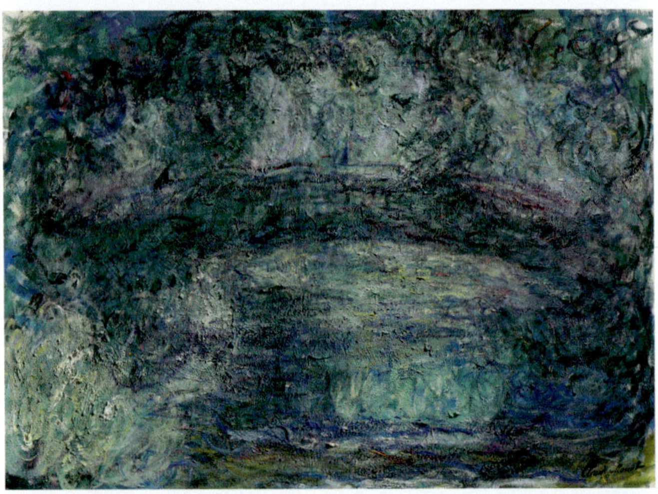

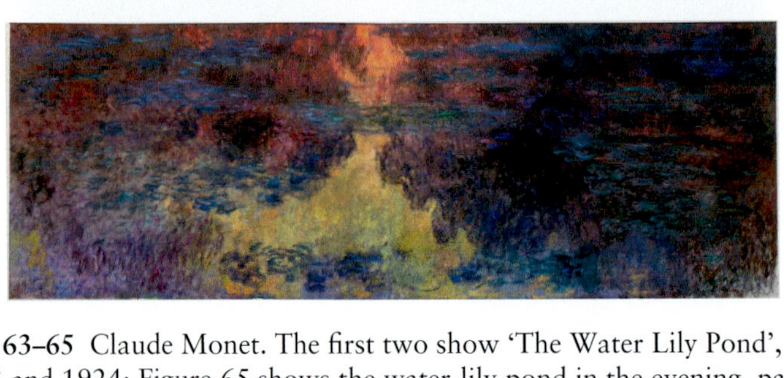

Figures 63–65 Claude Monet. The first two show 'The Water Lily Pond', painted in 1923 and 1924; Figure 65 shows the water-lily pond in the evening, painted in 1922. As Monet's eyes were still blighted by disease, when his cataracts were at their worst, a reddish yellow predominates; after the operation, blue takes over. Figure 65 was painted at a time when, according to Monet, he was unable to do anything well.

amounting to 'a revolution in the garden'.[6] But Monet himself knew better. While art historians admire the consistency and the assured brush-strokes they claim to see, the artist himself laments over 'the daubs I persisted in doing when I could see nothing but fog'.[7] As time went by, though, his sense of colour improved, partly aided by tinted spectacles: 'I'm delighted to be able to tell you that I've truly recovered my sight at last and did so virtually at a stroke. In short, I can live and breathe again, am overjoyed to see everything once more, and I'm working passionately.'[8] His peace of mind restored, he was able to finish his classic work, the paintings with ethereal water-lilies floating on a surface which reflects the sky and a celestial light.

* * *

It has now been clearly demonstrated that abnormal sight was not what caused El Greco to elongate his figures.[9] After all, since he saw his models and his paintings with the same eyes, surely the effect of any astigmatism would have been neutralised while he painted. The aesthetic evidence is equally compelling. In many of El Greco's paintings, human beings are markedly elongated in some parts of the picture but completely normal in others, which shows that he distorted his figures in order to enhance the artistic expression. This strategy is obvious in one of the finest works of art of all time, 'Burial of the Conde de Orgaz'. In the terrestrial region, where the corpse is being lowered into the ground, everybody is of ordinary human stature; but above, where Heaven opens dramatically, even the soul of the deceased man kneeling before God has the ecstatic, elongated shape that is characteristic of heavenly creatures in El Greco's work.

* * *

Ever since Classical Antiquity, loss of eyesight has been associated with prophesying powers and ability to compose poetry. Speaking about Demodocus, 'the sacred master of heavenly song', Homer wrote:

> Loved by the Muse was the bard: but she gave him of good and evil:
> Reft was the light of his eyes, but with sweetest song he was dowered.[10]

6 Paul Hayes Tucker, 'The Revolution in the Garden: Monet in the Twentieth Century', in Paul Hayes Tucker et al., *Monet in the Twentieth Century* (New Haven: Yale University Press, 1998), pp. 14–85.

7 Monet to Dr Charles Coutela, 13 September 1922, in Kendall, *Monet by Himself*, p. 260.

8 Another letter to Coutela, of 27 July 1925; p. 265 in Kendall, *Monet by Himself*.

9 G. P. Hodge, 'El Greco: On Ending the Myth of Distorted Vision', in *Abbottempo in Review* (Chicago: Abbott Universal, 1970), p. 88.

10 *Homer's Odyssey*, trans. H. B. Cotterill (London: G. G. Harrap, 1911), p. 96; *Odyssey* VIII, lines 63–64.

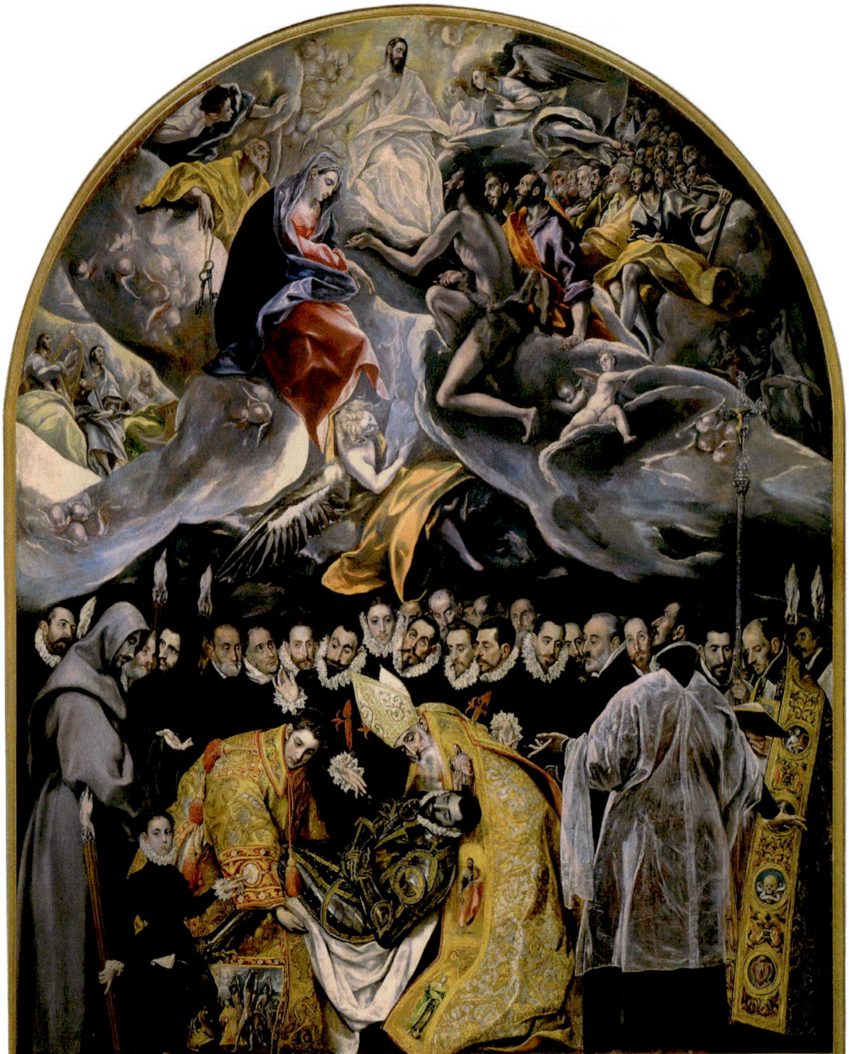

Figure 66 El Greco, 'Burial of the Conde de Orgaz', 1586–88. In this painting, earthly creatures possess normal stature, whereas the inhabitants of Heaven are ecstatically elongated.

'Sweetest song' often comes across as a sufficient consolation. John Milton completed *Paradise Regained* after going completely blind. In a famous sonnet, beginning 'When I consider how my light is spent', he refers to his blindness as a 'mild yoke':

> 'Doth God exact day-labour, light denied?'
> I fondly ask. But patience, to prevent
> That murmur, soon replies, 'God doth not need
> Either man's work or his own gifts; who best
> Bear his mild yoke, they serve him best.'

Even so, there were times when Milton experienced great sadness. When he married his second wife he was already completely blind and never saw his young wife except in fleeting dreams. When she died in childbirth two years later, he lamented his dual loss in a final, sublime line:

> Methought I saw my late espoused saint
> ...
> ... such as yet once more I trust to have
> Full sight of her in Heaven without restraint,
> Came vested all in white, pure as her mind;
> Her face was veil'd, yet to my fancied sight
> Love, sweetness, goodness, in her person shin'd
> So clear as in no face with more delight.
> But Oh! as to embrace me she inclin'd,
> I wak'd, she fled, and day brought back my night.

Milton found a brother in adversity in the Bible, Samson, blinded in Gaza. 'O loss of sight, of thee I most complain!' the giant lamented in Milton's *Samson Agonistes* (1671), line 67.

When Handel composed his oratorio to Milton's text, he, too was losing his sight and was able to interpret blind Samson's emotions with the same agitated fervour (lines 80–82):

> O dark, dark, dark, amid the blaze of noon,
> Irrecoverably dark, total Eclipse
> Without all hope of day!

To all three of them, Samson, Milton, and Handel, light – now a lost paradise – was the sublimest thing in creation (lines 83–85):

> O first created Beam, and thou great Word
> Let there be light, and light was over all;
> Why am I thus bereav'd thy prime decree?

When those in the audience who knew the background of the song heard these words and notes, they could not hold back their tears.

James Joyce regarded his blindness as one of the minor troubles in his life, and Jorge Luis Borges did not find gradual blindness, like 'a slow summer twilight', a tragedy.[11] Borges quoted Milton: 'I say again that I have lost no more / than the inconsequential skin of things'. But when he contemplated the full extent of his loss, his stoicism faltered: 'but then I think of letters and of roses'.[12] In another poem on blindness, he describes how other senses come to the blind man's aid:

---

11 From a television interview on The Dick Cavett Show in May 1980; printed in Willis Barnstone (ed.), *Borges at Eighty: Conversations* (Bloomington: Indiana University Press, 1982), p. 34.

12 From Borges's poem 'A Blind Man', trans. Alastair Reid, in Borges's *Selected Poems*, ed. by Alexander Coleman (New York: Penguin, 2000), p. 357. (The poem is originally from the collection named *The Unending Rose*.)

... I breathe a rose across the garden,
a wistful rose, my friends, out of the twilight.[13]

Inner vision helped Borges write some of his most beautiful passages during long years of blindness. The poet beholds the invisible without being confused by earthly delusions – just as the deaf composer is not disturbed by the noises of earthly existence.

***

There are times when the threat of a serious illness affects the individual as deeply as the disease itself. It has been established that Emily Dickinson had a squint and was threatened by partial blindness, 'a woe, the only one that ever made me tremble. It was the shutting out of all the dearest ones of time, the strongest friends of the soul – BOOKS.'[14] She was treated by a famous ophthalmologist in Boston, probably undergoing surgery. Dickinson was understandably upset by the idea of going blind: 'The medical man ... might as well have said, "Eyes be blind, heart be still" ...' – the same cry of distress that Beethoven had uttered when threatened with deafness.[15]

***

In a comparison between the consequences of reduced sensory functions in artists, it would appear that deafness is seen as a greater evil than blindness – apart from the natural exception that blindness makes figurative art impossible.[16] On closer reflection, it is easy to see that one becomes more isolated, more excluded from human companionship, when one can no longer hear one's fellow human beings and talk with them than when one can no longer see them. The disappearance of familiar constant small noises in one's surroundings produces a depressing feeling of deathly silence.

Jonathan Swift, Francisco de Goya, and Ludwig van Beethoven supply persuasive examples. Swift had been a good-humoured and sociable man until he lost his hearing in middle age. Affected by Ménière's syndrome, with increasing vertigo and deafness, he lamented:

See, how the Dean begins to break!
Poor gentleman, he droops apace!
You plainly find it in his face.

13 From 'The Blind Man', p. 311 in the edition mentioned in the preceding note. (This poem is originally from the collection named *The Gold of the Tigers*.)
14 Martin Wand and Richard B. Sewall, '"Eyes be blind, heart be still": A New Perspective on Emily Dickinson's Eye Problem', *New England Quarterly* 52.3 (1979), 400–406.
15 Ibid., 401.
16 F. Cawthorne, 'The Influence of Deafness on the Creative Instinct', *The Laryngoscope* 70 (1969), 1110.

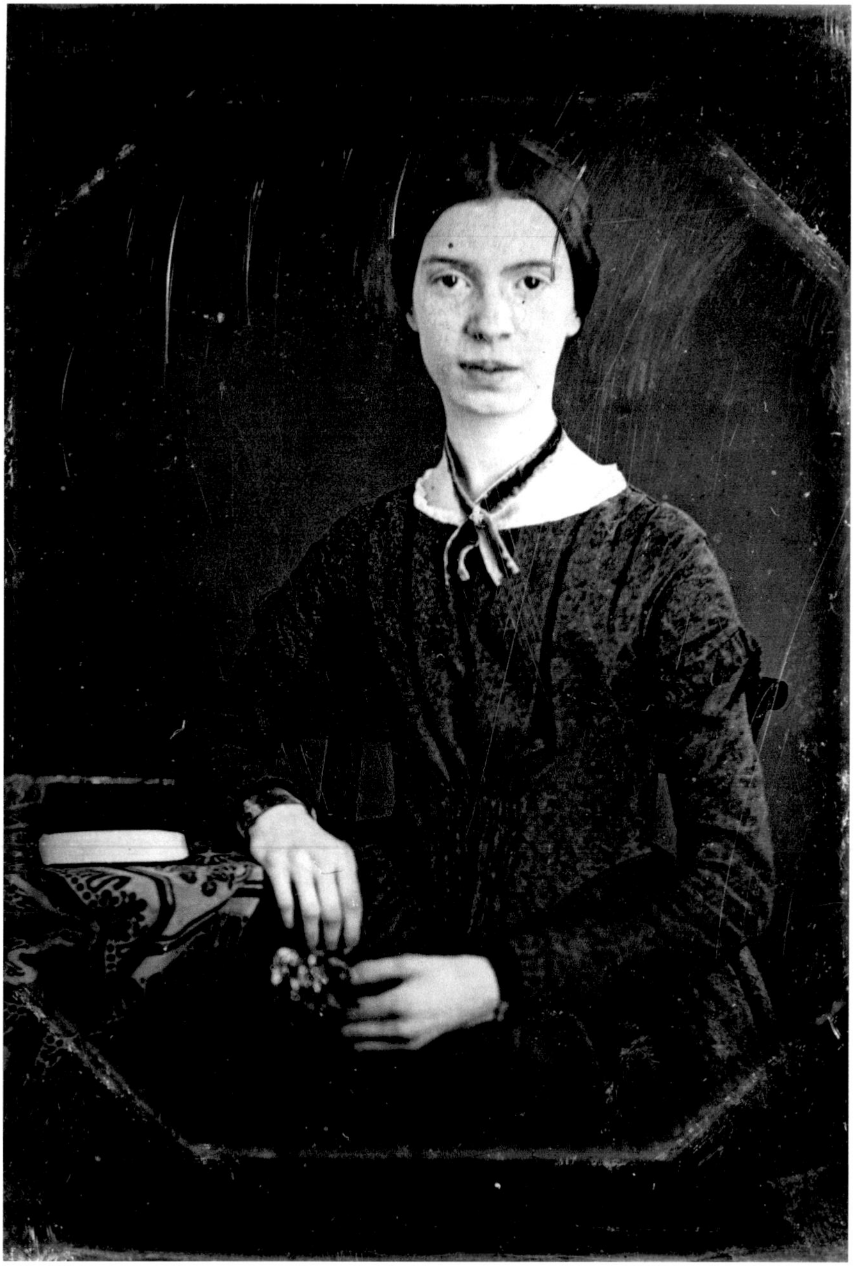

Figure 67 Emily Dickinson. In this daguerreotype portrait of the poet from 1846/47, the difference in position of the light reflections in the pupils shows that she has a squint.

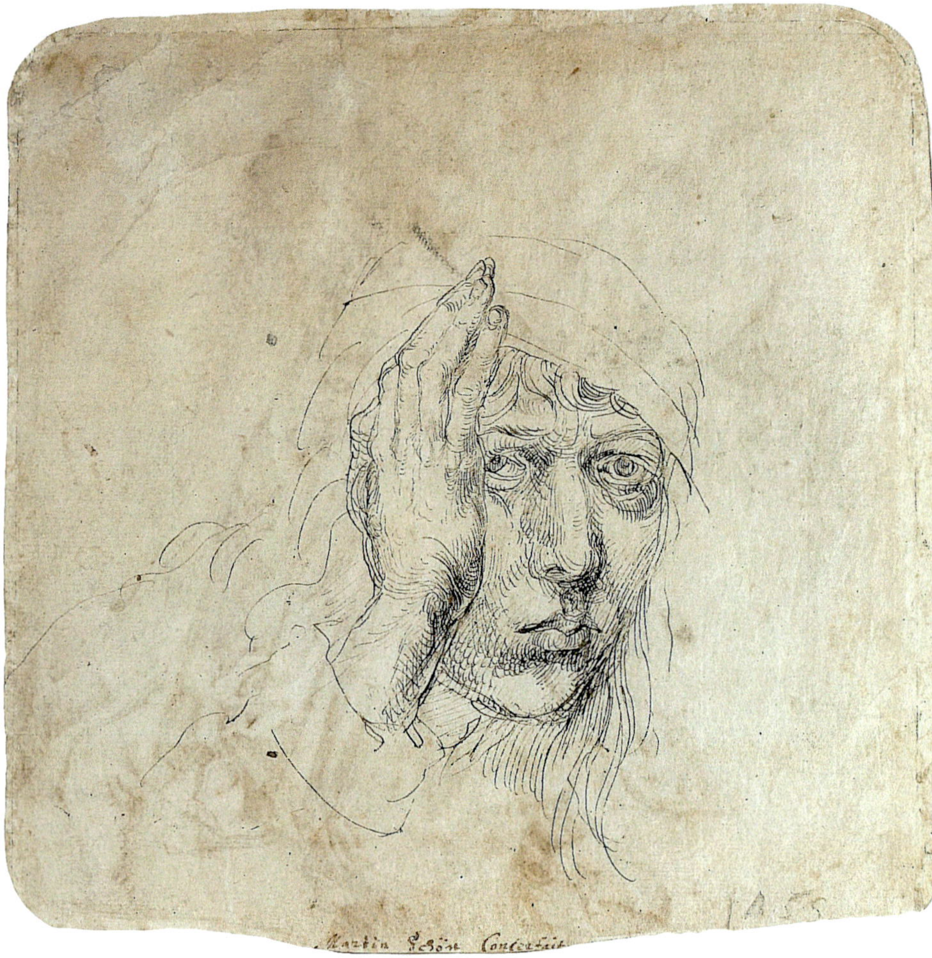

Figure 68 Dickinson's squint was as nothing compared to that of Albrecht Dürer; in this self-portrait from 1491/1492, he cuts off the vision in one eye with his hand in order to ward off the troubling double images.

That old vertigo in his head
Will never leave him till he's dead.[17]

In Swift, the slightly paranoid suspiciousness towards one's surroundings that sometimes affects deaf people grew into a profound mistrust of everything human, a distrust allegorically presented in *Gulliver's Travels*. It received its most drastic expression in his *Modest Proposal*, which suggests

17 From 'On the Death of Dr. Swift', p. 483 in the 1932 edition (1967 reprint) of *Satires and Personal Writings by Jonathan Swift*, ed. by William Alfred Eddy (London: Oxford University Press).

that starving Irish babies might be fattened in order to be exported to England as food.[18]

* * *

The misanthropy and dejection caused by sudden deafness are seen in the art of Francisco de Goya with unique emphasis and intensity. Though usually light-hearted in his youth, 'the world's happiest being' in both words and pictures, and a painter whose early works spread a radiant light over the beautiful figures in them, young Goya was not entirely spared those hours of melancholy that so often afflict exalted spirits. However, those were mere light summer skies in comparison with the heavy thunderclouds that were to come. At the age of 47, he fell ill with a disease that caused transient blindness and lifelong profound deafness.

Goya's illness might have been caused by a rare virus; but it is more likely that he was poisoned by lead, an essential component in his paints which he handled rather carelessly when attacking his canvas with his characteristic fervour. If we are to believe Théophile Gautier, Goya's working method was as unusual as his talent.[19] He would scoop paint from a tub and apply it with sponges, mops, rags, anything he could lay his hands on. According to Gautier, Goya would trowel and slap his paints on like mortar, smoothing them out with his thumb. Even allowing for the possibility that Gautier exaggerated, Goya must have been seriously exposed to the noxious effect of the paint. The resulting brain damage, lead encephalopathy, is known to cause deafness and personality changes, manifested as bitterness and depression.

Paralysed by his dire misfortune, Goya was initially quite incapable of engaging in any activity whatever; and, when he eventually did resume painting, his subjects changed from complaisant reverie to horrendous nightmares in which he gave vent to the deepest despair and mistrust in all things human. The latter culminated in the macabre 'black paintings' made during fits of melancholy in his later years.

In between those episodes, however, he was able to work in a lighter vein, and the misanthropic features are less apparent in the pictures he painted on commission. We might, for instance, compare the various roles he ascribes to Time as a symbol. In the large decorative painting usually referred to as 'Truth, Time and History', located in the Stockholm Nationalmuseum, the colour scale is bright and festive.[20] Time is represented by an amiable elderly man who does not allow the hourglass to run empty, but turns it in order to indicate a new era which would, it was hoped, be a happy one.

18 The full title of this 'ironical essay' is *A Modest Proposal for Preventing the Children of Ireland from Being a Burden to Their Parents or Country* (1729), pp. 21–31 in the edition mentioned in the preceding note.

19 Théophile Gautier, *Voyage en Espagne* (Paris: Charpentier, 1845), p. 129.

20 Eleanor A. Sayre, 'Goya: A Moment in Time', *Nationalmuseum Bulletin* 3 (1979), 28.

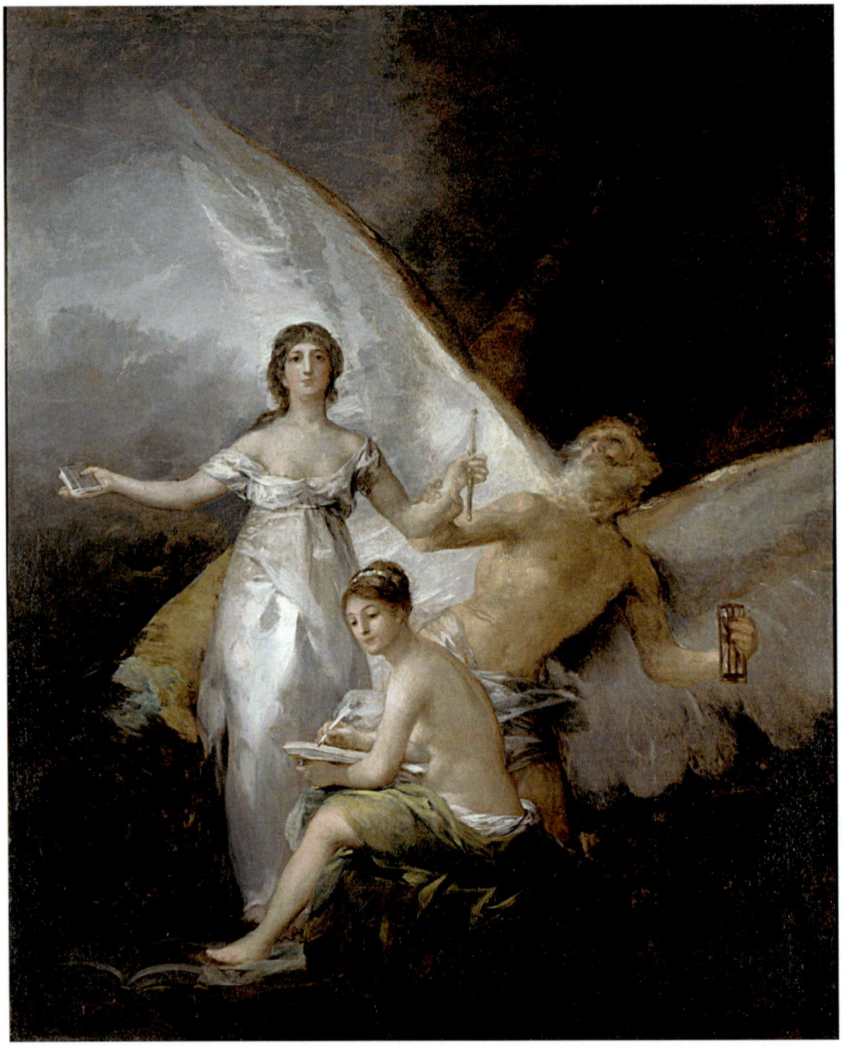

Figure 69 Francisco de Goya, 'Truth, Time and History', 1812–14. The painting is an allegory of Spain's receiving a new constitution in 1812.

The 'black painting' which Goya kept to himself is a completely different matter. In a letter to a friend, he wrote about attempting a couple of new paintings in order to occupy his imagination, which had been reduced to a state of torpor because of constant brooding over his troubles. In these pictures, he said, he had been able to express some ideas which it would have been difficult to include in commissioned work, giving free rein to his inventiveness in the process.[21] In the painting of Saturn the giant eating his

21 *Goya: A Life in Letters*, ed. by Sarah Symmons, trans. Philip Troutman (London: Pimlico, 2004), p. 237.

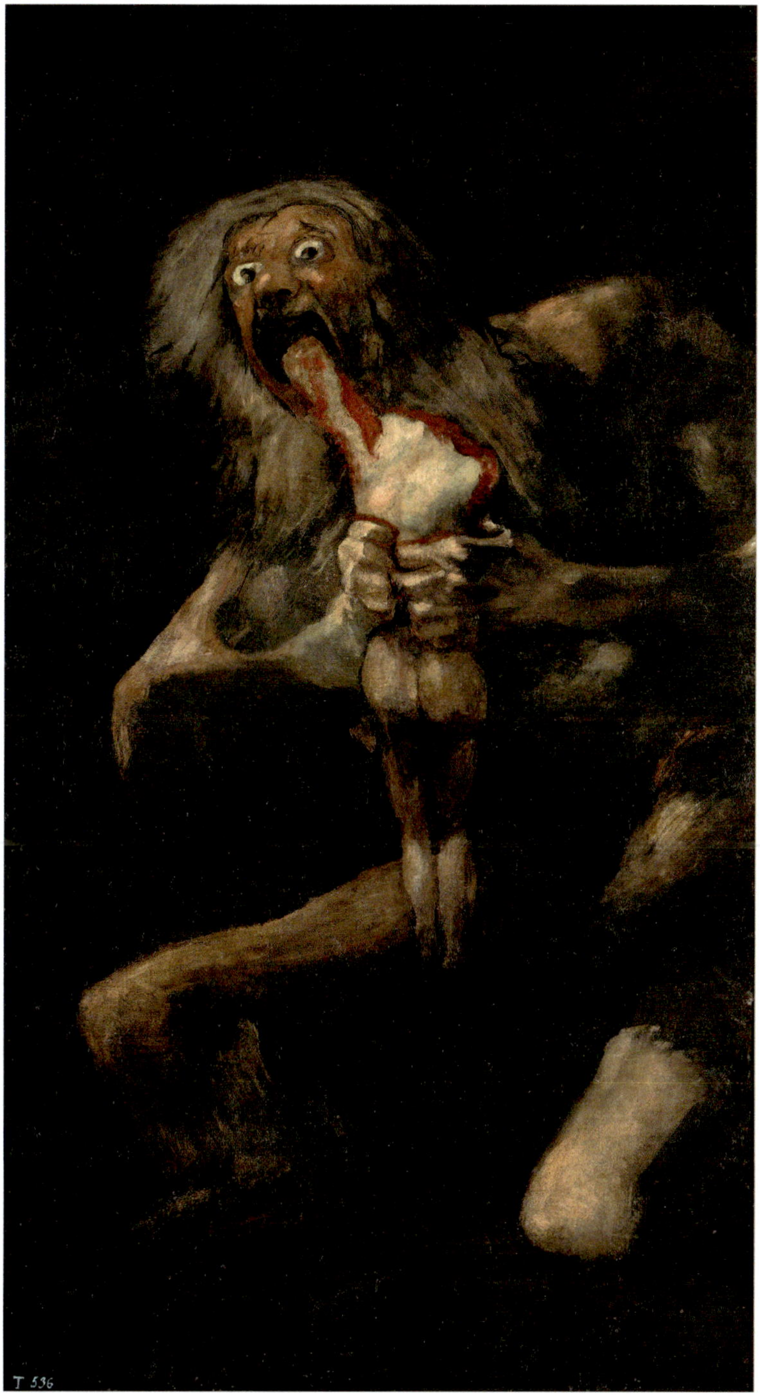

Figure 70 Francisco de Goya, 'Saturn devouring his son', 1820–23. In this 'black painting' Saturn creates moments in time – his own children, whom he then devours. In the Museo Nacional del Prado; see p. 215.

own children, which Goya hung in his dining-room, we see Time again, now indefatigably creating hours but at the same time insatiable, devouring and annihilating them just as rapidly, thereby rendering everything meaningless. This conception is akin to a view expressed by a modern physicist: 'The more the universe seems comprehensible, the more it also seems pointless.'[22]

* * *

The faculty of hearing is of course vital to those artists who create using sound. At about twenty years of age, Beethoven began to lose his hearing, and he spent the last years of his life stone deaf, in the loneliest of all lonely states.

To Beethoven this predicament was virtually unbearable, as is evident from his heartbreaking words in his 'Heiligenstädter Testament': 'Oh you men who think or say that I am malevolent, stubborn, or misanthropic, how greatly do you wrong me. You do not know the secret cause which makes me seem that way to you ... think that for six years now I have been hopelessly afflicted ... it was impossible for me to say to people, "Speak louder, shout, for I am deaf." Ah, how could I possibly admit an infirmity in the one sense which ought to be more perfect in me than in others ... I must live almost alone like one who has been banished ... If I approach near to people, a hot terror seizes upon me and I fear being exposed to the danger that my condition might be noticed ... what a humiliation for me when someone standing next to me heard a flute in the distance, and I *heard nothing*, or someone heard a shepherd singing, and again I heard nothing. Such incidents drove me almost to despair. A little more of that and I would have ended my life – it was only *my art* that held me back. Ah, it seemed to me impossible to leave the world until I had brought forth all that I felt was within me. So I endured this wretched existence – truly wretched ... *Patience*, they say, is what I must now choose for my guide, and I have done so. – I hope my determination will remain firm to endure until it pleases the inexorable Parcae to break the thread ... Forced to become a philosopher already in my twenty-eighth year, oh it is not easy, and for the artist much more difficult than for anyone else.'[23]

Beethoven was not always guided by patience, though. In his *Sonata Appassionata*, he bared his soul and gave free rein to his despair and to an irrepressible rebellion against his unhappy fate. On the whole, however, he was more successful when it came to taking his condition philosophically than his brothers in adversity, the unrestrained court painter in Madrid

22 Steven Weinberg, *The First Three Minutes: A Modern View of the Origin of the Universe* (London: Fontana, 1977), p. 149.

23 Quoted from https://debeethovencatalogus.wordpress.com/wp-content/uploads/2017/08/7273x_50_itow_heiligenstadt.pdf. This website, in its turn, quotes the 'Heiligenstädter Testament' from Alexander Thayer's *The Life of Beethoven*, ed. by Henry Krehbiel (New York: Beethoven Association, 1921). The 'testament', written in 1802 when Beethoven was 32 years old, was addressed to his brothers Carl and Johann.

and the venomous Dean in Dublin. It was under these circumstances that Beethoven composed the *Pastoral Symphony*, a work so elevated above human wretchedness and distress; indeed, he may have attained these heights solely thanks to his endeavour to endure his condition. It is moving to hear him rejoicing in the sweet notes from animated Nature, notes he was now only able to hear in memory. What he actually heard, day and night, was a nasty throbbing sound. In his Fifth Symphony, Beethoven lets us share and comprehend his suffering for a moment when reproducing the noise by means of monotonous beats on the kettle-drum against a subdued background of strings – a musical 'autopathography', one might say. Recognising Beethoven's stoic nature, we may imagine him smiling through tears as the tragic mood is dispersed by an outburst of exuberant joy in the finale.

An ear specialist has made the interesting experiment of manipulating tapes of Beethoven's music from this period, so that we can hear how it sounded to Beethoven with his limited auditory reception. While very enlightening, the experiment does not actually afford any explanation; and it remains an open, albeit intricate, question to what extent Beethoven's composing was affected by his impaired hearing. Might it have helped him break free from tradition and convention, thereby facilitating the creation of radically innovative works?

Hector Berlioz, who never learnt to play any instrument correctly, may afford us a clue to the answer: 'when I think of the appalling quantity of platitudes for which the piano is daily responsible – flagrant platitudes which in most cases would never be written if their authors had only pen and paper to rely on and could not resort to their magic box – I can only offer up my gratitude to chance which taught me to compose freely and in silence and thus saved me from the tyranny of keyboard habits, so dangerous to thought, and from the lure of conventional sonorities, to which all composers are to a greater or lesser extent prone'.[24]

In his later years, Beethoven was certainly delivered from 'ordinary sonorities' and could listen to his compositions only with his 'inner ear', the inaudible music that John Keats describes in his 'Ode on a Grecian Urn':

> Heard melodies are sweet, but those unheard
> Are sweeter; therefore, ye soft pipes, play on;
> Not to the sensual ear, but, more endear'd,
> Pipe to the spirit ditties of no tone ...[25]

It is unlikely that we will ever know for sure what caused Beethoven's deafness. It might have been an inherited genetic disease. Among possible chronic disorders, lead poisoning and sarcoidosis have been discussed. The latter, a chronic granulomatous illness, could account for the various infirmities that blighted his life, including chest pains and constant diarrhoeas as well as the liver cirrhosis which ultimately killed him. That is the

24 Hector Berlioz, *The Memoirs of Hector Berlioz*, trans. David Cairns (London: Gollancz, 1969), p. 47.

25 Stanza II.

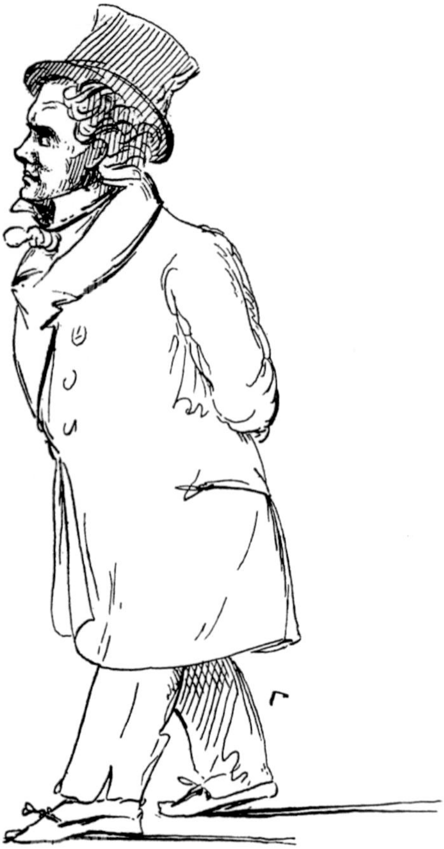

Figure 71 Johann Peter Lyser, drawing of Beethoven. Lyser's portrait demonstrates signs of Paget's disease, with an abnormally large head and a protruding forehead.

only diagnosis that covers all his symptoms, including the rarest, his early, progressive deafness.[26]

However, there are several strong indications that Beethoven suffered from Paget's disease. The symptoms affecting his hearing precisely correspond to those found in many cases of this bone disease, and he displayed other characteristics as well. His head grew to an impressive size with an Olympian forehead, massive jaws, and a jutting chin. Gioachino Rossini described how his eyes shone beneath bushy eyebrows as from the bottom of a well. These features are clearly discernible in portraits of Beethoven from his later years. One of them, a drawing made four years before his death, might be regarded as an illustration of an anecdote related by Bettina Brentano. Beethoven was walking with his friend Goethe when they encountered the Imperial family. The poet courteously stepped aside and bared his head while the headstrong composer pulled his outgrown hat firmer down on his head and continued walking straight ahead.

26 Thomas G. Palferman, 'Beethoven: A Medical Biography', *Journal of Medical Biography* 1 (1993), 35.

The composer Bedrich Smetana was able to make an exact reproduction of precisely the noise – ringing in his ears – that formed the first symptom of an ear disorder that ultimately made him deaf. In the last movement of his string quartet *Aus meinem Leben* (*From My Life*), there is a sudden shrill tone depicting this ringing sound which expresses the composer's misery caused by his infirmity.

It is hard to image a more cruel game that disease has played with an artist than Gabriel Fauré's ear complaint.[27] Not only did his hearing diminish; the quality of the tone changed so that he heard out of tune, perceiving treble notes one third above and bass notes one third below the right note. Consequently, he was never able to hear his late compositions as he had conceived them: 'I only hear horrors', the ageing master lamented.[28]

27 Patrick l'Echevin, *Musique et médecin*, a dissertation presented at Lille in 1980 and published by Éditions Stock in 1981; the passage on Fauré's (mis)hearing is on p. 112.
28 Philippe Fauré-Fremiet, *Gabriel Fauré* (Paris: Rieder, 1929), p. 70 ('je n'entendrais rien, que des choses affreuses!'),

Chapter 9
Severe pain

Severe pain is one of the worst scourges of humankind. When fully established, it becomes all-consuming and prevents any meaningful contact with the world around us. It compels us to endure the unendurable, reducing us to a state of hopeless despair. I know that myself, for as I write this I am bedridden with a broken spine, moaning and tossing and turning in fruitless attempts to escape from the agony.

Pain can never be rendered artistically in all its intensity, but it may make a more vivid impression when represented in the pictorial arts than when it is described in words (Figure 72).[1] Gotthold Ephraim Lessing had no doubts (see p. 11). In his discussion about expressions of pain, he chose the myth of Laocoon, who was killed by serpents. Lessing compared the representation in the well-known Greek sculpture with the account supplied by Virgil. In the sculpture, said Lessing, pain is expressed in an appropriate but not excessive manner; it is consequently recorded before the serpent bites and Laocoon is still merely groaning and sighing. In pictorial art, a mouth distorted by screaming – as dramatically described by Virgil – would infringe the laws of beauty and hence block the free play of the imagination. The idea of such a blockage appears to have been aesthetically unacceptable to Lessing – we can imagine how he would have condemned Munch's 'The scream' (Figure 33) or Picasso's 'Guernica' (Figure 73), while approving of Matisse's sensitivity (Figure 76).

* * *

Virginia Woolf deplored the poverty of language when it came to describing ill health and mental or physical pain. According to her, '[t]he merest schoolgirl, when she falls in love, has Shakespeare or Keats to speak her mind for her; but let a sufferer try to describe a pain in his head to a doctor and language at once runs dry'.[2]

Even so, many authors have interpreted pain with profound compassion, knowing that it forms an elementary factor in human life. Ralph Waldo

1 Cf. Ludwig Wittgenstein, *Philosophische Untersuchungen* (Frankfurt am Main: Suhrkamp, 1971), No. 295, p. 158.

2 Virginia Woolf, *On Being Ill* (Ashfield, MA: Paris Press, 2012), pp. 6–7.

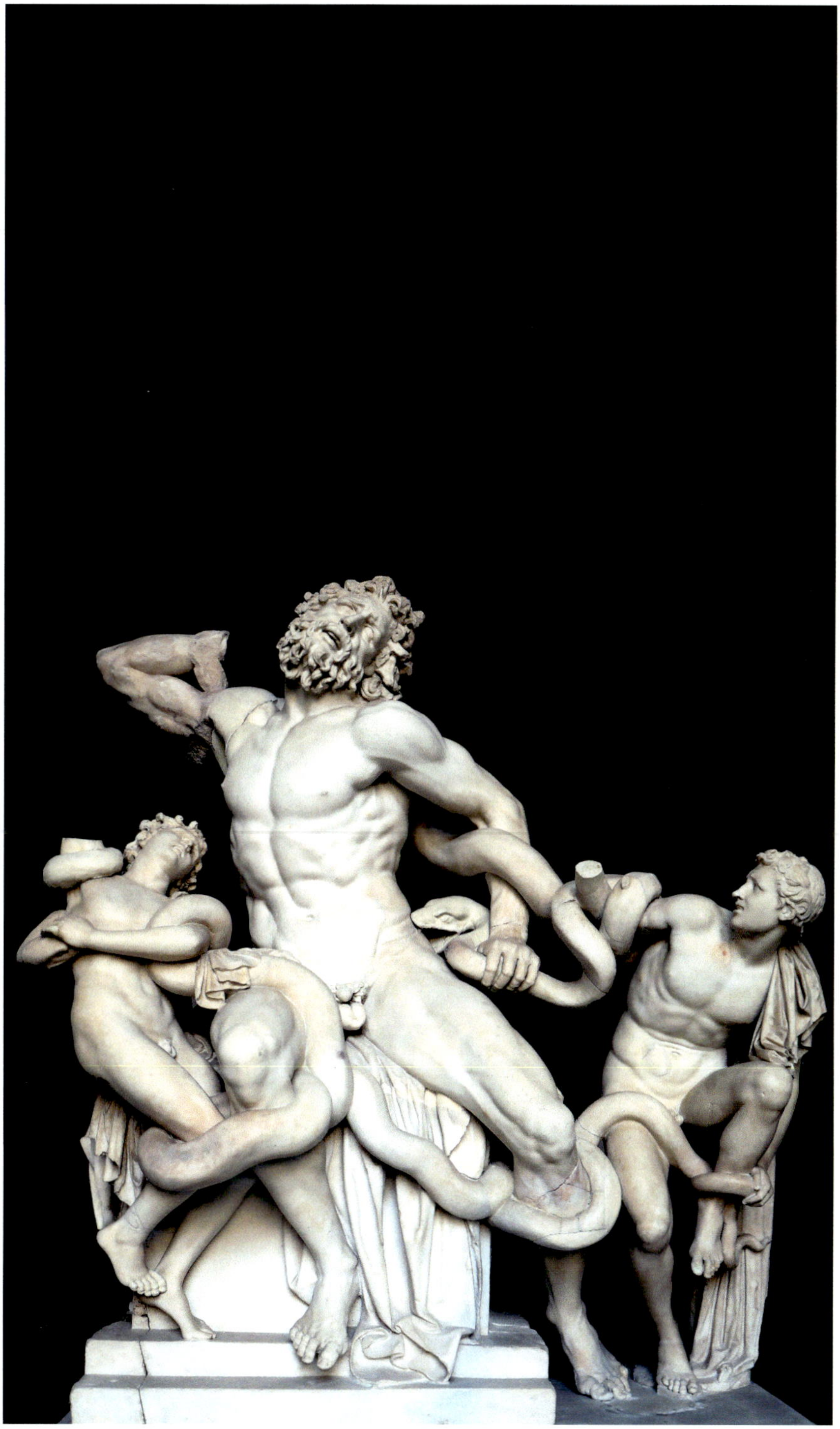

Figure 72 'Laocoon and his sons', Greece, 50 BC.

Emerson knew it well: 'He has seen but half the universe who never has been shown the house of Pain.'[3] I permit myself this antithetical statement: 'They do not know the height of happiness, above all earthly things, who have not on some occasion become rapt and beside themselves as a result of hearing sweet music.'

***

Pierre de Ronsard, the Renaissance poet, had hoped for a peaceful death at the end of his days:

> When my time comes, Goddess,
>   I ask of thee,
> Let me not languish long
>   In malady[.][4]

Ronsard's prayer went unheard, and he suffered severe pain for a long time, caused by gout, arthritis, and colic. However, his soul retained its greatness and strength. While his body degenerated, he transmuted his suffering into moving and beautiful poetry. What he found hardest to endure was sleeplessness:

> Bring back the sun, I lie harassed by pain,
> I die with open eyes, tossing and turning.
> For sixteen hours at least I storm
> From side to side, crying,
> Impatient, I cannot keep quiet.
> In vain I beg Death to come for me;
> Her ears are deaf – she does not come.[5]

It is the same lament that was once heard from Job in his misery. In the end, though, the goddess Death would come to Ronsard's aid:

> I hail thee, happy, welcome Death,
> Healer and comfort in extreme pain[.][6]

As Shakespeare found, there are other inescapable sufferings in human life besides those of unhappy love and jealousy:

---

3 Ralph Waldo Emerson, 'The Tragic', in *The Portable Emerson*, ed. by Mark van Doren (New York: The Viking Press, 1946 [renewed 1974]), p. 216.

4 From the final lines of Ronsard's poem 'Hymne de la Mort': 'Quand mon heure viendra, Déesse, je te prie / Ne me laisse longtemps languir en maladie'. Pierre de Ronsard, *Œuvres completes*, 2 vols, ed. by Gustave Cohen (Paris: Gallimard, 1950), Vol. II, p. 289.

5 The French original is found on p. 635 in the Ronsard edition quoted in the preceding note.

6 'Je te salue, heureuse et profitable Mort, / Des extremes douleurs medicin et confort', also from 'Hymne de la Mort', the lines just before 'When my time comes' quoted above. Ibid., p. 289.

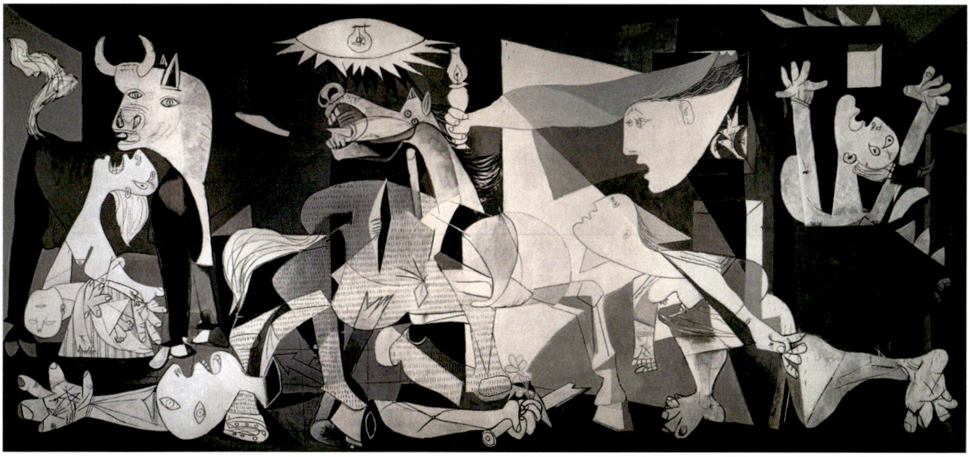

Figure 73 Pablo Picasso, 'Guernica', 1937. A terrifying expression of pain, an unrestrained, elementary reaction to violence.

> [T]here was never yet philosopher
> That could endure the toothache patiently,
> However they have writ the style of gods,
> And made a push at chance and sufferance.[7]

John Milton shared Shakespeare's view. In *Paradise Lost*, he makes Satan and his minions lose the battle against the angels because their own severe pain prevented them from fighting efficiently:

> But pain is perfect misery, the worst
> Of evils, and excessive, overturns
> All patience.[8]

Something those three poets could not foresee was the spiritual strength of Immanuel Kant. This philosopher was a pedant – the people of Königsberg would set their clocks by his morning walk – and had strict rules for his health. He would always breathe through the nose, never through the mouth, in order to avoid catching cold. Kant had regular hours for his meals and for bedtime, and he firmly stopped himself from thinking about complex or worrying subjects a quarter of an hour before going to bed, thereby ensuring that disturbing thoughts would not prevent him from falling asleep. It is easy to understand how distressed he must have been when severe pains began to impair his sleep as attacks of gout turned his toes a glowing red. In a stoic attempt to divert his thoughts from the agony, he forced himself to think intensively of some indifferent and trivial subject. Counting sheep was not appropriate for a learned philosopher, though;

7 From *Much Ado about Nothing* V.i.35–38.
8 *Paradise Lost*, Book VI, lines 462–464.

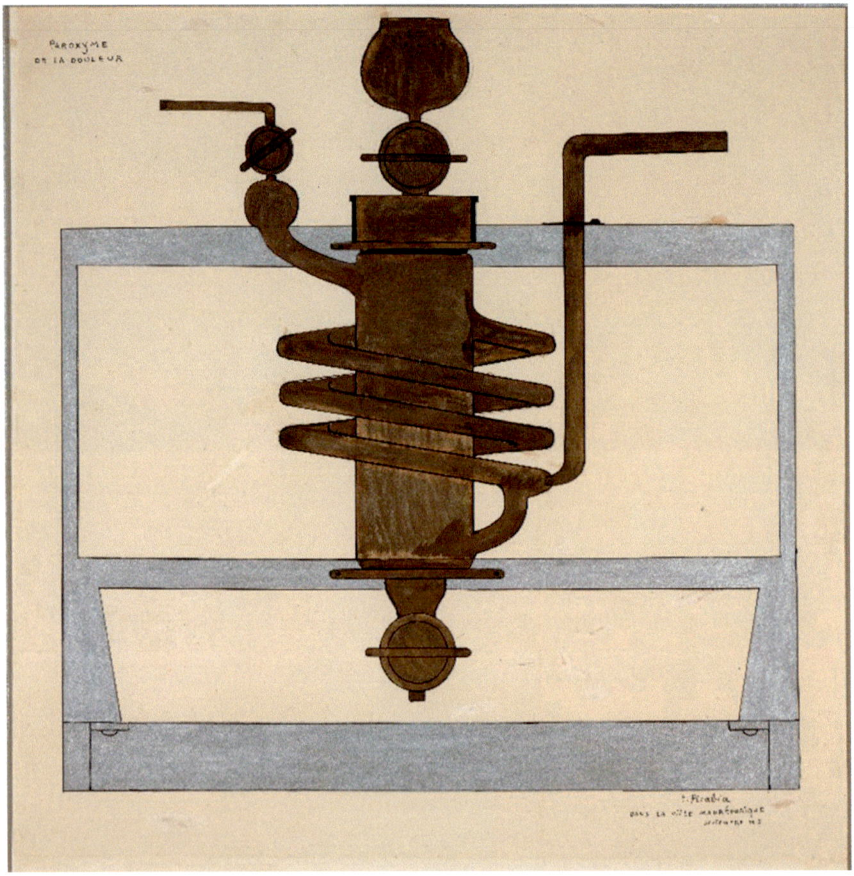

Figure 74 Francis Picabia, 'Paroxysm of pain', 1915. The artist's symbolic representation of pain is both grinding and drilling.

the simple everyday topic he chose to ponder was the name Cicero and the associations it roused in him.

Kant was successful; the pain subsided, and he fell asleep. He was subsequently convinced that even the worst pain may be controlled by willpower alone; but that did not of course apply to women and children, whom Kant – a bachelor and a child of his times – did not credit with willpower of that calibre.

Kant recorded his experiences in an account addressed to the Faculty of Medicine, in which he stated his view that the ability of a human being to achieve great things through willpower alone, even when in the throes of severe pain, was nothing short of incredible. In fact, he said, suffering might be the only thing that could arouse such a degree of willpower.[9]

9 Kant's account is found in *Von der Macht des Gemüths durch den bloßen Vorsatz seiner krankhaften Gefühle Meister zu seyn* (Jena: Die akademische Buchhandlung, 1798), pp. 26–29.

The Danish author Karen Blixen, alias Isak Dinesen, would later prove that a high degree of willpower is not a male prerogative. Her husband gave her good reason for jealousy but little consolation, since he also infected her with syphilis – unless it was the other way around; at any rate, the disease was to cause her infinite agonies. Even so, she declared that all sorrows can be borne so long as you can put them into a story.[10]

If Thomas de Quincy had been as stoic as Kant and Blixen and not surrendered to his trigeminal neuralgia, which caused intense pain in his jaw, he probably would not have become a drug addict, and we would have lost the best-written account that exists of the use as well as the abuse of opium (see pp. 55–56). His loathing of toothache is equally expressive: 'Two things blunt the general sense of horror, which would else connect itself with toothache – viz., first, its enormous diffusion; hardly a household in Europe being clear of it, each in turn having some one chamber intermittently echoing the groans extorted by this cruel torture. A second cause is found in its immunity from danger. [This latter ground of undervaluation is noticed in a saying ascribed (but on what authority I know not) to Sir Philip Sidney] – [viz., that] supposing toothache liable in ever so small a proportion of its cases to a fatal issue, it would be generally ranked as the most dreadful amongst human maladies.'[11]

When pain is at its most intense, the torment at its apex, there can no longer be any question of creative work, a fact eloquently described by George Gissing after an attack of migraine: 'The very I, it is too plain, consists but with a certain balance of my physical elements, which we call health. Even in the light beginnings of my headache, I was already not myself; my thoughts followed no normal course, and I was aware of the abnormality. A few hours later, I was but a walking disease; my mind – if one could use the word – had become a barrel-organ, grinding in endless repetition a bar or two of idle music' – amounting to schizophrenic perseveration, this is a sign of illness which we all experience at some point.[12]

* * *

Abdominal pain is frequently a symptom of more serious illness. In the 1820s, two poets in different parts of Europe suffered badly from gallstone

10 Blixen in an interview with Bent Mohn, 'Talk with Isak Dinesen', *The New York Times*, 3 November 1957, p. 49.

11 Thomas De Quincey, *Confessions of an English Opium-Eater* (1856 edition), reprinted in *The Works of Thomas De Quincey, Vol. 2: Confessions of an English Opium-Eater 1821–1856*, ed. by Grevel Lindop (London: Routledge, 2000), p. 105. The words within square brackets are from a footnote written by De Quincey and hence not in the running text.

12 George Gissing, *The Private Papers of Henry Ryecroft* (Westminster: Archibald Constable & Co., 1903), pp. 189–190.

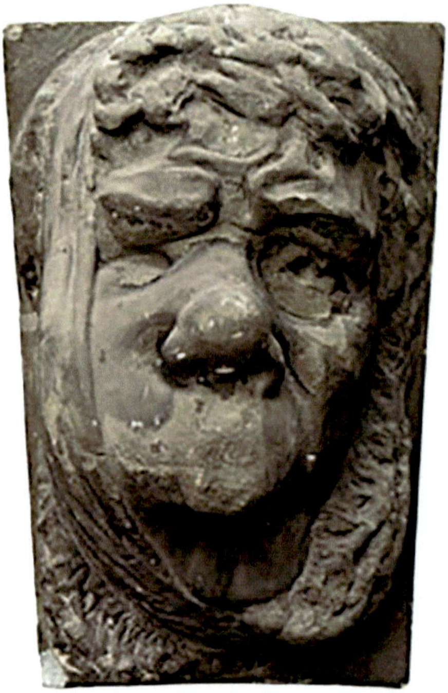

Figure 75 Arnold Böcklin, 'Mask' ('Fratze'), 1871. This 'grimace' represents the agony of pain in a realistic mode. The Swiss master was furious with an art jury that had failed to show him due appreciation. He avenged himself on its six members by making sculptured caricatures of their faces. This one must have aroused his particular ire.

disease – Walter Scott and the Swedish poet Esaias Tegnér.[13] They form examples of the ways in which the same illness may find different kinds of expression in dissimilar personalities. Their case histories were remarkably similar from a medical point of view; but what a disparity with regard to reaction and response between the robust Scotsman, lame but self-assured, and the emotional Swede!

Walter Scott was not overly concerned. During attacks he would roar like a bull, so people could hear him quite a distance down the road; and one night when he feared he was about to die, he bade farewell to his children. As soon as the pain ceased, however, he forgot his suffering.

Conversely, Tegnér was profoundly disturbed. Though witty as usual, he prepared for an early death: 'On New Year's Day I suffered a Colic which I believed would put an end to both my poetical and my theological life, thereby teaching me a variety of things about which both Poetics and the Symbolic Books have left me in some uncertainty'. In a letter written three years earlier, he had written, 'I know that we must all die. Nevertheless, under the circumstances it would be somewhat inconvenient, if not for me, then at least for my family. ... However, only a fool complains about the inevitable. Resignation is the sum of life's wisdom; and the

13 See Hesketh Pearson, *Walter Scott* (London: Methuen, 1954), and Philip Sandblom, 'Esaias Tegnérs kroppsliga ohälsa', *Tegnérstudier* 1951 (published by Tegnérsamfundet, The Tegnér Society, in Lund).

slightest consideration should teach us to put a brave face on the cruel game we call life, a game we are bound to lose in any case.'[14]

Both patients learnt that even friends in need may be a nuisance. Scott had such a friend in Lord Buchan. His lordship promised to devote Christian zeal to arranging Scott's funeral, which Scott could confidently entrust to him, down to the last detail.[15] An example of similarly tactful compassion is supplied by Tegnér's disciple Samuel Abraham Leijonhufvud: 'God be thanked that you are well again, Doctor. The news of your illness frightened me a great deal, and I had reason to be frightened, having lost three close acquaintances from the years of my youth during this year alone.'[16] No wonder the addressees became discouraged.

As was pointed out above, the two writers responded very differently to the illness. Scott bore up courageously and wrote, 'I should be a great fool, and a most ungrateful wretch, to complain of such inflictions as these. My life has been, in all its private and public relations, as fortunate perhaps as was ever lived, up to this period; and whether pain or misfortune may lie behind the dark curtain of futurity, I am already a sufficient debtor to the bounty of Providence to be resigned to it.'[17]

Poor Tegnér was more pathetic, and more poetic: 'I can no longer hope for health and happiness, but I do hope I will in days to come, up to the very end, be able to retain that strength of mind which must so often in this optimistic world of ours serve as a substitute for Providence ... If my slight personality will return to whence it came a few months sooner or later, conscious or not, in order to drown in the large fountain-head or float around like a bubble for some time yet, reflecting the sky and an alien light – this seems to me an increasingly indifferent matter.'[18] Even his most sombre ideas are dressed in ethereal and beautiful images.

The same illness thus made essential contributions to the experiences of the two writers: suffering in their lives, but useful material for their works. Their creative energy and capacity for work were very differently affected. Scott continued to work through his attacks with 'the strength of a team of horses', but was able to observe that the quality of his writing was adversely affected. Reading what he had dictated during his attacks, he found himself unable to recall anything about the plot or the dialogue: 'When I was so dreadfully ill that I could hardly speak five minutes without loss of breath,

14 The first quotation is from a letter to C. G. von Brinkman of 29 January 1825, in Vol. III of Tegnér's letters, ed. by Nils Palmborg (*Esaias Tegnérs brev III: 1824–1825*, Malmö: Allhems förlag, 1954), p. 182, and the second from a letter to Martina von Schwerin of 17 March 1822 in Vol. II, also edited by Palmborg and published the same year, p. 230.

15 Pearson, *Walter Scott*, p. 140.

16 Unfortunately it was not possible to locate a source for this quotation.

17 Letter to Robert Southey of 4 April 1819, in *The Letters of Sir Walter Scott 1817–1819*, ed. by H. J. C. Grierson (London: Constable & Co., 1933), p. 338.

18 Letter to C. G. von Brinkman of 31 January 1833, in *Esaias Tegnérs brev VII: 1833–1835*, ed. by Nils Palmborg (Malmö: Allhem förlag, 1960), p. 25.

I found that the exertion of dictating the nonsense ... suspended for a time the sense of my situation.'[19]

Although Scott himself could not recollect anything about the events he invented while suffering from illness, and though he regarded what he had dictated as nonsense, it is hard for us, his readers, to agree with him. On the contrary, *Ivanhoe* – written while he was particularly afflicted – turned out to be one of his best-loved novels: a beautiful demonstration of mind over matter. It is not surprising that Scott, repeatedly in dreadful pain, turned the healer Rebecca into the true hero of his tale.

The effect of the illness on the sufferer's ability to write was far more pronounced in Tegnér's case. While he was able to write poetry during periods of illness, his magnum opus, *Frithiofs saga*, had to be put aside for a while. He lamented that his illness blocked his poetic inspiration: 'I suppose that ill health and perennial worry about one's livelihood may depress stronger minds than mine. No profession calls for so much liberty of mind and freedom from trouble as that of the poet. I am well aware that the true Poets overcome all external obstacles, but the rest of us middle-class people want to be fed in our cage if we are to sing.'[20]

Tegnér also began to utilise medical similes from his own experience: 'Even in my better and healthier days I would ... often form Epigrams, but that happened *par gaité du coeur*. They were usually thought to be as harmless as they meant to be; but now they are hardened, petrified bile and therefore hurtful.' The disease was not the least important of the circumstances that caused a change in the poet's style and the character of his poetry. Tegnér became disillusioned, frequently cynical: 'Personally, I believe the whole thing is haemorrhoidal. The pelvic cavity is the sounding-board of life. It is preposterous that everything good about our being should be dependent on such a – sewer.'[21]

Thomas Carlyle was equally indignant: '[T]o-day the *guts* are all wrong again, the headache, the weakness, the black despondency are overpowering me. I fear those paltry viscera will fairly dish me at last. And do but think what a thing it is! that the ethereal spirit of a man should be overpowered and hag-ridden by what? by two or three feet of sorry tripe full of ... Were it by moral suffering that one sunk – by oppression, love or hatred or the

19 The 'strength of a team of horses' reference is from the 4 April 1819 letter to Robert Southey quoted in note 17 and the second quotation from a letter to Archibald Constable of 30 September 1821; both letters are quoted, in reverse order, in Pearson, *Walter Scott*, p. 141.

20 Letter to C. G. von Brinkman of 17 February 1822, pp. 220–221 in the second volume of Tegnér's letters mentioned in note 14.

21 The first quotation is from a letter of Tegnér's to M. Lagerlöf, of 22 December 1833, in Vol. VII of his correspondence, mentioned above in note 18, p. 128; the second is from a letter to L. Lemchen written on [2]7 January 1826, in *Esaias Tegnérs brev IV: 1826–1827*, ed. by Nils Palmborg (Malmö: Allhems förlag, 1955), p. 29.

thousand ways of heartbreak – it might be tolerable, there might at least be some dignity in the fall; but here!'[22]

One of Tegnér's most personal poems, 'Spleen', bears witness to his desperation. It was written at a time when he was tormented by frequently occurring attacks of pain and fever, caused by stones in his inflamed bile ducts:

> I stood at the summit of my life
> Where the waters are divided, flowing
> In frothy waves in different directions ...
>
> I looked upon the earth, she was green and lovely,
> And God was good, and mankind was honest.
>
> Then a splenetic imp arose, and suddenly
> The black creature sank his teeth into my heart:
> And lo, at once all things were waste and empty,
> And sun and stars went dark in haste. ...
>
> A smell of rotting corpses floats through life,
> Poisoning the air of spring and summer's glory. ...
>
> Tell me now, watchman, how far night has passed!
> And will there ever be an end to it? ...
>
> My pulse beats fast, just as it did when I was young,
> But does not have the time to count the hours of agony.
> How long, how endless is the pain of every heartbeat!
> O my consumed heart, bled to death!
>
> My heart? There is no heart within my breast,
> Merely an urn that holds the ashes of life.

Scott and Tegnér also had very dissimilar opinions regarding the medical care they received. The former expressed a high opinion of physicians and their activity from his early life onwards. In his tale 'The Surgeon's Daughter', Scott made use of his own observations when describing the toils and travails of a Scottish country doctor. In spite of his troubles, the physician is devoted to his profession and has no wish to exchange it for a comfortable position in the town. Scott came to realise – and he did not change his mind after he was treated for his illness – that love for fellow human beings is the chief virtue of a doctor.[23]

---

22 Letter of 10 February 1821 to John A. Carlyle, quoted from *The Collected Letters of Thomas and Jane Welsh Carlyle*, Duke–Edinburgh edn, Vol. 1: 1812–1821, ed. by Charles Richard Sanders (general editor) and Kenneth J. Fielding (associate editor) (Durham, NC: Duke University Press, 1970), p. 325.

23 Marie DuMont Low, 'Self in Triplicate: The Doctor in the Nineteenth-Century British Novel', diss. University of Washington, 1973. Available at ProQuest, https://www.proquest.com/openview/80468254c22b7adb5d337ae17ae2a21b/1?pq-origsite=gscholar&cbl=18750&diss=y.

Conversely, Tegnér was suspicious and sarcastic. One of his friends had fallen ill but was dissatisfied with his physician, who had previously sent him some verses, adding that he was better at writing prescriptions than poetry. The friend had not had any difficulty believing this; but now, he said, he was afraid the doctor might have been unfair to his poems – a well-grounded suspicion, in Tegnér's view.[24] Friends of Oliver Goldsmith had expressed similar doubts when Goldsmith averred that he would no longer write prescriptions for his friends, suggesting that it would indeed be best if he saved his prescriptions for his enemies.[25]

***

A century later, a great French painter was racked by the same kind of torment. As Matisse stubbornly refused to undergo an operation for his gallstones, he came to suffer as much and as long as his brothers in misfortune.[26] It was, in fact, the fourth serious illness that had a profound impact on this master's life and work – first the appendicitis in his youth which was the reason why he became an artist in the first place; then the bronchitis which brought about a change in his style of painting (see pp. 24–25); after that the cancer of the colon in his seventies; and soon afterwards his gallstones.

For more than a year, Matisse endured frequent attacks of severe pain, fever, and jaundice. He was, however, more stoical than even Walter Scott. His proud nature did not permit him to complain; only the people closest to him knew about his agonies: 'As for me, I am still here in bed except for one hour a day when I get up. I don't enjoy that much, for I've lost the habit – I'm always glad to be back in bed, I work there regularly. Painting in the afternoon'. In this manner, his strict self-discipline enabled him to continue to create serene masterpieces, 'the calm and powerful expression of pain overcome'.[27] Only in the illustrations for Montherlant's *Pasiphae*[28] does he afford us a glimpse of his suffering. In 'L'angoisse qui s'amasse en frappant sous ta gorge' ('The gathering anguish that strikes in your throat'), the agony of pain itself wields the etching-needle with fine-spun subtlety.

Matisse's case history is an excellent example of the dangers of consulting several doctors, each of them with his or her own opinion. 'Dear Louis Aragon – I shan't go to Switzerland this summer: I am too much taken up

24 Letter of Tegnér's to Martina von Schwerin of 2 April 1826, in the fourth volume of Tegnér's correspondence mentioned above in note 21, p. 55.

25 From James Prior's *Life of Oliver Goldsmith* of 1837, reprinted in E. H. Mikhail (ed.), *Goldsmith: Interviews and Recollections* (New York: St Martin's, 1993), p. 38.

26 Louis Aragon, *Henri Matisse: Roman*, Vol. I (Paris: Gallimard, 1971), p. 183. (For an English translation, see the following note.)

27 Louis Aragon, *Henri Matisse: A Novel*, trans. Jean Stewart, Vol. I (New York: Harcourt Brace Jovanovich, 1972), pp. 183 and 184.

28 A book containing 51 linoleum cuts, published in Paris 1944 by Fabiani.

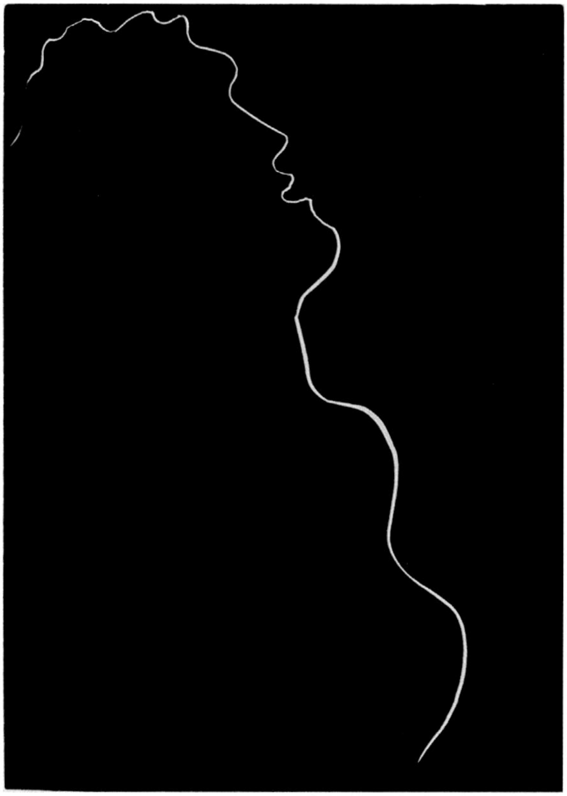

Figure 76 Henri Matisse, 'L'angoisse qui s'amasse en frappant sous ta gorge', 1943–44. The agony of pain, subtly simplified. From Henry de Montherlant's *Pasiphae: Chant de Minos (Les Crétois).*

with illness and doctors; I have two teams of them. (1) One wants me to be operated on. (2) The other doesn't – the one that doesn't is presided over by a *surgeon* – my own surgeon from Lyons, who knows what risks I ran and is not anxious to expose me to the same risks again.'[29]

One evening the medical consultations turned into a loud quarrel, and through the closed door even the patient himself was able to hear the furious Professor Wertheimer shouting that the patient's heart would not be able to stand an operation. No wonder Matisse declared that he had some right to his own skin, and that since he lacked character, he preferred having an occasional attack of pain to being operated on, feeling certain that he would not survive it. In the letter containing that declaration, Matisse expressed his envy of Ronsard, who had not had to worry about doctors, recalling – adding a polite 'forgive me' – a song from a play in which it was argued that all doctors were murderers.[30]

Matisse could also have quoted the lines written by Shakespeare's contemporary Ben Jonson who had also, three centuries earlier, been ill and

29 Pages 175–176 in the English translation of Aragon's book mentioned in note 27.
30 Ibid., p. 176.

dissatisfied with the medical treatment he received. He vented his anger in the poem 'To Dr Empirick':

> When men a dangerous disease did 'scape
> Of old, they gave a cock to Aesculape.
> Let me give two, that doubly am got free:
> From my disease's danger, and from thee.

Chapter 10
Digression: Artists' views on medicine and physicians

It may seem perverse for a doctor to discuss the views held by the great creators of art on the subject of medicine, since they have usually been extremely critical. But I have good reason to share their opinions, having been the victim of a medical error at the age of 13: my abdominal discomfort was wrongly interpreted as having been caused by a gastric ulcer because the doctor had found a tender spot at the pit of my stomach, and I underwent months of treatment with bed rest and a severe diet consisting of egg gruel four times a day.

Many years later, making rounds as a young resident, I suddenly found myself having a profuse haemoptysis ('blood cough'). An X-ray revealed an old, now healed pulmonary tuberculosis, the source of my childhood complaint. My sister and I recalled that we had had a nursemaid who died of consumption, and it appeared likely that we had caught the disease from her. The treatment to which I had been subjected may have contributed to curing my lung, but it certainly left me with an allergy to eggs and a lifelong scepticism towards doctors.

***

The irony of Matisse and the sarcasms of Ben Jonson are echoes of innumerable expressions of dissatisfaction with physicians through the centuries. There were ample reasons for that, at least in the rather more distant past. The healthcare available to Scott and Tegnér reminds us that they lived during a period in which the ideas of the Enlightenment, whose lines of thought were grounded in the natural sciences, had not yet assumed ascendancy in medicine, which was consequently still dominated by many medieval delusions. The idea was that illness was caused by tainted and impure matter in the blood and that that matter had to be removed. That notion was behind the widespread use of bleeding, leeches, emetics, and enemas. In the course of a single year, King Louis XIII was treated with 47 bleedings, 212 doses of purgatives, and 215 enemas. The King had to pay dearly for this special attention – he died young.

Lord Byron's life was also cut short by excessive blood-letting, despite his angry attempts to defend himself. When his doctor insisted, he was indignant, voicing his belief that more people had died from doctors'

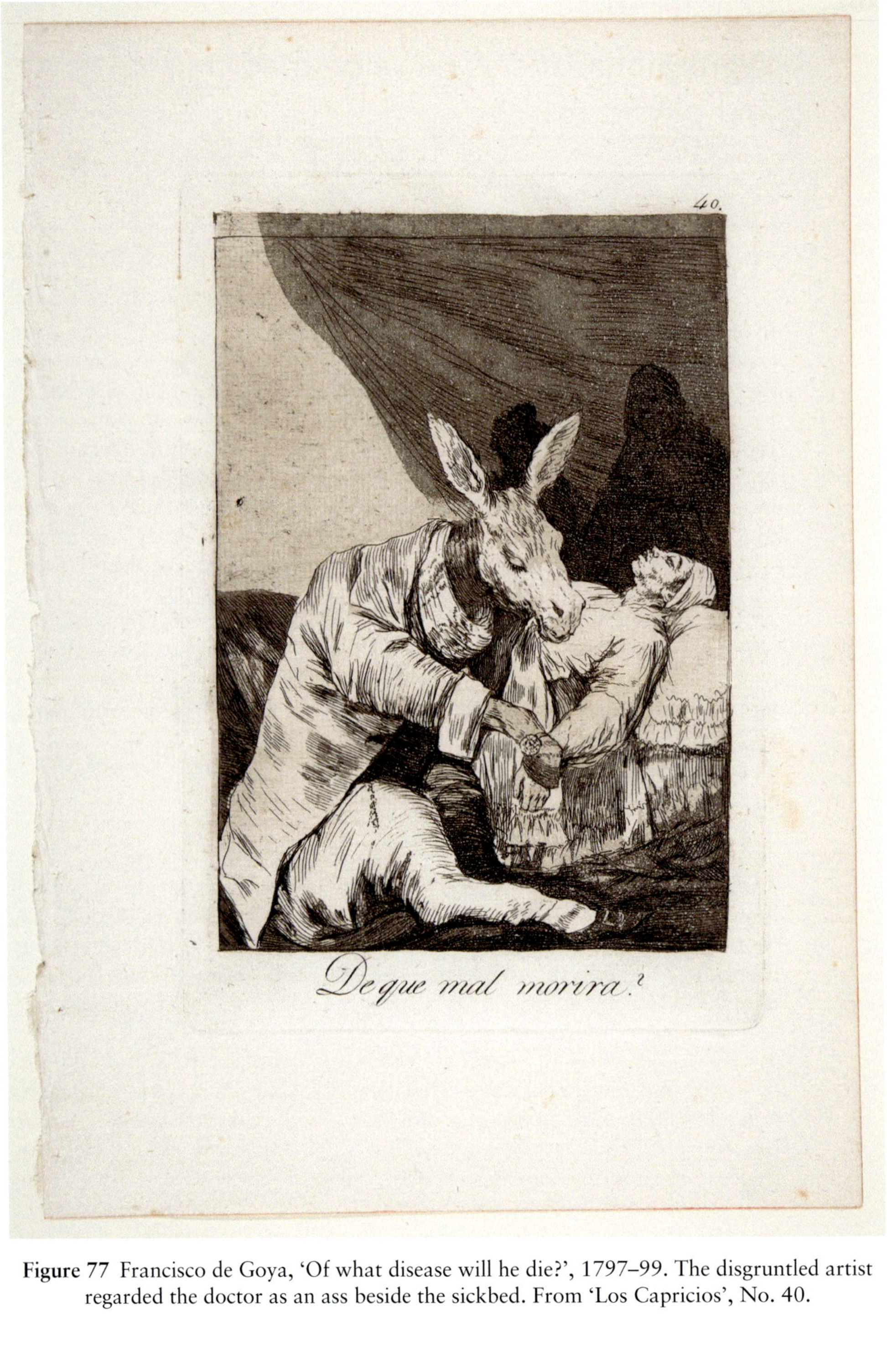

Figure 77 Francisco de Goya, 'Of what disease will he die?', 1797–99. The disgruntled artist regarded the doctor as an ass beside the sickbed. From 'Los Capricios', No. 40.

lancets than from soldiers' lances.[1] Other bodily fluids needed to be safeguarded as well: 'As I have just escaped from a physician and a fever which confined me five days to bed, you won't expect much "allegrezza" in the ensuing letter ... What can a helpless, feverish, toasted and watered poor wretch do? In spite of my teeth & tongue, the English Consul forced a physician upon me, who in three days vomited and clystered me to the last gasp.'[2]

* * *

In the course of the centuries, enlightened and erudite personages have expressed doubts as to the abilities of physicians, jokingly, sarcastically, or bitterly, depending on the degree of their disappointment. Voltaire regarded wars, priests, and doctors as the worst scourges of humanity.[3] Montaigne and Molière were implacable critics, too.[4] Suffering from protracted illnesses, both men prized good health. The former expressed his appreciation of it as follows: 'Health is precious. ... Without health all pleasure, scholarship and virtue lose their lustre and fade away'.[5]

Montaigne was a stoic: 'We must quietly suffer the laws of Man's condition. Despite all medicine, we are made for growing old, growing weaker and falling ill.'[6] The sage and sensible essayist had greater confidence in the healing powers of Nature than in the medicines prescribed by physicians. Despising doctors, he questioned not only their competence but also their honour: 'Did you ever find a doctor taking over a colleague's prescription without putting in something extra or cutting something out? That gives their Art away and reveals that they are more concerned with their own reputation (and therefore with their fee) than with the well-being of their patients.'[7] He went as far as suspecting that some doctors do not hesitate to impair the condition of their patients in order to earn more money, summarising his attitude in the following terms: 'Contrary to other people, I always despise that Art [medicine] when I am well but never make a truce with it when I am ill: I then begin to hate it and to fear it. I tell those who urge me to take medicine at least to wait until I am well and have got my strength

1 Harold Nicolson, *Byron: The Last Journey, April 1823–April 1824* (London: Constable, 1924), p. 252.
2 Letter to Francis Hodgson of 3 October 1810, in *Byron's Letters and Journals*, ed. by Leslie Marchand, Vol. 2 (Cambridge, MA: Belknap, 1973), pp. 18–19.
3 No source for this statement was found.
4 Kurt Heller, 'Michel de Montaignes Einfluss auf die Aerztestücke Molières', diss. (Jena, 1908); and Georges Bordonove, *Molière génial et familier* (Paris: Robert Laffont, 1967). Unfortunately, page references could not be located.
5 From essay No. II:37, 'On the Resemblance of Children to Their Fathers'; Montaigne's *Essays*, trans. M. A. Screech (London: Penguin, 1987), p. 865.
6 From essay No. III:13, 'On Experience', p. 1236 in the edition mentioned in the preceding note.
7 From the essay mentioned in note 5 above; p. 871 in the Screech translation.

back in order to have the means of resisting the hazardous effects of their potions.'[8]

The mordant jest that it takes good health to be able to endure medical treatment was appropriated by Molière, one of the fiercest adversaries of medicine. In *Le Malade imaginaire*, he says about himself that he was too feeble to stand the medicinal remedies; it was all he could do to bear the illness itself. When Molière speaks about doctors, there is no trace of his habitual joviality, only the bitterest mockery: 'Why does he need four doctors – is not one enough to kill a patient?'[9]

Molière's hatred was well founded: 'Vain and foolish doctors you / Have no balm can cure my ills, / Not your Latin nor your skills / Can ease my heart's pain and grief: / Your art commands no belief.'[10] The suffering that was making him desperate, the disease he tried to bear, was tuberculosis. His doctors insisted on a therapy that only made him weaker, and ultimately he succumbed. Coughing and shortness of breath made stage performances increasingly difficult. A born comedian, he exploited his symptoms in his acting, passing them off as intentional comic turns and making the effect as irresistible as the coughing attack.

Towards the end of the fourth performance of *Le Malade imaginaire*, in which Molière himself played the part of Argan, he was attacked by a violent bloody cough. The sudden drop of the curtain ended not only the play but the stage life of an actor who could no longer make believe. Anyone familiar with that story will always discern the faint sound of a sob behind the boisterous laughter after this comedy.[11]

Antoine Watteau also died young from tuberculosis. In his painting, the artist shared the low opinion of the medical profession that Montaigne and Molière expressed in words; their physicians are vividly presented in one of his pictures. He also depicts himself, already at the cemetery, wrapped in his dressing-gown, trying to escape from his tormentors at the Faculty of Medicine who pursue him with their enema syringes. The threat of death is hanging over him, barely concealed by his customary enchanting imagination. Only in the inscription does the cry of distress, pain, and agony break from his lips without restraint: 'What have I done, confounded assassins, to so incur your wrath?' In order to fully appreciate the scenes described by Molière and represented by Watteau, we might listen to an accompaniment by Rossini where the composer makes fun of Dr Bartolo, the basso-buffoon in *The Barber of Seville*.

8 From essay No. I:24, 'Same Designs: Differing Outcomes', p. 143 in the Screech translation.

9 Act II, Scene 1 in *L'Amour médecin* (*Love's the Best Doctor*).

10 From the second Prologue to *The Hypochondriac* (*Le Malade imaginaire*), p. 228 in Molière, *The Hypochondriac*, in *The Miser and Other Plays*, trans. by John Wood and David Coward (London: Penguin, 2000).

11 Jacques Arnavon, *Le Malade imaginaire de Molière* (Geneva: Slatkin Reprints, 1970), p. 16.

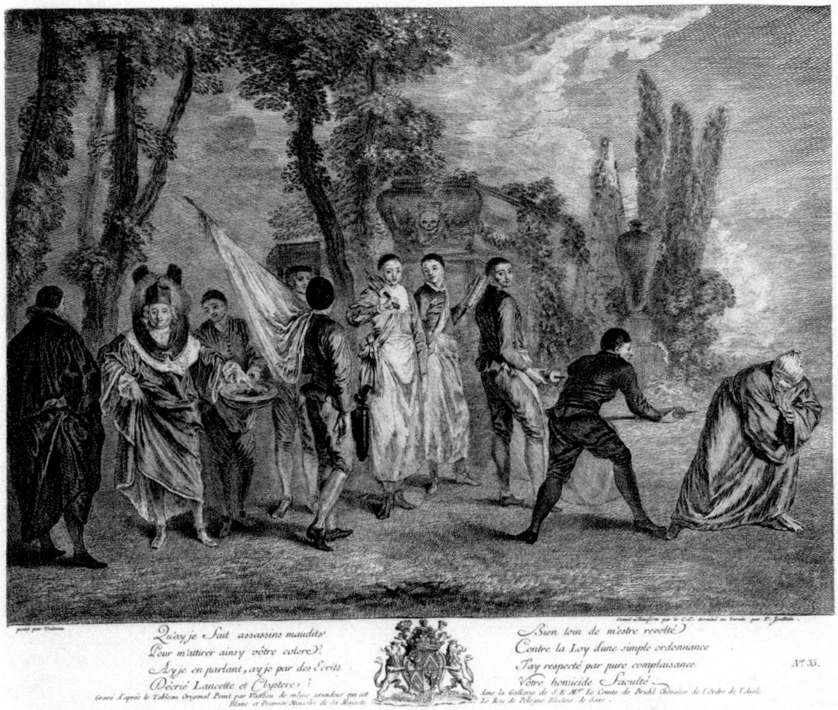
Qu'ay je fait assassins maudits
Pour m'attirer ainsy vôtre colere?
Ay je en parlant, ay je par des Ecrits
Décrié Lancette et Clystere?
Bien loin de m'estre revolté
Contre la Loy d'une simple ordonnance
J'ay respecté par pure complaisance
Votre homicide Faculté.
N°. 35.

Figure 78 Antoine Watteau, 'Satire on physicians', c. 1708. 'The confounded assassins', the members of the Faculty of Medicine, examine the blood of the artist after having bled him and attack him with their enema syringes.

Poor Frédéric Chopin, who suffered from a protracted pulmonary disease, resorted to grim humour, pouring ridicule on his doctors whose main interest appeared to be in his sputum: 'One sniffed at what I spat, another tapped at the place whence I spat it, the third poked and listened while I spat. The first said I would die. The second, that I was dying, and the third said I was dead already!'[12]

* * *

Across the chorus of dissatisfied and irate voices from disillusioned patients, some notes of cheerful gratitude may be heard, as we shall see, from two seventeenth-century gentlemen who had had their bladder-stones removed.

12 John O'Shea, *Music and Medicine: Medical Profiles of Great Composers* (London: Dent, 1990), p. 145.

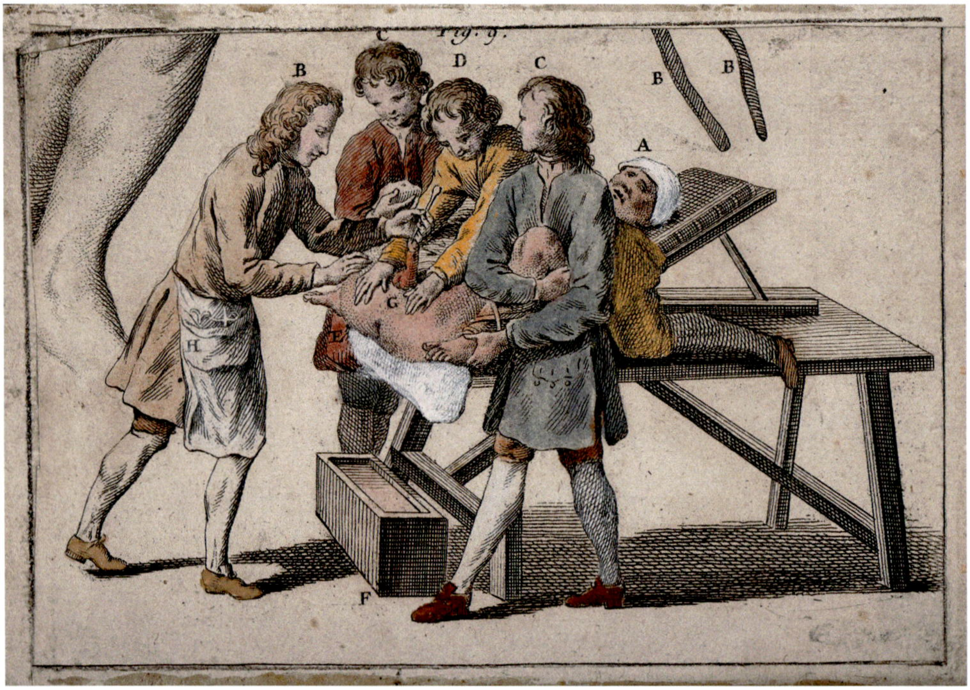

Figure 79 James Mynde, c. 1747. An illustration of an eighteenth-century operation to remove a bladder-stone.

The formation of stones in the bladder was a common and extremely painful disorder at this time. It could be surgically remedied by barber-surgeons, who travelled from one fair to another and conducted their operations in public. The procedure was so dramatic that tickets were sold to people who wished to witness the horrific spectacle. Two strong servants would hold the victim's legs while a third sat astride across his chest, holding up the scrotum. The 'surgeon' introduced a metallic catheter through the urinary duct into the bladder and then made a rapid incision through the perineum. When the bladder had been opened, the stone was extracted with forceps. The mortality rate of the procedure was 60 per cent.

The famous diarist Samuel Pepys evinced rapturous delight on having been liberated from a bladder-stone the size of an apple in the 1660s. He had an abundantly sculptured casket made in order to house it in a worthy manner, subsequently celebrating each anniversary of the operation with an opulent dinner for a number of brothers in misfortune. In the course of the meal, the guests would circulate their magnificent trophies, bladder-stones of varying proportions, around the table for general admiration: 'And were very merry all the afternoon, talking and singing and piping on the Flagelette.'[13]

13 *The Diary of Samuel Pepys: Vol. III: 1662*, ed. by Robert Latham and William Matthews (London: G. Bell and Sons, 1970), p. 53 (Wednesday 26 March 1662).

It would seem that the composer Marin Marais, having put his last will and testament on paper, underwent the same operation. In any case, he created a wonderful suite for viola called 'Description of a cystotomy', one of the earliest examples of instrumental programme music. He still sounds agitated when describing the agonising and perilous procedure step by step, in rapid sequences of notes: '(A) The appearance of the surgical apparatus (B) Shuddering while seeing it (C) Resolving to climb into it (D) Reaching for the top (E) Descending into said apparatus (F) Serious thought; (G) Tying the silks around the arms and legs (H) Here the incision is made (I) Then the forceps are introduced; (J) Then the stone is withdrawn (K) Then there is screaming until the voice is lost (L) Blood gushes (M) Then the silks are untied (N) Then you are transported in the bed (O) Recovery (P) Happy.'[14] No wonder the composer, after such an adventure, felt the need to compose no fewer than three merry dances in order to lend full expression to his relief.

***

On the whole, however, the medical profession was still held in low esteem; but, in some cases, profound dissatisfaction might be replaced by gratitude when medical treatment did eventually restore a person's health. That was the case with two artists: Claude Monet, when his doctor had improved his eyesight, and Francisco de Goya, who had good reason to doubt his physicians from the start, depicting them as donkeys sitting by the sickbed.

Gradually, medicine evolved into a science, and Goya had reason to change his mind. Aged about 70, he was close to death with a serious illness but recovered thanks to skilful medical care. As sarcastic as he used to be towards the medical profession, as grateful he now became to his physician, to whom he dedicated a portrait. It represents the artist, gravely ill, plucking at the bedcovers in order to make breathing easier, as he had seen other patients do.

In the nineteenth century, 'water cures' dispensed at special spa resorts formed a popular treatment for all sorts of diseases. The essential attraction at these watering-places was the social life they offered; the cure itself was a boring routine. That becomes easy to understand in the company of the credulous Alfred Tennyson: 'Of all the uncomfortable ways of living, sure an hydropathical is the worst: no reading by candlelight, no going near a fire,

14 See Jubin E. Matloubieh, Manizheh Eghbali, and Ronald Rabinowitz, 'Blood Gushing and Musical Screaming in Marin Marais' Cystolithotomy', *Urology* 141 (July 2020), 60–63 (p. 62). There is a detailed account in French of the operation and Marais's works in Jean-Charles Léon, '*Le Tableau de l'Opération de la Taille* de Marin Marais', *Épistèmocritique*, 13 May 2016, available at https://epistemocritique.org/le-tableau-de-loperation-de-la-taille-de-marin-marais. Sandblom's own source may have been Georges Raymond, 'La Lithotomie musicale ou le théatre d'opération de la taille', *Histoire des Sciences Médicales* 22.2 (1988), 141–150 (p. 148).

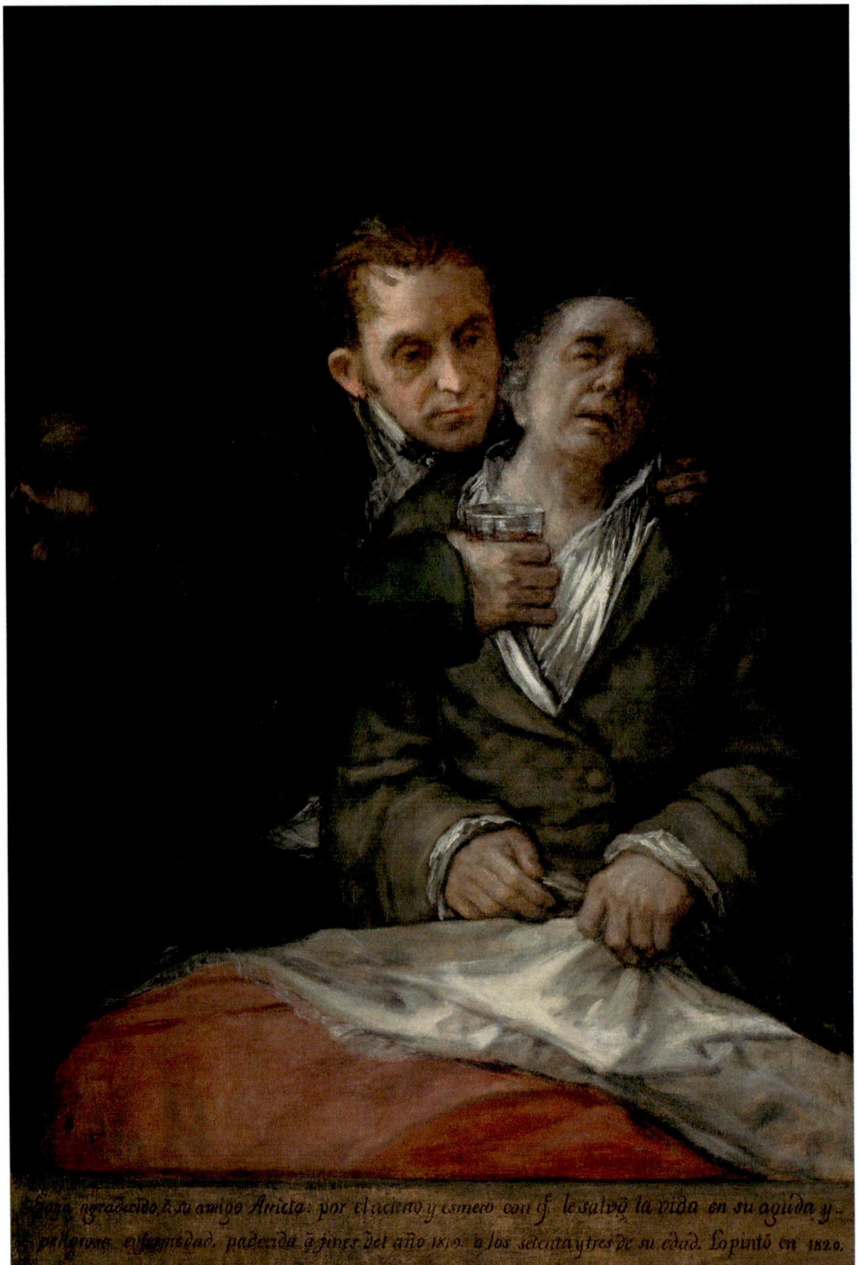

Figure 80 Francisco de Goya, 'Self-portrait with Dr Arrieta', 1820. Goya's painting expresses gratitude towards Dr Arrieta, whose skilful treatment saved him from a serious illness by which he was afflicted at the age of 73.

no tea, no coffee, perpetual wet sheets & cold bath & alternation from hot to cold: however I have much faith in it.'[15]

A later, but no less rancorous, doctor-hater was George Bernard Shaw. The origin of his hostility was that he was afflicted by caries in one leg. This is usually a very protracted illness, especially when, as was the case with Shaw, fragments of dead bone are formed and gradually expelled by the body. On many occasions, physicians have to resort to amputation. Shaw's patience was limited and he became utterly disgusted with his doctor, or, rather, furious with him: 'The tragedy of illness at present is that it delivers you helplessly into the hands of a profession which you deeply mistrust.'[16]

In *The Doctor's Dilemma*, and in the preface to the play, he vented his scorn and anger. What particularly upset him was the circumstance that doctors have a pecuniary interest in the patient's illness: 'I cannot knock my shins severely without forcing on some surgeon the difficult question, "Could I not make a better use of a pocketful of guineas than this man is making of his leg? Could he not write as well – or even better – on one leg than on two? ... artificial legs are now so well made that they are really better than natural ones."'[17]

It is hard to say whether Shaw would have written better had he been deprived of one of his legs, but he would certainly have become desperate. The fury that was once kindled in Montaigne and Molière boils up again in his statement, '[i]t is simply unscientific to allege or believe that doctors do not under existing circumstances perform unnecessary operations and manufacture and prolong lucrative illnesses'.[18] Shaw's acrid criticism of the 'existing circumstances', which meant that doctors benefited financially from their patients' illnesses, led to the first steps towards socialised medicine in Great Britain.

That was far from being the last time such sarcastic statements were uttered – disappointment with the medical treatment of incurable diseases is still around, and sadly not without reason. Marcel Proust's experience was that people recover from natural illnesses, but that this never happens with a disorder caused by medical science, as that science does not know the secret of the art of healing.[19] The prescription of potent drugs can be like trying to exorcise the Devil with Beelzebub. Dying, Flannery O'Connor

15 Alfred Lord Tennyson, letter to Edward FitzGerald of 2 February 1844, quoted in Robert Bernard Martin, *Tennyson: The Unquiet Heart* (Oxford: Clarendon Press, 1980), p. 280.

16 George Bernard Shaw, 'Preface on Doctors', in *The Doctor's Dilemma: A Tragedy*, ed. by Dan H. Laurence (London: Penguin, 1987), p. 10.

17 Ibid., p. 9.

18 Ibid., p. 11.

19 Marcel Proust, *The Captive*, trans. by C. K. Scott Moncrieff (New York: The Modern Library, 1956 [1929]), p. 243.

was forced to realise that 'the medicine and the disease run neck & neck to kill you'.[20]

***

Since mental illness affects and interferes with the essence of creativity in particular ways, it is not surprising that authors suffering from such illness have an especially sharp eye for the failings of their doctors. Virginia Woolf was full of contempt for psychiatry. In *Mrs Dalloway*, she poured her scorn on an ordinary family doctor as well as on a shrewd specialist.

The general practitioner 'brushed it all aside – headaches, sleeplessness, fears, dreams – nerve symptoms and nothing more ... Take up some hobby ... did he not owe his own excellent health ... to the fact that he could always switch off from his patients on to old furniture?' She described the tragic situation of being grossly misunderstood in which a person with a mental illness not infrequently finds himself or herself: '"So you're in a funk", he said agreeably, sitting down by his patient's side ... "Wouldn't it be better to do something instead of lying in bed?"'[21]

The specialist saw at once that the case was an extremely serious one: '[W]hen a man comes into your room and says he is Christ (a common delusion), ... and threatens, as they often do, to kill himself ... you order rest in bed ... rest without friends, without books, without messages, six months' rest.' In addition, the specialist took pleasure in his professional success: 'Not only did his colleagues respect him, his subordinates fear him, but the friends and relations of his patients felt for him the keenest gratitude for insisting that these prophetic Christs ... should drink milk in bed.'[22]

Rejoicing at his recovered health after a near-fatal depression, William Styron could reflect with amusement on some now very popular therapeutic methods. They may have helped him in an unintended manner, by making him laugh heartily, and us with him: 'The best I can say for Group Therapy is that it was a way to occupy the hours. More or less the same can be said for Art Therapy, which is organized infantilism. Our class was run by a delirious young woman with a fixed, indefatigable smile, who was plainly trained at a school offering courses in Teaching Art to the Mentally Ill.'[23] In Styron's view, not even a teacher of small retarded children could have been made to utter such affected chuckling and cooing noises without direct instruction.

20 Letter to Maryat Lee of 1 July 1964, in Flannery O'Connor, *The Habit of Being*, ed. by Sally Fitzgerald (New York: Farrar, Straus, & Giroux, 1979), p. 590.

21 Virginia Woolf, *Mrs Dalloway*, pp. 119–120 in Claire Tomalin's World's Classics edition of the novel (Oxford: Oxford University Press, 1998 [1992]).

22 The two quoted passages are found on pp. 129 and 130 in Tomalin's edition of Woolf's novel.

23 William Styron, *Darkness Visible: A Memoir of Madness* (New York: Vintage Books, 1992), p. 74 (originally published by Random House in 1990).

Styron describes how the art teacher would 'tell us to take our crayons and make drawings illustrative of themes that we ourselves had chosen. For example: My House. In humiliated rage I obeyed, drawing a square, with a door and four cross-eyed windows, a chimney on top issuing forth a curlicue of smoke. She showered me with praise, and as the weeks advanced and my health improved so did my sense of comedy. I began to dabble happily in colored modeling clay, sculpting at first a horrid little green skull with bared teeth, which our teacher pronounced a splendid replica of my depression. I then proceeded through intermediate stages of recuperation to a rosy and cherubic head with a "Have-A-Nice-Day" smile. Coinciding as it did with the time of my release, this creation truly overjoyed my instructress (whom I'd become fond of in spite of myself), since, as she told me, it was emblematic of my recovery and therefore but one more example of the triumph over disease by Art Therapy.'[24]

* * *

Having observed with equanimity how my professional brethren in past ages were blamed and ridiculed for their efforts, I was indignant when, as an appropriate conclusion to this digression, I found myself being laughed to scorn. I was thoroughly disgruntled when I came upon some sarcastic remarks on 'what happens when doctors start dabbling in the arts', how they impose all sorts of bold diagnoses on the creative geniuses of the past, whereupon they make laboured attempts to find symptoms of the presumed disorders in the works of these great creators.[25] An art historian who resented amateurs encroaching on his academic field compares the intruder to Polonius, taunted by Hamlet for seeing changing shapes in the clouds: a camel, a whale, or a weasel. A mere three species! I must have released a whole zoo in the sky.

24 Ibid., pp. 74–75.

25 Judith Shulevitz, 'Second Opinions', *The Art News* 2 (1991). Unfortunately, it was not possible to provide a page reference.

Chapter 11
Tuberculosis

In the history of creative work there are many who, like Molière and Watteau, had their efforts influenced and their lives shortened by tuberculosis. It is quite obvious that this disease has frequently exercised a peculiar influence on the creative imagination of artists. The slight temperature enlivens thoughts and infuses the sufferer's fancy with dreamlike images. A heightened appetite for life which cannot be satisfied in real life because of the weariness engendered by the disease is instead fulfilled in the life of the imagination.

The consumptive poet Sidney Lanier from the American South, whose last poem was written in a cheerful mood despite the shortness of breath caused by his reduced pulmonary capacity, supplied an enchanting account of his feverish dreams: 'Were it not for some circumstances wh. make such a proposition seem absurd in the highest degree, – I wd. think today that I am shortly to die, and that my Spirit hath been singing its swan-song before dissolution. All day, my Soul hath been cutting swiftly into the great space of the Subtle Unspeakable Deep, driven by wind after wind of heavenly melody. The very inner spirit and essence of all wind-songs, bird-songs, passion-songs, folk-songs, country-songs, sex-songs, soul-songs and body-songs, hath blown upon me in quick gusts like the breaths of Passion, and sailed me into a sea of vast dreams whereof each wave is at once a vision and a melody.'[1]

***

John Keats had had medical training and was hence fully aware of the fate awaiting him after having nursed his brother, who died young of tuberculosis.[2] In a letter to his fiancée he described the ominous turning-point in his own illness, a sudden haemorrhage of the lungs, as follows:

---

1 Letter to Mary Day Lanier of 24 February 1873, in *Sidney Lanier: Letters 1869–1873*, ed. by Charles R. Anderson and Aubrey H. Starke, The Centennial Edition of the Works of Sidney Lanier, 10 vols (Baltimore: Johns Hopkins Press, 1945), Vol. VIII, p. 332.

2 See Lionel Trilling's Introduction to *The Selected Letters of John Keats*, ed. by Lionel Trilling (New York: Farrar, Straus & Young, 1951), p. 13; see also p. 131.

'On the night I was taken ill – when so violent a rush of blood came to my Lungs that I felt nearly suffocated – I assure you I felt it possible I might not survive, and at that moment [thought] of nothing but you.'

Watching the progress of his illness and the appearance of his expectorations with the trained eye of the medical man, he commented, 'I know the colour of that blood, it is arterial blood; I cannot be deceived in that colour, that drop is my death warrant. I must die.' Nevertheless, he tried to reassure Fanny, his 'dearest girl', by using a moderate language; 'this is unfortunate'. He even attempted to fool himself with the aid of the euphoria that is characteristic of the disease: ''Tis true that since the first two or three days other subjects have entered my head. I shall be looking forward to Health and the Spring and a regular routine of our old Walks.'[3]

During the last year of his life, consumed by a hopeless passion and wasting away, he mused upon the connection between creativity and illness: 'How astonishingly does the chance of leaving the world impress a sense of its natural beauties on us.'[4]

'Ode to a Nightingale', that hymn of praise to the ecstasy and eternal joy of life, is imbued with a paradoxical yearning for death, for following the nightingale

> ... into the forest dim:
> Fade far away, dissolve, and quite forget
> What thou among the leaves hast never known,
> The weariness, the fever, and the fret
> Here, where men sit and hear each other groan;
> Where palsy shakes a few, sad, last grey hairs,
> Where youth grows pale, and spectre-thin, and dies,
> Where but to think is to be full of sorrow
> And leaden-eyed despairs,
> Where Beauty cannot keep her lustrous eyes,
> Or new Love pine at them beyond to-morrow.
> ...
> Already with thee: Tender is the night,
> And haply the Queen-Moon is upon her throne ...
> ...
> Thou wast not born for death, immortal Bird!

... since the nightingale's song remains the same throughout the centuries:

> Perhaps the self-same song that found a path
> Through the sad heart of Ruth, when, sick for home,
> She stood in tears amid the alien corn[.]

3 Ibid., pp. 250–251. The words on the colour of the blood were apparently directed to Keats's friend Lord Houghton; see the note on p. 250.

4 Letter to James Rice of 14 and 16 February 1820, in John Keats, *Letters of John Keats*, ed. by Stanley Gardner (London: University of London Press, 1965), p. 203.

Humankind was born to die, since our songs are our own and our personalities expire with us.

* * *

In the course of the nineteenth century, tuberculosis continued to reap a terrible harvest among the young, and many promising artistic careers were cruelly cut short. The Keats brothers were followed by the Brontë sisters.

A predisposition for illness and periods of melancholy, as well as poverty and an isolated life among the dreary moors, form the gloomy background of their melodramatic tales which reflect the contemporary sentimental taste so well. After the two eldest girls had died of consumption in their early years, it fell to the third, Charlotte, to help raise and soon enough also nurse the two youngest sisters. They were extremely different. Emily, who had been able to finish *Wuthering Heights*, a solitaire of strange and singular lustre, before succumbing to the disease was reticent and headstrong, a solitary wanderer on the moors, and in her own words

In life and death, a chainless soul,
    With courage to endure.[5]

Conversely, the youngest sister, Anne, who wrote ethereal verse such as the hymn to resignation quoted on p. 19, was gentle and submissive.

This difference between the sisters can also be seen in their respective attitudes to their illness. Proud Emily sought solitude like an injured animal, declining compassion as well as nursing, whereas Anne gratefully accepted both. Tears rise to the reader's eyes at the simple words in which Charlotte revealed the full measure of her tragic fate as tender bonds were severed: 'One by one I have watched them fall asleep on my arm – and closed their glazed eyes.'[6]

Watching her sisters die, Charlotte became thoroughly acquainted with the symptoms of progressing pulmonary tuberculosis. Her description in the chapter called 'The Valley of the Shadow of Death' in the novel *Shirley* (1849) is more expert and eloquent than any doctor's. There is the ominous loss of appetite – 'palatable food was as ashes and sawdust to her' – and a tormenting thirst, '[y]ou wish to drink? Your lips are parched.' The sick girl 'wasted like any snow-wreath in thaw; she faded like any flower in drought'.[7] Charlotte makes fun of the helpless doctors: 'One came, but that one was an oracle: he delivered a dark saying of which the future was to solve the mystery, wrote some prescriptions, gave some directions – the whole with an air

5 The last stanza of the poem called 'The Old Stoic', p. 31 in Janet Gezari's Penguin Classics edition of Emily Jane Brontë, *The Complete Poems* (London: Penguin, 1992).

6 Letter to W. S. Williams of 13 June 1849; p. 220 in Margaret Smith's edition of *The Letters of Charlotte Brontë*, Vol. 2, 1848–1851 (Oxford: Clarendon Press, 2000).

7 Charlotte Brontë, *Shirley* (Oxford: Oxford World's Classics, 2007 edition with an Introduction by Janet Gezari), pp. 351 and 352. Subsequent page references supplied in parentheses in the text.

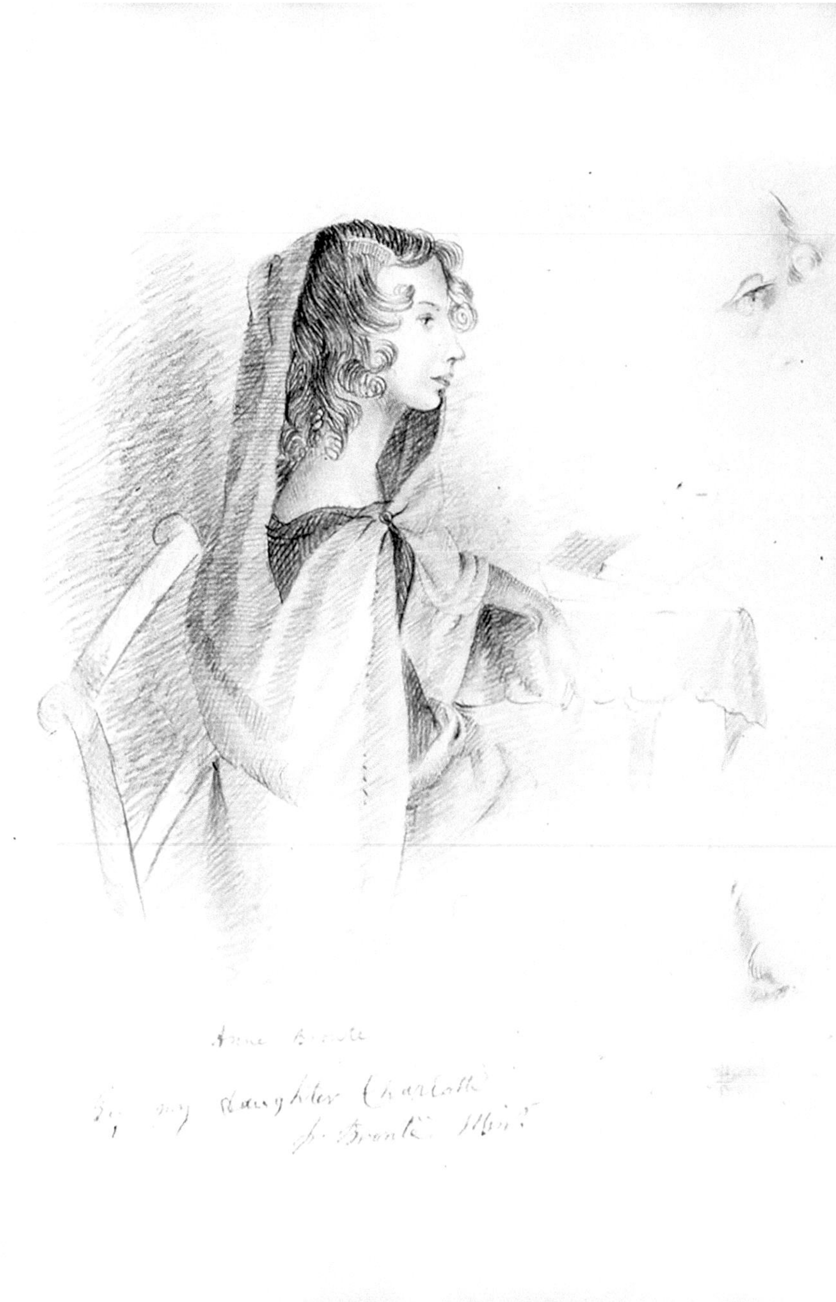

Figure 81 Charlotte Brontë, 'Anne Brontë', 1833. The author has drawn a delicate portrait of her gentle and submissive consumptive sister Anne.

of crushing authority – pocketed his fee, and went. Probably, he knew well enough he could do no good; but didn't like to say so' (pp. 353–354). But Charlotte knew how easily an undermined edifice may suddenly collapse.

The exhausted patient is torn between weariness of life and fear of death: 'she usually buried her face deep in the pillow, and drew the coverlets close round her, as if to shut out the world and sun, of which she was tired: more than once, as she thus lay, a slight convulsion shook the sick-bed, and a faint sob broke the silence round it' (p. 354). '"God grant me a little comfort before I die!" was her humble petition' ... 'Sustain me through the ordeal I dread and must undergo!' (p. 356).

Feverish dreams and failing strength seem to presage the end: 'Oh! I have had a suffering night. This morning I am worse. I have tried to rise. I cannot. Dreams I am unused to have troubled me.' The desperately helpless nurse-mother prays humbly but insistently, 'with that soundless voice the soul utters when its appeal is to the Invisible': '"Spare my beloved ... Rend not from me what long affection entwines with my whole nature."'[8] Terrified, she recognises the symptoms that foretell the final annihilation: 'the watcher ... approaches the patient's pillow, and sees a new and strange moulding of the familiar features, feels at once that the insufferable moment draws nigh ... and subdues his soul to the sentence he cannot avert, and scarce can bear' (p. 369).

Towards the end of her hard life, Charlotte was at last allowed to experience a great but brief joy in a late marriage. But in keeping with her misfortunes, the very seal of her happiness, her pregnancy, proved fatal; the vomiting and the other strains that pregnancy entailed made her tuberculosis flare up and put an end to her life.

Robert Louis Stevenson, who was 'Ordered South' as a way of treating his tuberculosis, observed that the exhausting effect of advanced illness made it easier for him to accept his weakened condition: after some feverish efforts and the impatient anxiety of the first few days, he adapted, satisfied with the reduced activity that was the consequence of his feebleness. He has described the stages in the course of which the tubercular patient is 'tenderly weaned from the passion of life, thus gradually inducted into the slumber of death'.[9]

* * *

Two Nordic women poets who died young form examples of how this disease begins by generating an intense zest for life but subsequently brings increasing lassitude and apathy. In her early poetry, the Fenno-Swedish poet Edith Södergran expresses an ecstatic and defiant *joie de vivre*:

8 The author's original Swedish text refers to the nurse as a 'sister', but in fact the nurse whose care brings the sufferer back to life is her mother.

9 Robert Louis Stevenson, 'Ordered South' (March 1874), in *Virginibus Puerisque and Other Papers*, ed. by J. H. Fowler (London: Macmillan, 1925), pp. 77–91 (p. 87).

We should love life's long hours of illness
And narrow years of yearning
As we love the brief moments when the desert is in bloom.[10]

Södergran's late poetry is characterised by cool resignation and an exalted acceptance of the thought of dying:

I long for the land that never was,
For whatever is, I am tired of desiring.[11]

Harriet Löwenhjelm was touchingly lonely in her illness:

Am I tired unto death,
Rather tired,
Very tired,
Sick and tired and mournful.[12]

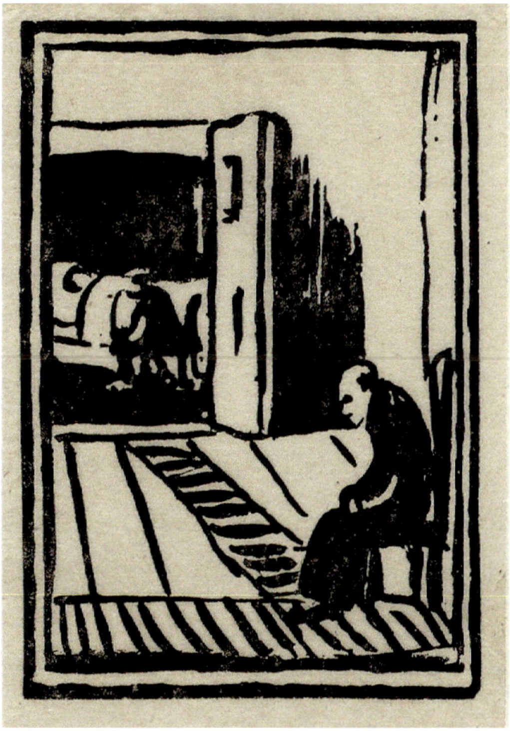

Figure 82 Harriet Löwenhjelm. Death waits for the artist who is ill in a sanatorium. From the 1919 edition of Löwenhjelm's poems, *Dikter*.

10 Edith Södergran, 'Ingenting', in *Landet som icke är* ['The Land That Never Was']: *(Efterlämnade dikter)* (Helsinki: Holger Schildts Förlag, 1925), p. 29.

11 Ibid., p. 71.

12 Harriet Löwenhjelm, *Harriet Löwenhjelms dikter* (Stockholm: P. A. Norstedt & Söner, 1927, 2nd edn), p. 104.

In her despondency, she yearns for tenderness:

> Take me. – Hold me. – Caress me gently.
> Embrace me with caution a little while.[13]

* * *

The febrile, occasionally over-excited streak in the Swedish twentieth-century writer Sven Stolpe's very personal literary style took shape during his stay in 'death's waiting-room'.[14]

A more playful, but equally defensive, attitude was adopted by the German poet Christian Morgenstern around 1900. Having caught tuberculosis from his mother, he spent his short life in and out of sanatoria. Morgenstern faced his illness and maintained his independence with dark humour. In the spirit of François Villon, he made fun of his tragic fate in grotesque *Gallows Songs*, discovering that you see the world differently from the hill on which the gallows stand, as well as seeing things that other people do not perceive. In his poems, he indicates what those things are:

> It's springtide at my gallows' beams!
> O time of joy and blessing!
> A bladelet in a knothole dreams
> of sunlight's sweet caressing.
> The breezes rock it tenderly,
> they rock it to and fro –
> I almost feel alive, although
> I am no longer me.[15]

Morgenstern's address to the imagined female assistant to the executioner, a girl he calls Sophie, invites her to kiss and caress his skull despite its gruesome appearance, the mouth a black pit and hair and eyes missing, since she is such a kind and noble creature.[16]

---

13 Ibid., p. 107.

14 The title of the Swedish novel is *I dödens väntrum* (Stockholm: Albert Bonniers Förlag, 1930).

15 Christian Morgenstern, *Galgenlieder: A Selection*, trans. by Max Knight (Berkeley: University of California Press, 1963), pp. 66–67. The German original, called 'Galgenbruders Frühlingslied', runs, 'Es lenzet auch auf unserem Spahn, / o selige Epoche! / Ein Hälmlein will zum Lichte nahn /aus einem Astwurmloche. / Es schaukelt bald im Winde hin / und schaukelt bald drin her. / Mir ist beinah, ich wäre wer / der ich doch nicht mehr bin[.]' From *Alle Galgenlieder* (Wiesbaden: Insel-Verlag, 1947), p. 32.

16 'Galgenbruders Lied an Sophie, die Henkersmaid': 'Sophie, mein Henkersmädel, / komm, küsse mir den Schädel! / Zwar ist mein Mund / ein schwarzer Schlund – / doch du bist gut und edel! / Sophie, mein Henkersmädel, / komm, streichle mir den Schädel! / Zwar ist mein Haupt / des Haars beraubt – / doch du bist gut und edel! / Sophie, mein Henkersmädel, / komm, schau mir in den Schädel! / Die Augen zwar, / sie fraß der Aar – / doch du bist gut und edel!'. Knight's translation is on p. 49 in the edition mentioned in the preceding note.

Like John Keats, Anton Chekhov, another victim of tuberculosis, had had medical training: 'Medicine is my lawful wedded wife, and literature my mistress. When one gets on my nerves, I spend the night with the other.'[17] The parable indicates where his true love resided, and the 'lawful wife' was soon abandoned – but never completely forgotten: 'There is no doubt in my mind that my study of medicine has had a serious impact on my literary activities. It significantly broadened the scope of my observations and enriched me with knowledge whose value for me as a writer only a doctor can appreciate.'[18] Maybe it also contributed – along with his illness – to forming that attitude of resignation which he shared with a number of indecisive and irresolute doctors in his writings? 'With me, a physician, there are ... few illusions. Of course, I am sorry for such an approach to existence ... since it somehow deprecates life.'[19]

Chekhov developed his tuberculosis at an early age. As is sometimes the case with doctors, he stubbornly refused to accept his colleagues' diagnosis, carefully concealing the telltale specks of blood on his handkerchief from the anxious eyes of his parents. Nevertheless, a secret preoccupation with his condition finds expression in many of his works, imbued with nostalgia and a melancholic foreboding of death, as in the closing lines of 'The Black Monk': 'Blood began to flow from his throat straight on to his breast ... He fell on the floor and ... called "Tania!" He called to Tania, he called to the great gardens with their lovely flowers sprinkled with dew, he called to the park, to the pines with their rugged roots, to the fields of rye, to his wonderful science, to his youth, courage, joy, he called to life that was so beautiful. He saw on the floor close to his face a large pool of blood, and from weakness he could not utter another word, but an inexpressible, a boundless happiness filled his whole being.'[20]

Dr Chekhov appreciated, and was thoroughly familiar with, the euphoria which makes our last farewell easier by spreading a merciful veil across a painful reality. Shostakovich, who spent long periods of time in a sanatorium, must have had a fellow-feeling for his brother in adversity; he stated that 'The Black Monk' was the theme of his Fifteenth Symphony, just as fear of death had been the theme of the Fourteenth.

* * *

17 Letter from Anton Chekhov to Alexei Suvorin of 11 September 1888, in *Letters of Anton Chekhov*, trans. by Michael Henry Heim (London: The Bodley Head, 1973), p. 107.

18 Letter from Chekhov to Grigory Rossolimo of 11 October 1899, p. 367 in the edition mentioned in the preceding note.

19 Thomas Gaiton Marullo, 'Editor's Introduction' to Ivan Bunin, *About Chekhov: The Unfinished Symphony*, ed. and trans. by Thomas Gaiton Marullo (Evanston: Northwestern University Press, 2007), p. xxvii, n. 57.

20 Anton Chekhov, 'The Black Monk', in *Selected Stories* (New York: Walter J. Black, 1943 [1929]), p. 87.

In the spirit of Chekhov, the consumptive author Katherine Mansfield wrote melancholy short stories while she was slowly wasting away: '[t]here is a little boat, far out, moving along, *inevitable* it looks and *dead silent* – a little black spot, like the spot on a lung'.[21] For a couple of years she filled her life with erotic adventure, exulting, 'we made love like two wild beasts'. By speaking of 'the spirit which fascinates me in flesh', she may have attempted to impart a measure of dignity to her conduct.[22]

Progressive tuberculosis tamed Mansfield. She related her female experiences to her friend D. H. Lawrence, supplying material for some of his erotic descriptions which he could not very well have invented on his own (he also had other, less heated, sources). He is sure to have benefited from Mansfield's impressionistically vivid accounts, which competed with those of Degas in respect of graphic intimacy.

Even so, revulsion against the disease they had in common, and the sexual weakness that attends it, may have been the reason why Lawrence insulted her by telling her that she was repulsive, stewing in her consumption.[23] Maybe he was sickened and revolted by her breath, the same tubercular smell that the Goncourt brothers noticed when calling upon the dying author of *Scènes de la vie de Bohème*, 'the odour of rotting flesh in his bedroom'.[24] Lawrence also attempted to conceal his tuberculosis up to the very end by giving it different names – influenza, bronchitis, common cold. He transformed it into fiction by transferring it to Lady Chatterley's lover, the gamekeeper, who was 'curiously full of vitality, but a little frail and quenched' – but not to such an extent that he would have been incapable of sharing the most intemperate physical excesses with the lady, who was herself ill with boredom and sexual starvation. The candid and detailed description of their sexual activities, trembling with excitement, was regarded as offensive at the time and marketed as 'shamelessly uninhibited'.[25]

This new literary naturalism was coloured by – or, rather, a direct consequence of – Lawrence's illness. The novel was written during the final stages of his tuberculosis as the toxins circulating in his blood made him weary and despondent. Might his latent homosexuality have facilitated his understanding of female sexuality?[26] In any case, it is with the voice of Lady Chatterley that Lawrence laments his indifference – 'Why don't I really care?' – and his

21 Anthony Alpers, *The Life of Katherine Mansfield* (Oxford: Oxford University Press, 1982), p. 300.

22 'Wild beasts': Journal, 6 September 1911, in *Journal of Katherine Mansfield*, ed. by J. Middleton Murry (London: Constable & Co., 1962), p. 46.

23 See Claire Tomalin, *Katherine Mansfield: A Secret Life* (London: Viking, 1987), p. 188.

24 Edmond and Jules Goncourt, *Journal des Goncourt; Mémoires de la vie littéraire*, Vol. I: 1851–1861 (Paris: Bibliothèque Charpentier, 1891), p. 362 ('l'odeur de viande pourrie qui est dans sa chambre – et qu'il ignore être la sienne').

25 D. H. Lawrence, *Lady Chatterley's Lover* (London: Vintage, 2011), p. 66.

26 William B. Ober, *Boswell's Clap and Other Essays* (Carbondale: Southern Illinois Press, 1979), pp. 92, 116, and 109–117.

fear of approaching death, of the 'ghastly white tombstones ... detestable as false teeth, which stuck up on the hillside'.[27]

Lawrence's own sexual activity was reduced by the disease, which actually made him impotent. As so often happens, unsatisfied lust engendered erotic fantasies whose feverish intensity is reminiscent of the dreams of puberty. There is no end to all the flowers threaded among pubic hairs, 'forget-me-not flowers in the fine brown fleece of the mount of Venus' and 'a bit of creeping-jenny round his penis', to quote a few selected localities.[28]

* * *

Lady Chatterley's Lover may be regarded as the very pattern of a consumptive creation. It has features in common with works by Aubrey Beardsley, who also gave artistic vent to a sexual appetite restrained by illness. A concentrated atmosphere of *fin de siècle* and *art nouveau* assaults the viewer of the drawings created by this master draughtsman. Tubercular since childhood, Beardsley was strongly marked by his suffering and perfectly aware of his fate: 'yesterday I was laid out like a corpse with a haemorrhage. For me and my lung there seems to be little hope'; 'I shall not live longer than did Keats', he said, and made a drawing which represented himself dying in bed while his co-actors on the stage of life assemble to bid farewell. In spite of this, he continued to work like a man condemned – which, after all, is what he was.[29]

Beardsley's refined, decadent art reflects both his sexual hunger and his arrogance, haunted as he was by feverish erotic fantasies. His friend William Butler Yeats has said that Beardsley's sexual appetite had become insatiable under the pressure of his disease;[30] and indeed Beardsley himself admits this in representing himself tied to Priapus. Beardsley implies that his illness had rendered him impotent. Instead, he tried to satisfy his desires by means of erotic drawings. With progressing disease and tiredness, his art became increasingly obscene – but at the same time it achieved new heights of elegance, artistry, and skill. The last sheets, the illustrations of *Lysistrata*, came into being in between frequent lung haemorrhages.[31] It is a pity that they were deemed to be too pornographic for publication; rarely has more charming and lovable, innocently candid, erotic art been created.

* * *

27 D. H. Lawrence, *Lady Chatterley's Lover; A propos of Lady Chatterley's Lover*, ed. by Michael Squires (London: Penguin, 2006 [1993]), pp. 255 and 76.

28 Ibid., pp. 223 and 228.

29 Stanley Weintraub, *Aubrey Beardsley: Imp of the Perverse* (University Park: Pennsylvania State University Press, 1976), pp. 200 and 121.

30 W. B. Yeats, *Memoirs*, ed. by Denis Donoghue (London: Macmillan, 1972), p. 92.

31 Weintraub, *Aubrey Beardsley*, p. 195.

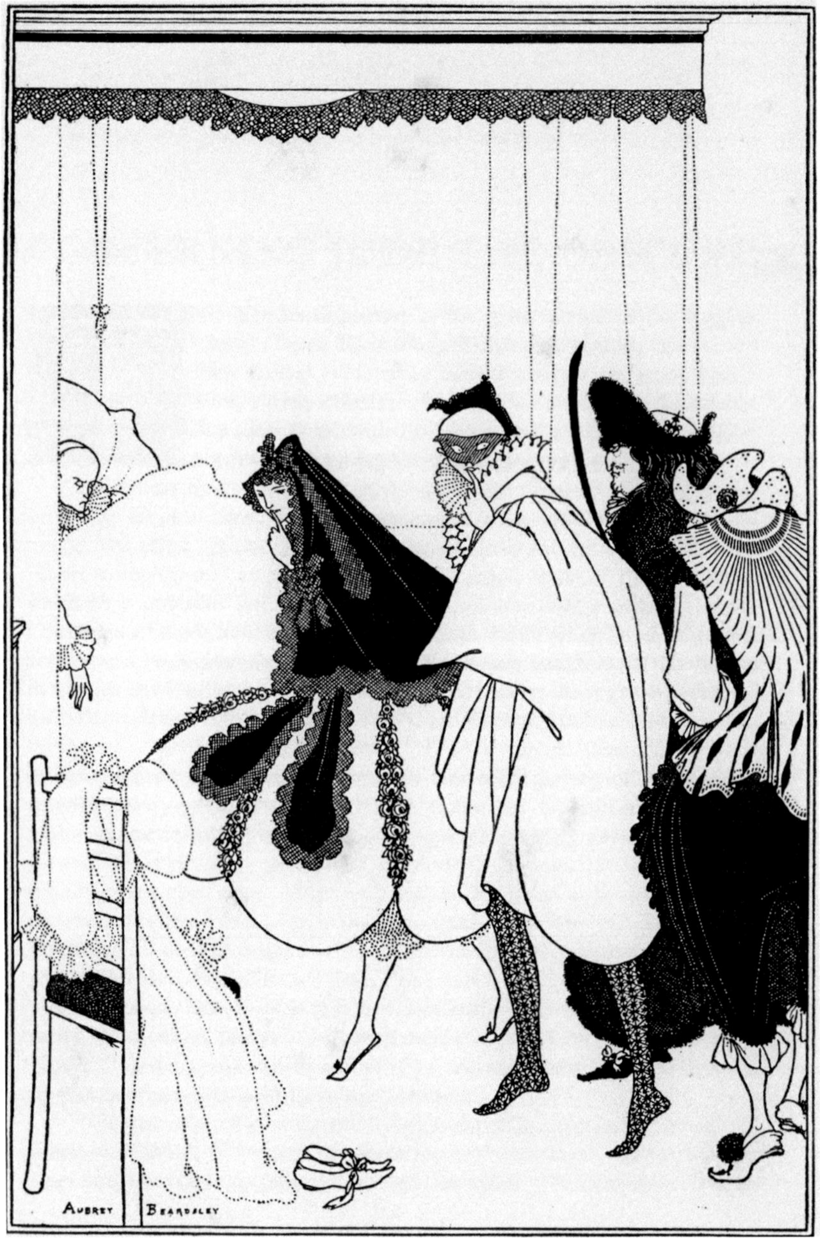

Figure 83 Aubrey Beardsley, 'The death of Pierrot', 1896. 'As dawn broke, Pierrot fell into his last sleep. Then upon tip-toe, silently up the stairs, noiselessly into the room, came the comedians, Arlecchino, Pantaleone, Il Dottore, and Columbina, who with much love carried away upon their shoulders the white-frocked clown of Bergamo; whither, we know not.'[32]

32 *Aubrey Beardsley: Selected Drawings* (New York: Grove Press, 1967), illustration No. 89 (unpaginated).

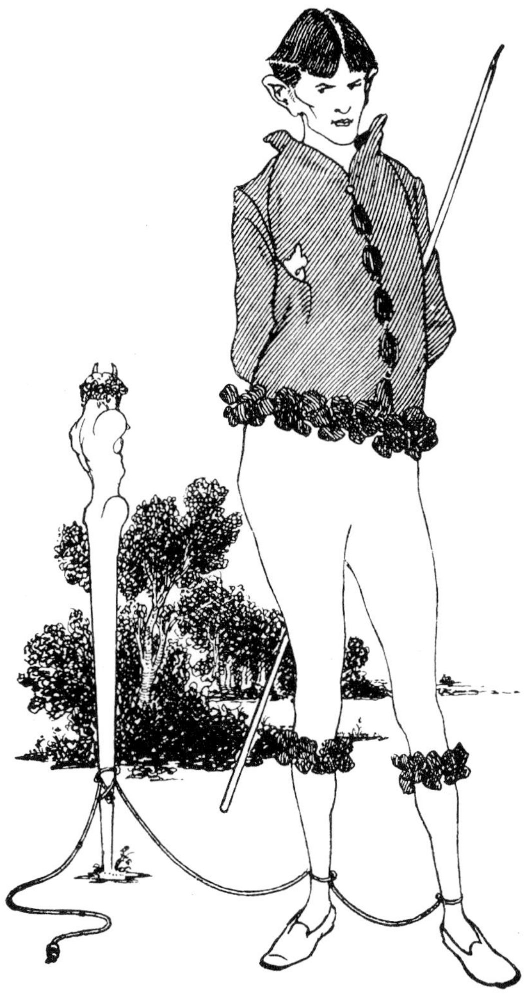

Figure 84 Aubrey Beardsley, 'A foot-note', 1896. The artist tethered to Priapus, symbol of sexuality. From *The Savoy*, No. 2, 1896.

To the Catalan artist Antoni Tàpies, tuberculosis was a transient but intense period of illness in his youth, introduced by a violent heart attack that nearly cost him his life.

Tàpies was compelled to break off his law studies in order to spend time in a sanatorium. Treatment with pneumothorax, the insertion of gas into the patient's pleura, restored his health after four years. The feeling of being ill, as well as the painful therapy he endured, came to make a great difference to his art. Involuntary isolation in the mountains offered him the opportunity to meditate, and awareness of physical decay and the depressing closeness of death imparted profundity to his views on human life.

As was the case with Schlegel (p. 18) and others, the disease did not detract from Tàpies's mental powers. According to him, his life would

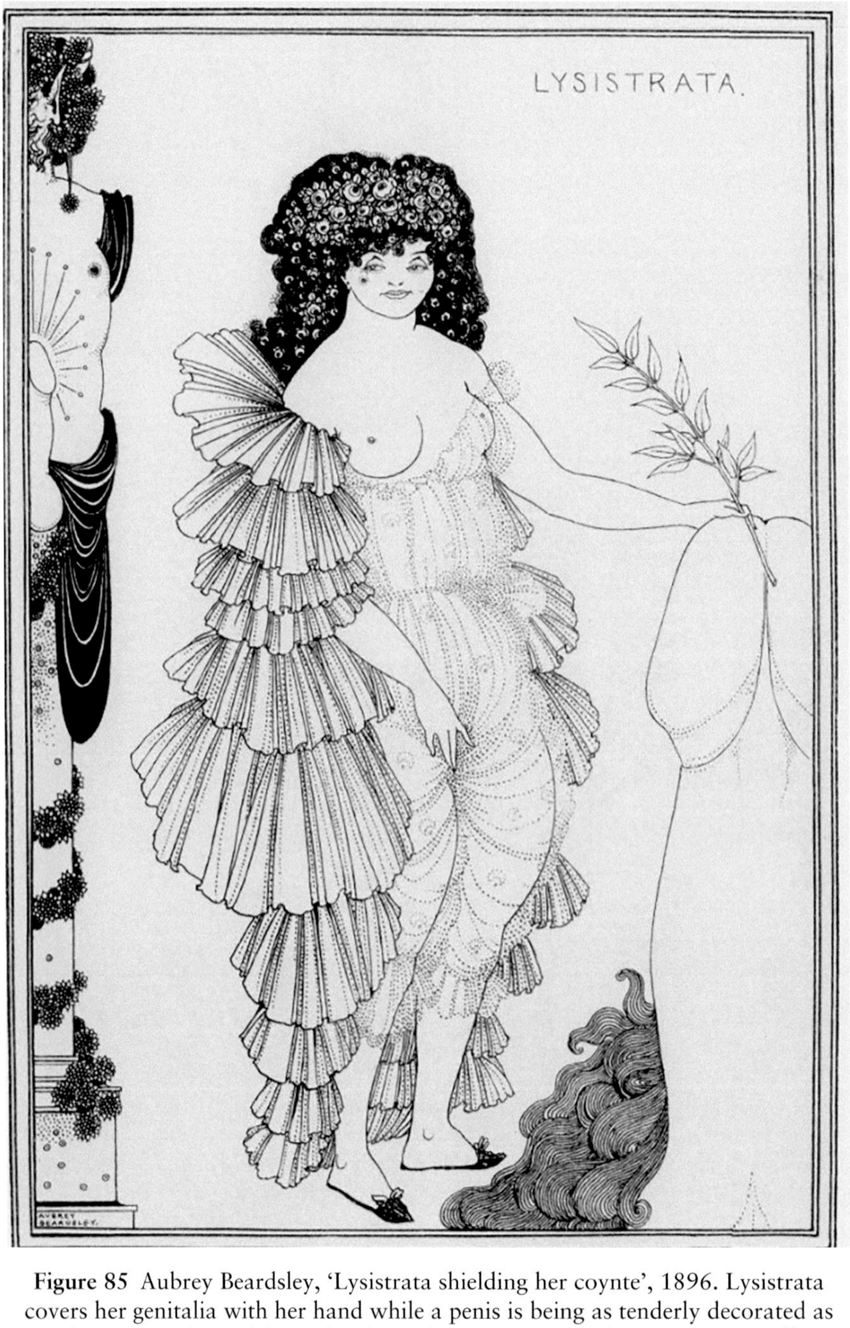

Figure 85 Aubrey Beardsley, 'Lysistrata shielding her coynte', 1896. Lysistrata covers her genitalia with her hand while a penis is being as tenderly decorated as the one worshipped by Lady Chatterley. From Aristophanes' *Lysistrata*.[33]

33 Ibid., illustration No. 96 (unpaginated).

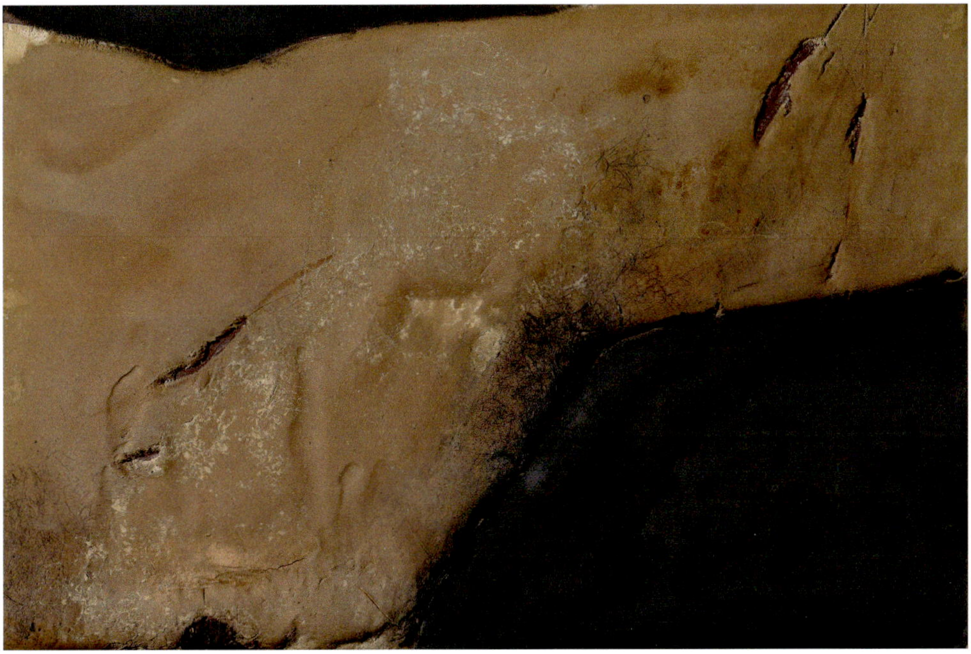

Figure 86 Antoni Tàpies, 'Matter in the form of an armpit', 1968. Sores around an armpit.

certainly have developed differently if he had not been ill. He was surprised to find that the illness did not diminish his mental activity in the least; on the contrary, it gave him a feeling of exaltation which made him feel that he was better able to appreciate the meaning of life than healthy people. In particular, he observed that the difficulty breathing and the ways in which that could be overcome improved his mental acuity.[34] Like his brother in misfortune Sam Francis, Tàpies distracted himself by drawing and painting – for which he had a decided aptitude – and soon wished to express himself by means of artistic pursuits. Having studied modern art – especially Picasso and Miró – on his own, he began a successful career in the course of which he made a name for himself as an independent and original personality.

Tàpies developed a great desire to make his paintings works of art in their own right. He did not wish them to be mere windows, he said, possibly aiming a kick at Realism. Consequently, he worked with solid materials, wood, textiles, and especially sand mixed with acrylic. He was fond of representing stone walls in varying stages of decay; Francis's words about the scratches and rifts in his works originating in his own state of brokenness spring to mind.

34 Barbara Catoir, *Conversations with Antoni Tàpies*, trans. by John Ormrod (Munich: Prestel, 1991), p. 71.

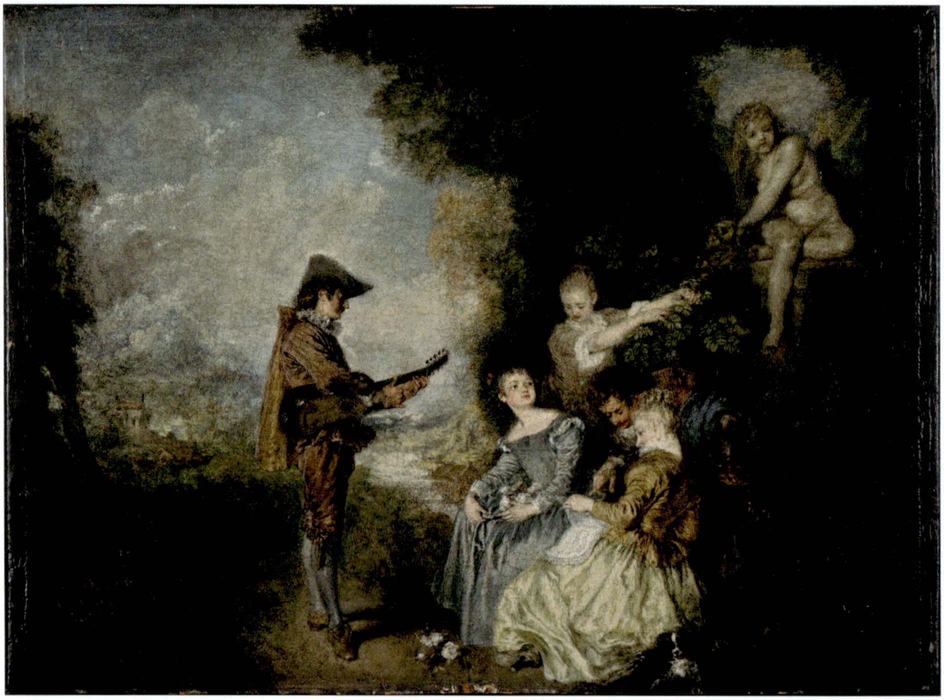

Figure 87 Antoine Watteau, 'The lesson of Love', 1716/1717. The guitar-player might be a symbolic self-portrait – the melancholy consumptive.

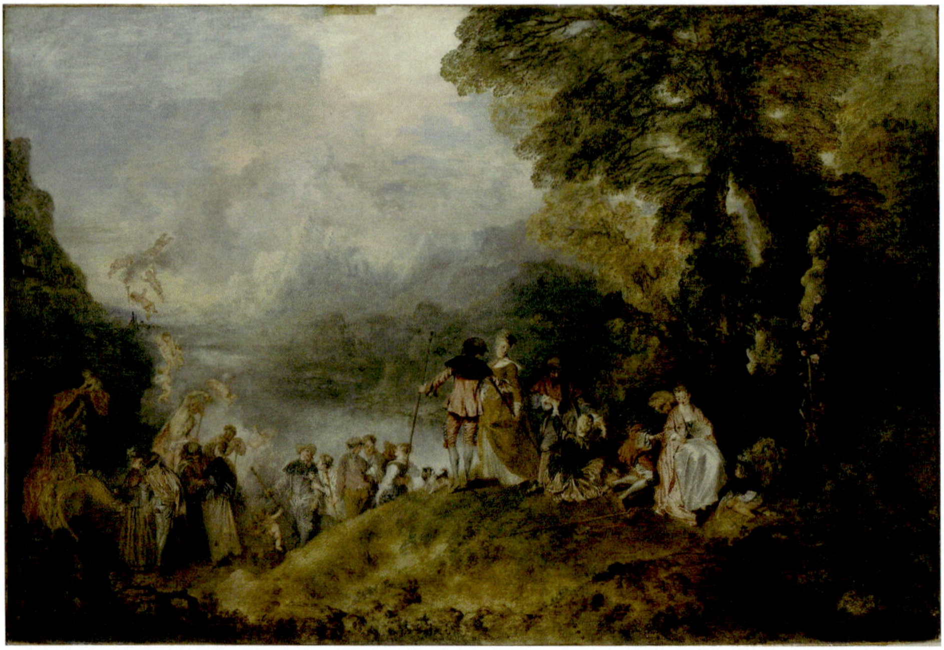

Figure 88 Antoine Watteau, 'Pilgrimage to Cythera', 1717.

No wonder Tàpies, with his experience of pain and of physical ruin, was given to depicting sick and injured body parts, expressions of the dramatic situation that arises when the body is exposed to trials and suffering. The upsetting representation of sores around an armpit moved Miró so much that he acquired it for his own collection.

According to Tàpies, the depictions of these body parts do not merely reproduce their infirmities; the images also encompass the beginnings of a restoration to health – indeed, he went so far as to state that his own representations form part of recovery. He claimed that an artistic vocation is typically instigated by a form of suffering that presents itself as a particular experience, sometimes vehemently in connection with an accident, at other times as a slowly draining disorder. When recovery begins, says Tàpies, the artistic impulse comes into being: there is no other way of accounting for the origin of an artist's vocation.[35] Those words tell us something about the process of artistic creation, and we devour them as greedily as we do similar utterances by Matisse (p. 25).

* * *

In the late paintings of Antoine Watteau, we find moving and passionate endeavours to hold on to the fast-vanishing joys experienced during the pleasures of love, so that we may linger on Cythera, the island where there is neither sorrow nor pain.[36] The picture named 'The lesson of Love' features a lone musician playing to a pretty girl who turns away from him. Carl Nordenfalk assumes that this guitar player is a symbolic self-portrait, a melancholy consumptive who is never allowed to drain the cup that holds the pleasures of life – a cup which he instead offers us, up to the brim, in his art.[37]

In 'Pilgrimage to Cythera', Kenneth Clark sensed a kinship with the ailing Mozart, who knew a great deal about the ephemeral nature of human pleasures: 'The delicate relationships between these men and women who have spent a few hours on the Island of Venus and must now return reminds one of those rapturous stirrings that precede the departure of the confident lovers in *Così Fan Tutte*.'[38]

We register the same feeling of sweet pain and gentle sadness in the Nocturnes of Chopin, those melancholy fever dreams. Poor deserted Chopin worked himself to death during the last stages of pulmonary disease. He was at that time in London, the city to which Carl Maria von Weber had once journeyed, feverish, out of breath and coughing blood, in order to attend the première of his opera *Oberon*, soon followed by his exit from life. In the Sonata in B Minor, Chopin gave vent to the anguish that

35 Ibid., p. 122.
36 Arthur-Martin Dinaux, *Watteau* (Paris: A. Prignet, 1834), p. 10.
37 Carl Nordenfalk, 'The Stockholm Watteaus', *Nationalmuseum Bulletin* 3 (1979), 185.
38 Kenneth Clark, *Civilisation* (London: BBC and John Murray, 1971), pp. 232–235.

seized him on leaving the monastery of Valldemossa after his last sojourn there with George Sand. The famous 'Funeral March' is interrupted for the space of a couple of bars expressing nostalgic memories of happier days; but the break is soon followed by a presto which has been compared to the flutter of the night breeze among tombstones – the concert where no encores are granted.

Chapter 12
Various physical illnesses

The Swedish poet Hjalmar Gullberg (1898–1961) was afflicted by a horrible disease, progressive myasthenia or muscular debility, which causes increasing paralysis. In harrowing words, he showed how extreme physical misery, caused by an illness so severe that it can hardly be borne, may still find expression in beautiful poetry. One of his poems has the form of a letter of reply to a young man who had lamented over the mental distress that his own poetical endeavours had cost him:

> But I am old, and have
> read a hundred letters of this kind.
> And now I am so tired.
> I'm going through a crisis.
> Maltreated flesh is real in a way
> that differs from the distress
> of a suffering soul. I found
> confirmation of this thesis
> in a stench of flowing phlegm.
> Now I catch the smell of bird cherry.
> You are a healthy young man ...[1]

Gullberg's dreadful illness left profound marks in his late poetry. He expressed a yearning for annihilation:

> Deeper within, through bone and marrow,
> days and nights so long:
> one wish only, only one –
> some people have so many.

Gullberg's poetry contains shocking and moving insights into the terrifying final decomposition of our physical being. The waterman who found Ophelia drowned in the reeds becomes his mouthpiece:

> I found Ophelia. She surfaced in the reeds
> her hair undone. She was much changed
> ...
> Death by the pouring of water

---

1 The Swedish poem is entitled 'Till en amatör', 'To an amateur'. It comes from Gullberg's last collection of poems.

was what I saw in my nets: a swollen
mermaid put to fermentation by the brook.
...
What was the first thing that I did
on finding a court lady in the mire?
Saw what I saw, and then vomited in the reeds.[2]

When Gullberg was obliged to face a relapse of his illness, with renewed 'stench of the flowing phlegm', he chose to follow Ophelia into the wet mire, fulfilling the premonition he had had many years before:

There is a lake and nothing beyond it,
the river levelling out in the grey mirror
that no shore frames, no strokes of oars
will shatter.[3]

* * *

Rainer Maria Rilke displayed heroic fortitude during the illness, leukaemia, which ended his life after years of suffering, with unbearable pain towards the end; he is said to have declined analgesics so as not to quench his creative power. Having composed a draft of his first two 'Duino Elegies', he fell silent as a poet for a couple of years and must have wondered whether he would ever finish them. But then, in a sudden flash of inspiration, he completed '[a]ll in a few days, it was a nameless storm, a hurricane of the spirit'.[4] Not only were the ten elegies completed; he also wrote ecstatic musings about poetry and death – never far away – in his 'Sonnets to Orpheus':

Be – and yet know the demands of not-being,
the infinite basis of your inner vibration,
so that, this once, you bring it to perfect completion.[5]

It is an esoteric sigh which consoles us with its intimate tone and its feeling of fellowship in a fate shared by all human beings. Not long afterwards, the first signs of his illness appeared:

Come, you, the last to be recognized by me,
Terrible pain in the tissue of my body[.][6]

---

2 From the poem 'Död i dyn eller Han som fann Ofelia', 'Dead in the mire, or He who found Ophelia'.

3 From the poem 'Det finns en sjö och sedan aldrig mer', 'There is a lake and nothing beyond it'. Gullberg died by suicide in a lake south of Lund.

4 Letter from Rainer Maria Rilke to Princess Marie von Thurn und Taxis of 11 February 1922; quoted from *The Letters of Rainer Maria Rilke and Princess Marie von Thurn und Taxis* (London: The Hogarth Press, 1958), p. 214.

5 No. XIII in the second part of the 'Sonnets to Orpheus'. German original: 'Sei – und wisse zugleich des Nicht-Seins Bedingung, / den unendlichen Grund deiner innigen Schwingung, / daß du sie völlig vollziehst dieses einzige Mal.'

6 German original: 'Komm du, du letzter, den ich anerkenne, / heilloser Schmerz im leiblichen Geweb'. The poem is the final entry in Rilke's last notebook.

Rilke loved flowers and was transported by roses; in the end they transported him to death, as he was pricked by a thorn at a point in time when the disease had robbed him of every defence against infection and death. His sole consolation – in so far as it is one – was to have a rose named after him.

The remarkable coincidence of illness and creativity has given rise to much speculation about a causal relationship. According to one imaginative theory, excess of creativity would lead to disease in a psychosomatic process; 'every fibre and tissue in me was strained to breaking-point'.[7]

The opposite process has been proposed as well, namely that illness will have been transformed into creativity, as Novalis once imagined (p. 00) From a medical point of view, however, the most probable link (if indeed there is one at all) is that the poet, consciously or subconsciously, sensed the closeness of 'not-being' and made haste to complete his work while there was still time. This explanation is supported by Rilke himself: 'But now it is done. Done. Done. Amen. Thus I have survived this, through everything. Through it all. And it was this that was needful. *Only* this.'[8]

* * *

Béla Bartók, who died from the same 'diseased blood', grieved at having to bid farewell with so much still to say. Increasingly exhausted, and fired by a persistent fever, he composed his swan song, the Third Piano Concerto. In the shadow of death, tragically in exile, he called to mind the fullness and richness of life in melodies whose source was in the folk-songs of his father.

Another victim of leukaemia was the Swedish artist Lage Lindell. In a suite of elementarily expressive images, he traced the successive stages of the sick person's annihilation.

A female counterpart was the fatally ill but strong-minded Flannery O'Connor.[9] She fought against a natural self-pity with grim humour and looked evil straight in the eye, in her life as well as in fiction, where 'A Good Man Is Hard to Find' and where a good girl is easily duped, especially if she has a disability.[10] Her illness, *lupus erythematosus*, starts by affecting the sufferer's joints, but later on it attacks one organ after another. 'My father had it – but at that time there was nothing for it but the undertaker; now it can be controlled with the ACTH.'[11] This anti-inflammatory drug gave O'Connor another 15 precious years of life and work.

The English term for O'Connor's illness, 'butterfly rash', encompasses the same carefree manner of expressing grim realities that we find in her writing.

7 From the letter mentioned in note 4.
8 Ibid. Italics in original.
9 See Flannery O'Connor, *The Habit of Being*, ed. by Sally Fitzgerald (New York: Farrar, Straus, & Giroux, 1979).
10 'A Good Man Is Hard to Find' is a short story from 1953.
11 Letter from Flannery O'Connor to Elizabeth and Robert Lowell of 17 March 1953, p. 57 in *The Habit of Being*.

'I have never been anywhere but sick. In a sense sickness is a place, more instructive than a long trip to Europe, and it's always a place where there's no company, where nobody can follow.'[12] She even made a pun on the medical term for her illness, *lupus* (Latin for 'wolf'), as she finally succumbed to it, describing the process as 'the wolf ... inside tearing up the place': 'I had a blood transfusion Tuesday so I am feeling sommut better and for the last two days I have worked one hour each day and my my I do like to work. I et up that one hour like it was filet mignon.' In her miserable state, she found that 'what you have to measure out, you come to observe closer, or so I tell myself'.[13]

O'Connor presented her close observations in a mature, distinctive personal style in her last stories, finished when she was dying. Her profound religious faith in combination with the continuous threat of a fatal disease may have created the basis for her intense interest in ruthless fate and in merciless people and doomed individuals.

***

The Swedish painter of fairy-tales Ivar Arosenius died of haemophilia, 'the bleeding disease', a mere 30 years old.[14] The congenital disorder had already robbed him of his elder brother, who bled to death aged 14 after having a tooth extracted. Consequently, Arosenius was tragically aware of the constant mortal danger hanging over him, and he depicted it with gory realism – never did a dragon bleed so furiously as the one that confronted the artist fighting his illness in the guise of St George. His haemorrhages were followed by severe pain, and they restricted his mobility; whenever he hurt himself, there were large bruises and a painful swelling of the joints.

This circumstance both promoted and modified Arosenius's artistry. During the long periods in childhood when he was obliged to lie in bed, he amused himself by painting and drawing. He acquired a remarkable manual dexterity as a result – few artists ever had such a short distance between idea and hand. Not only the form but also the content of his art was affected by his illness. At first it found expression in a desperate rebellion against fate, a wild desire to extract from life what it had to offer as quickly and intensely as possible. He depicted himself, weary and exhausted, riding his Pegasus in pursuit of comfort with a girl and a bottle.

In his miserable condition, he revealed another sentiment as well: contempt, mixed with envy, towards the fat and prosperous bon vivant – frequently depicted as an arrogant prince of fortune – who selfishly and ruthlessly picks flowers from the wayside and girls for his bed.

12 Flannery O'Connor to 'A', p. 163 in *The Habit of Being*.

13 Ibid. First quotation: Flannery O'Connor to Sister Mariella Gable, 5 July 1964, p. 163; second quotation: O'Connor to Maryat Lee, 15 May 1964, p. 577; third quotation: O'Connor to Elizabeth and Robert Lowell, 17 March 1953, p. 57.

14 Per Bjurström, *Arosenius*, Nationalmuseum's exhibition catalogue No. 410 (1978), p. 6.

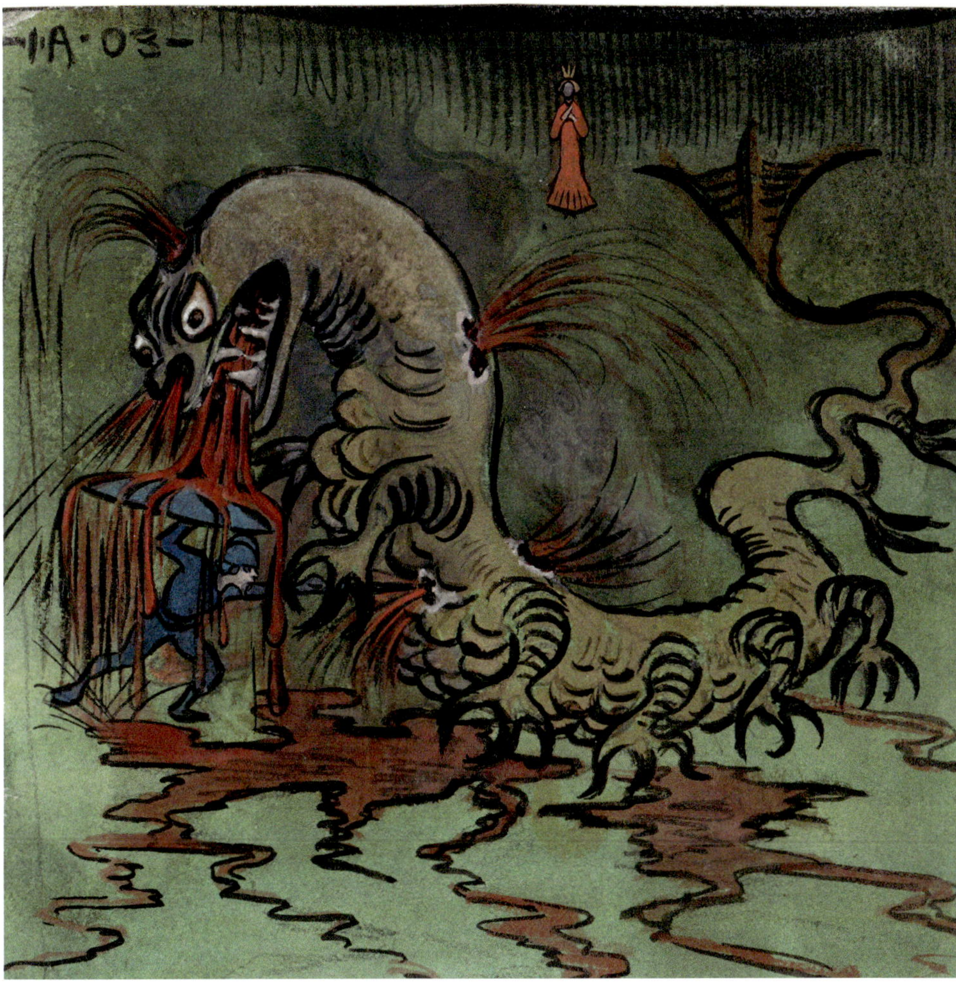

Figure 89 Ivar Arosenius, 'S:t Göran och draken' ('St George and the dragon'), 1903. The artist struggling against his haemophilia.

Arosenius was saved from the wear and tear of wild Bohemian life by a marriage which afforded him a couple of years of pure and unalloyed happiness. His greatest joy was his small daughter, for whom he painted fairy-tale pictures which belong among the most beautiful, most imaginative, and most expressive illustrations ever created. His happiness was not free from anxiety, though, for the dangerous disease was constantly waiting for an opportunity to strike its victim. Having once been close to dying from a nosebleed, he worked with double zeal, realising that his working day would soon be at an end. Death will suddenly take its seat at the merriest feast – a feared guest, a macabre companion. A couple of lines from the eighteenth-century Swedish poet Carl Michael Bellman make up an appropriate motto:

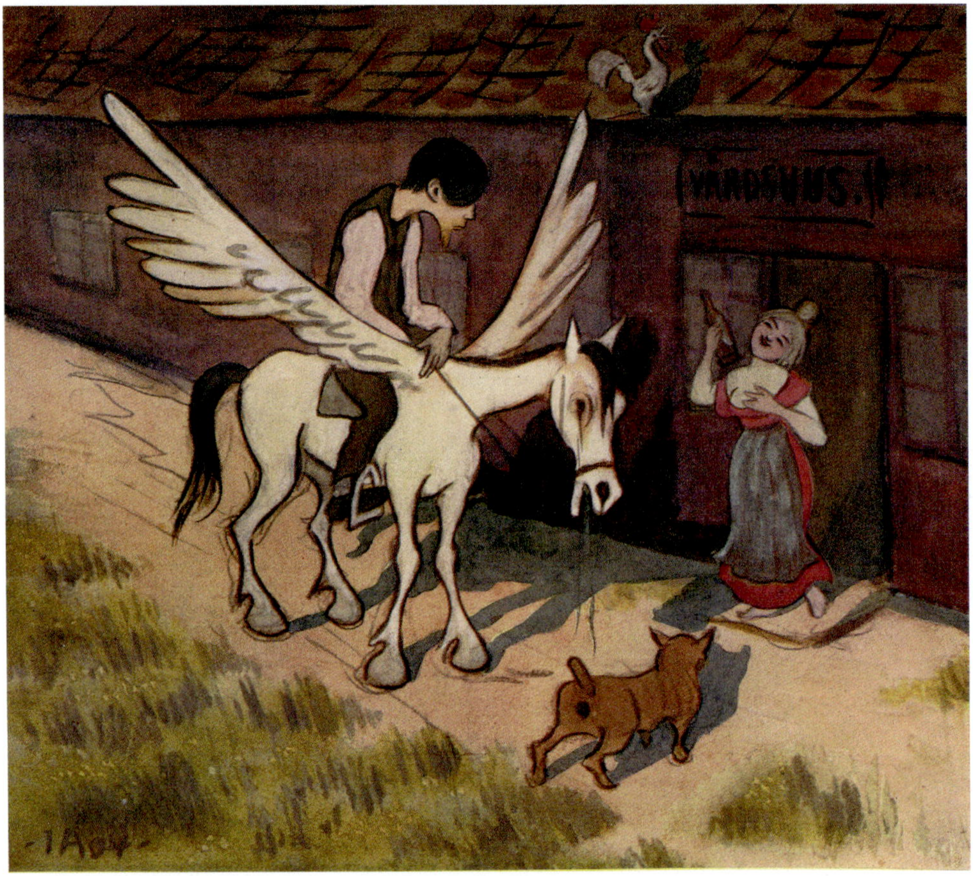

Figure 90 Ivar Arosenius, 'Värdshuset' ('The tavern'), 1904. Weary and exhausted, the artist comes riding on his Pegasus.

> Drain your glass, see, Death is waiting for you ...
> Now pluck the octave,
> tune your strings, and sing of the springtime of life![15]

Death did not tarry long in reality either. One New Year's Eve, Arosenius's wife had gone to bed while he sat up working although he had a sore throat. She suddenly awoke and found him blue in the face, struggling to breathe. Before any help could arrive, he had been suffocated by a haemorrhage in his throat and his beautiful, too brief life was over.

* * *

15 'Drick ur ditt glas, se döden på dig väntar ... Knäpp nu oktaven: / stäm dina strängar, sjung om livets vår!' From the first stanza of the song named 'Till fader Movitz, under dess sjukdom, lungsoten. Elegi'.

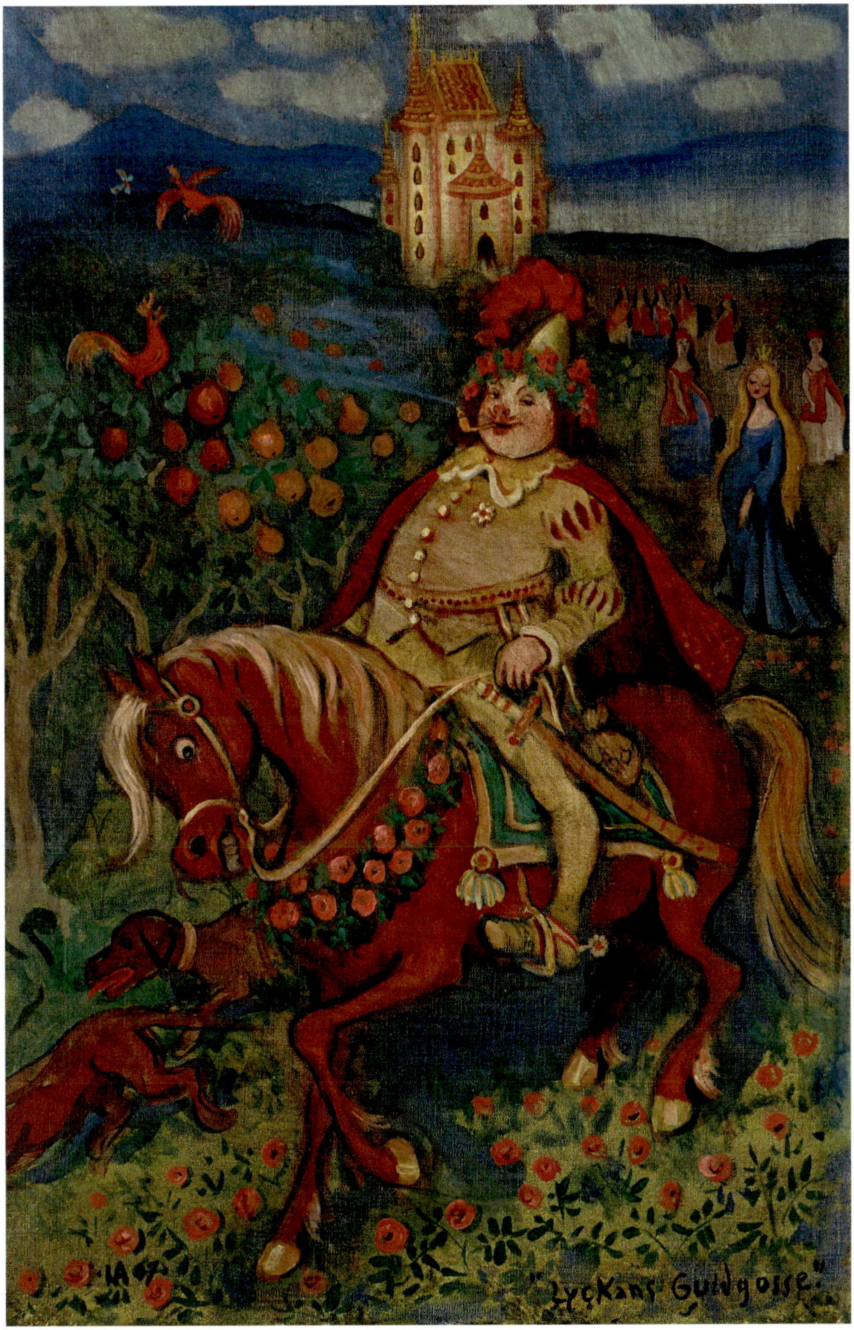

Figure 91 Ivar Arosenius, 'Lyckans guldgosse' ('Fortune's favourite'), 1907.

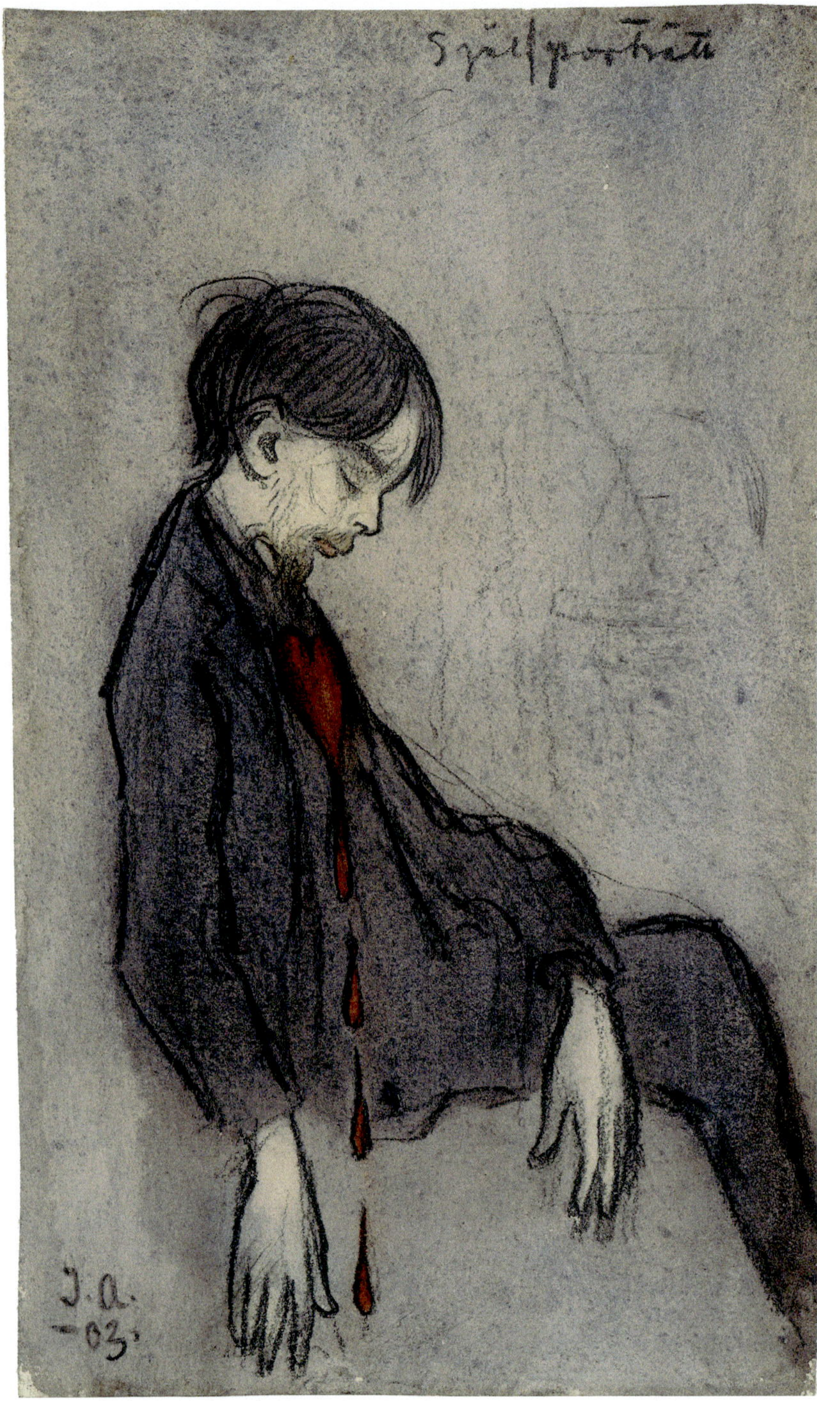

Figure 92 Ivar Arosenius, 'Självporträtt' ('Self-portrait'), 1903.

One of the most original artists of our time was Paul Klee. Musical and highly talented, he sought and found new modes of expression for pictorial art, modes that transmitted the spontaneous joy of the soul as well as the hand in shaping new images in new colours, as well as in new intricate and unprecedented constellations. He loved 'going for a walk with a line'. His imagination was one of a kind and endlessly inventive. He evidently enjoyed himself a great deal when constructing the strange and fantastic castle to which he gave the name *Sängerhalle* ('Great Hall for Singers', Figure 93). It must have been a very cheerful artist who wielded pencil and brush in that picture and hoisted the flag at the end.

The good times did not last. At the age of 40, Klee began to show signs of a serious illness, scleroderma, which entails shrinkage of the skin and of underlying muscles. There is still no cure, and it usually leads to death in five to ten years. The progress of the disease is inexorable, and it extends inward as well. Its development is tragically evident, also to the patient himself; he can tell how death is approaching practically day by day.

It is true that most of us are already developing those pathological changes that will ultimately end our lives, but fortunately they are concealed from us; we are rarely able to observe our own degenerative processes. This helps us to forget the brevity of life. The disease that destroyed Klee could not be concealed, however, and it was not long before he found that it affected not only his state of mind but also his art. Owing to increasing stiffness in his joints, it became difficult for him to execute his small, detailed pictures. He shows us his plight in the drawing of a mournful figure, 'Ein Gestalter' ('A creator'; Figure 94), who wields a pencil in his crippled hand – the same situation that Renoir and Dufy found themselves in with their arthritic hands. The difference is that Klee's disorder was hopeless.

At this stage, Klee's pictures lost their cheerful character. Thoughts of death and annihilation were his constant companions, almost the only ones, as he spent his last years in extreme mental isolation. He expressed his agony only through his work, claiming that he never drew so much or so intensely in his life before, and confessed that he created in order not to weep.[16]

His late drawings form a peculiarly tragic suite, with titles such as 'Will dabei sein' ('Wishes to participate') and 'Trennt sich schwer' ('Finds it hard to leave').[17] One of the last of them, a drawing named 'Durchhalten!' ('Endure!'), forms a powerful expression of the artist's endeavour to keep up his courage in the course of life's tragedy and follow Montaigne's

16 Felix Klee, *Paul Klee: His Life and Work in Documents*, trans. by Richard and Clara Winston (New York: George Braziller, 1962), p. 72. The statement 'ich schaffe pour ne pas pleurer, das ist der letzte und erste Grund' is quoted from Esther Dreifuss-Kattan, *Art and Mourning: The Role of Creativity in Healing Trauma and Loss* (London: Routledge, 2016), pp. 40–41.

17 J. Glaesemer, *Paul Klee: Handzeichnungen III* (Bern: Kunstmuseum, 1979).

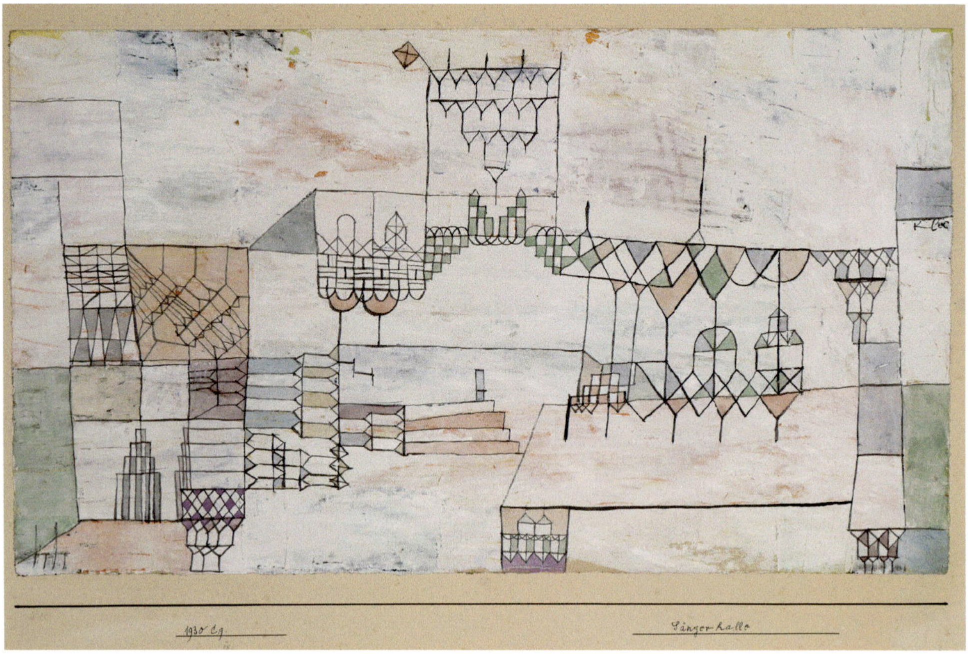

Figure 93 Paul Klee, 'Great Hall for Singers', 1930. The artist loved 'going for a walk with a line'.

exhortation: 'endure, suffer, and be quiet'.[18] The marked lines around the mouth resemble the artist's own, sadly stiffened features, marked by his illness. Before long, 'Der Kranke im Boot' ('The sick one in the boat') would be transported by Charon (Figure 97).

* * *

At the end of this dance of death with poets, painters, and composers, Paul Klee is followed by Juan Gris and Gustav Mahler.

Juan Gris was the third of the great Cubists, somewhat younger than Braque and Picasso. He was their friend and comrade, as well as their equal with regard to creative power, becoming perhaps the most discerning of the three. He often went for a richer and warmer colour scale than the other two, especially during the early stage of Cubism when Braque and Picasso excelled in exquisite harmonies of greys and browns. Juan Gris was entirely preoccupied with opportunities to extract new values from reality by contemplating objects from different perspectives at the same time, as Cézanne

18 'Endure, souffre, et tais toy', from the essay called 'De l'expérience'; Michel de Montaigne, *Essais: Livre III*, ed. by Alexandre Micha (Paris: Garnier-Flammarion, 1969), p. 300.

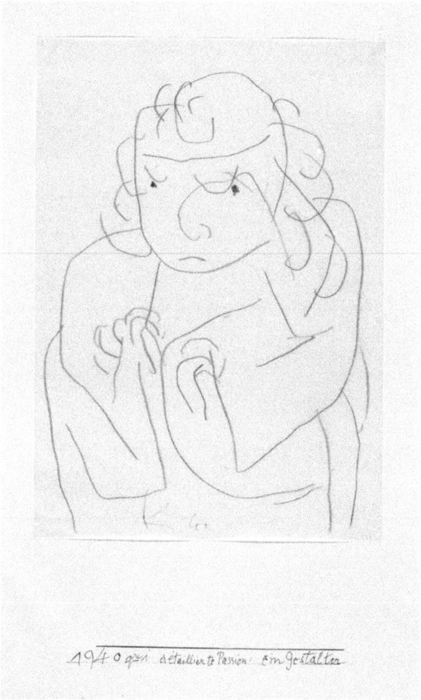

Figure 94 Paul Klee, 'Detailed passion: an artistic creator', 1940. The artist continues to create even after a serious illness has deformed his hands and made it hard for him to grasp the pencil.

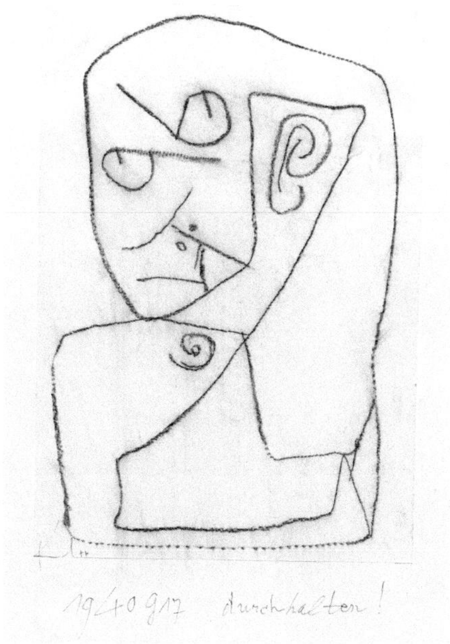

Figure 95 Paul Klee, 'Endure!', 1940. The face is reminiscent of the artist's own, marked by his illness.

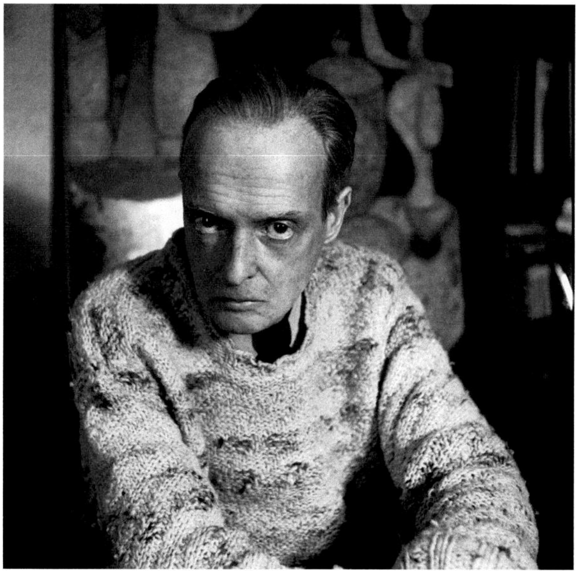

Figure 96 Paul Klee, photographed by Walter Henggeler in December 1939.

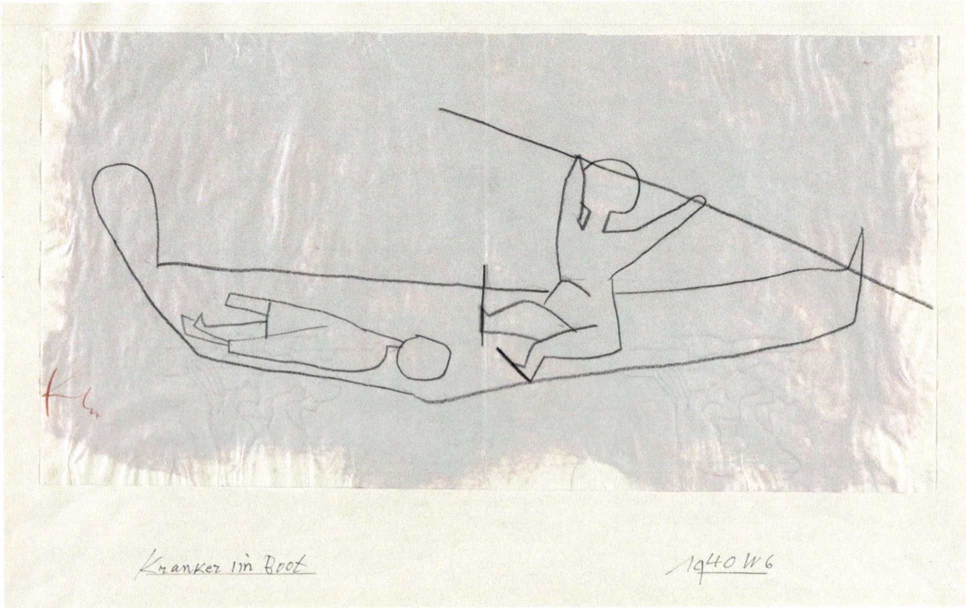

Figure 97 Paul Klee, 'The sick one in the boat', 1940. The traveller will soon arrive on the other side, conveyed by Charon.

had done, and unfolding them so as to form intricate patterns with overlapping angles and triangles (Figure 98).

By nature, Juan Gris was a melancholy and reserved man. For some time in the 1920s, he felt that his painting had become too chilly and intellectual; like others before him, he then made an effort to reach beyond his capabilities. In his endeavour to convey more in the way of human warmth, he repressed his personality. There is, it is fair to say, general agreement to the effect that his art lost some of its artistic vigour and intensity as a result. The figures and objects seem somehow inflated and the colours drier, and the high artistic merit of his early artworks has vanished. At this time, Gris showed the first signs of the disease that would cost him his life a couple of years later. His kidneys had been damaged by scarlet fever and gradually lost more and more of their function. The diagnosis of uraemia was not made at once; he suffered increasingly severe attacks of breathlessness, which were wrongly interpreted as allergic asthma, and he was treated with injections, sedatives, and a change of climate.

It became increasingly difficult for Gris to work for extended periods, and he complained that his pictures had acquired something of a sickly tone. Even so, he pushed on with his painting with great willpower. The works from his last few years show that the disease had made him relinquish every ambition to reach beyond himself: in them, he once more gave full expression to his original, vigorous personality (Figure 99).

Many art critics have misunderstood the situation, maintaining that Gris's illness rendered his entire late artistry inferior. I would, along with his

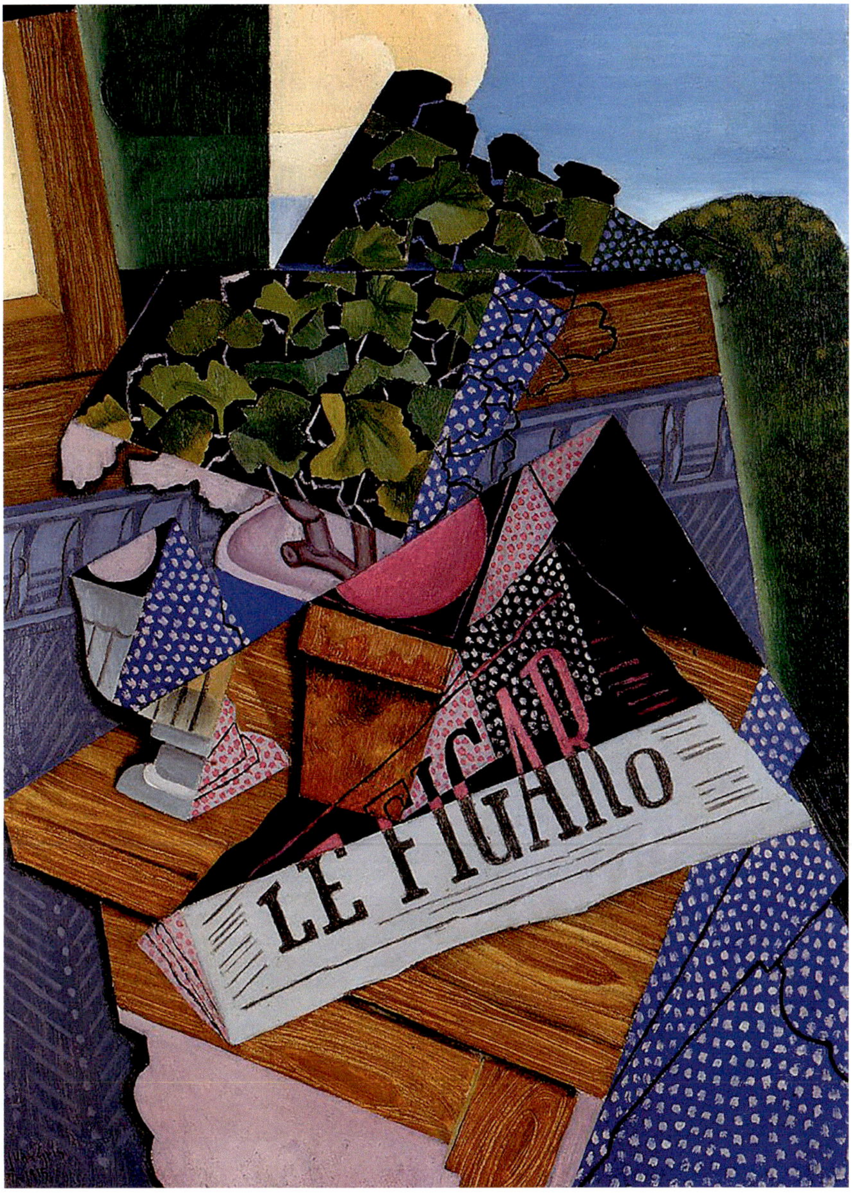

Figure 98 Juan Gris, 'The pot of geraniums', 1915. A Cubist painting from the artist's healthy years.

friend and patron Daniel-Henry Kahnweiler, argue that the opposite is true: the disease liberated him from an aspiration that had harmed his work in the 1920s. In fact, Gris's illness restored his original greatness, a greatness which remained in evidence until the artist's death.

Contemplating the fruits of Juan Gris's last efforts, the infinitely beautiful and mournful chords in Gustav Mahler's *Das Lied von der Erde* seem

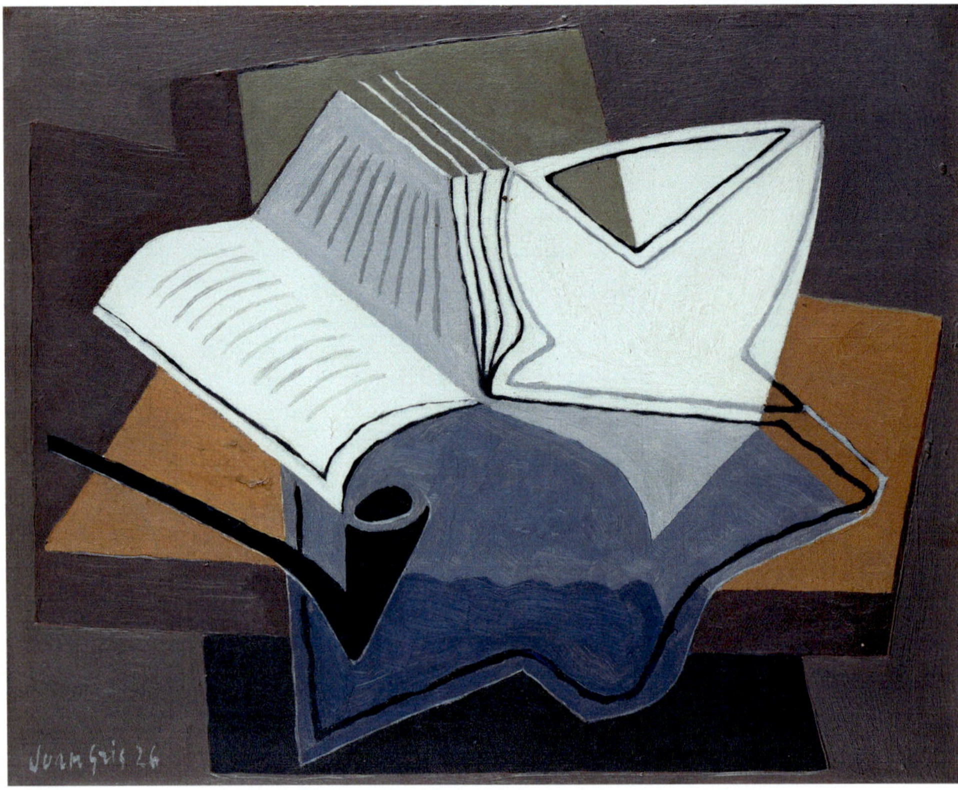

Figure 99 Juan Gris, 'The pipe and the open book', 1926. From the artist's final years, when he had recovered his original artistic power in spite of his illness.

to echo in the background. The inexorability of death and the hope for resurrection had been a constantly recurring theme in the composer's music ever since a slight heart murmur had been discovered (see p. 73). When the dangerous streptococci settled on his heart valves after a throat infection, the disease took a serious turn. Now that his death seemed imminent, his music became even more serene and solemn, a final farewell to life.

Mahler expressed the change in a letter to Bruno Walter: 'you do not know what has been and still is going on within me; but it is certainly not that hypochondriac fear of death, as you suppose. I had already realized that I shall have to die. – But without trying to explain or describe to you something for which there are perhaps no words at all, I'll just tell you that at a blow I have simply lost all the clarity and quietude I ever achieved; and that I stood *vis-à-vis de rien*, and now at the end of life am again a beginner who must find his feet.'[19]

19 Letter from Gustav Mahler to Bruno Walter of 18 July 1908, in *Selected Letters of Gustav Mahler*, ed. by Knud Martner, trans. by Eithne Wilkins, Ernst Kaiser, and Bill Hopkins (New York: Farrar, Straus, Giroux, 1979), p. 324.

The psychoanalyst Theodor Reik discusses Mahler's frame of mind in the following terms: 'One can trace through his letters, through certain things he said, but most of all through his music how his reaction to the near end was changing, how he himself changed, how he discarded everything that was alien to him. When he confronts perdition naked, there is no more sentimentality, no false emotionality, no false tones. Here a man rises highest at the moment he is crushed ... There, where others sink, he soars to an unsurpassable height.'[20]

20 William G. Niederland, 'Psychoanalytic Approaches to Artistic Creativity', *Psychoanalytic Quarterly* 2 (1976), 185.

Summary

In this book, I have collected and studied 140 masters of creation – 36 poets, 40 prose writers, 12 philosophers, 32 pictorial artists, and 20 composers – from whose works it is apparent that ill health played a part in their creativity.[1] It may seem surprising that illness has exercised a favourable influence on creativity in a majority of cases (134), because the creation of the work in question was directly *inspired* by ill health (90) and/or because the nature of the illness *caused* it (48), circumstances precluding any other kind of activity for the sufferer.

With regard to a large number of artists (127), their experiences enabled them to describe their symptoms with feeling and understanding, as was the case with Chekhov, Charlotte Brontë, Dostoevsky, Woolf, Proust, and Goya.

By virtue of their peculiar and salient characteristics, diseases have also proved serviceable as metaphors for multifarious conditions and processes. In the old days, the symptoms of tuberculosis were most often utilised for such purposes; they were later superseded by cancer.[2]

Illness may affect creativity in many different ways. Its effect is indubitable in cases where it formed the main reason for the artist's choice of activity; Pierre de Ronsard, for instance, devoted himself to poetry because his deafness made him useless as a diplomat, and Vivaldi began to compose when he was no longer able to perform Mass because of his asthma. Matisse, who began to paint when his legal career was interrupted by appendicitis, is on record as saying that his creative urge was roused when he observed the manifestations of light in Nature.

L'art brut, 'insane art', has left profound traces in the development of the arts, and Hölderlin's schizophrenia gave new impulses to poetry by enriching it with thitherto unknown ways of producing effects.

In respect of direct influence on artistic pursuits, technical execution may be affected by ill health. This phenomenon is striking in the late paintings of semi-blind Monet, with their rough brush-strokes and disturbed sense of colour.

---

1 In the Swedish original, the author modestly refers to the present volume as an 'essay'.

2 Susan Sontag, *Illness as Metaphor* (New York: Farrar, Straus & Giroux, 1978).

That example shows that ill health might actually open new and different paths for cultural development, independently of the originator's own intentions. With the confused mode of drawing and the strange colouring in his late works, Monet unwittingly took a step away from the generally accepted idea of reality towards a subjective vision in abstract, non-figurative art.

Disease may also serve as a direct inducement. The humiliating feeling of physical malformation drove Byron and Toulouse-Lautrec to compensate themselves by means of artistic creativity. Awareness that the working day of life is approaching its end has often produced a final blaze of the artistic flame, as is seen in the cases of Beardsley and Klee. Montaigne said, 'Above all now, when I see my span so short, I want to give it more ballast; I want to arrest the swiftness of its passing by the swiftness of my capture, compensating for the speed with which it drains away by the intensity of my enjoyment.'[3]

All this does not mean that suffering is in any way a prerequisite for artistic creation, nor does it follow that an artist must be sick in order to represent the pains of illness in a vivid manner. Thomas Mann went through both tuberculosis and syphilis – but only in his work – and Hieronymus Bosch painted gruesome pictures of torment he never suffered.

It might be added that art has occasionally provided medicine with valuable elucidation. There has never been a better picture of the course of tuberculosis than that supplied by Charlotte Brontë, nor have there ever been any more agonisingly detailed accounts of depression than those of Virginia Woolf and William Styron.

Conversely, it has become apparent that artistic activity frequently promotes both bodily and mental health; as a result, it has been put to increasing use in healthcare.

3 From the latter part of 'De l'expérience'; the English translation is from Michel de Montaigne, *The Complete Essays*, ed. by M. A. Screech (London: Penguin, 2003 [1987]), p. 1263.

Epilogue

> Song rises out of sorrow
> But out of song comes joy.
>
> Zacharias Topelius

Now and then in the past, a special feature in an artist's work has erroneously been ascribed to ill health; for instance, as was pointed out above, El Greco's elongated figures have been assumed to be due to a visual defect. Even so, this book has, I hope, persuaded readers that many authors, artists, and composers have had illnesses that have indeed had a profound, sometimes decisive, impact not only on their lives but on their works as well.

Virginia Woolf wondered why *illness* is not one of the major themes of literature. A searing attack of pain is enough to convince its victim that suffering and agony change everything (see pp. 13–14 on Shaw and Updike); and many masters have themselves grasped the vital role played by their illnesses, as is seen from the quotations from Byron, Proust, and Van Gogh (pp. 110, 68, 96)

H. C. Andersen, teller of fairy-tales, gives suffering a prominent place in cultural history. His 'Auntie Toothache' argues mercilessly *ad hominem*: '"Well, you're a poet", she said. "All right, I'll teach you poetry in all the metres of pain ...!" It was as if a red-hot awl went through my cheekbone ... "Will you admit that I'm mightier than poetry, philosophy, mathematics, and all music?" she said. "Mightier than all the feeling that went into paint and marble? I'm older than all of them. I was born close to the Garden of Eden but outside, where the wind blew and moist toadstools grew. I got Eve to wear clothes when it got cold and Adam too. I'm telling you, there was power in the first toothache."'[1]

Many people over the years have joined Heinrich Heine, Karen Blixen, and Graham Greene in ascribing a healing power to creative pursuits, a power which helps sufferers to bear the evils of human life. In *The Birth of Tragedy*, Friedrich Nietzsche argues that '*art* ... alone can turn these

---

1 Hans Christian Andersen, 'Auntie Toothache', in *The Stories of Hans Christian Andersen*, trans. by Diana Crone Frank and Jeffrey Frank (London: Granta, 2004), pp. 257–258.

thoughts of repulsion at the horror and absurdity of existence into ideas compatible with life'.[2] Gustave Flaubert had the same idea, maintaining that '[t]he only way of leading an acceptable life is to drown oneself in literature as in an endless orgy'.[3]

Samuel Johnson assures us that he never experienced a single day without pain ever since a childhood illness transformed him into a trembling wreck (p. 71). He concluded that 'the only end of writing is to enable the readers better to enjoy life, or better to endure it'. The Doctor himself, a victim of severe periodic depression, was helped by his writing: 'Employment, Sir, and hardships, prevent melancholy.'[4]

Medical knowledge of an artist's ill health may enhance our understanding of his or her works. We saw examples in Frida Kahlo's realisation that her ailment was incurable – a realisation which explains the desperation in her view of suffering – and in the ways in which Claude Monet's decreasing eyesight changed his painting style. That insight was the fundamental impetus of this book.

A reaction to ill health which we find in almost all these artists, notwithstanding the nature of their respective illnesses, is a pronounced equanimity, even a heroic fortitude, in the face of the blows dealt by fate. The urge and endeavour to complete their works, to lend the final touch to the expression of their personal ideas, is able to conquer severe ill health.

The most significant and profound impression that illness can make on a work of art is seen in the cases where it has an impact on its basic tone, making that tone clearer, deeper, or more powerful. Such experiences have contributed to the lasting value of Charlotte Brontë's novels, Keats's poetry, the late paintings of Cézanne and Rothko, and Chopin's and Mahler's music.

Realising that much of what is best and finest in the arts was born out of suffering and pain leads to the conclusion that illness has sometimes enriched the artist and his or her time as well as benefiting succeeding generations: 'Pain inspires the artist, imparting greatness, sincerity, gravity, and

---

2 Friedrich Nietzsche, *The Birth of Tragedy*, trans. by Shaun Whiteside, ed. by Michael Tanner (London: Penguin, 1993), p. 40, end of §7. The German original text, quoted from *Die Geburt der Tragödie aus dem Geiste der Musik* (Munich: Goldmann, 1994), p. 58, runs, 'die *Kunst* ... allein vermag jene Ekelgedanken über das Entsetzliche oder Absurde des Daseins in Vorstellungen umzubiegen, mit denen sich leben läßt.' (Italics in the originals.)

3 Letter from Gustave Flaubert to Mademoiselle Leroyer de Chantepie of 4 September 1858, in *Correspondance (1854–1861)* (Paris: Louis Conard, 1927), p. 277: 'Le seul moyen de supporter l'existence, c'est de s'étourdir dans la littérature comme dans une orgie perpétuelle'.

4 On Johnson's ill health, see James Boswell, *The Life of Samuel Johnson*, ed. by David Womersley (London: Penguin, 2008), pp. 40–41 and 847; the quotation on 'the end of writing' is from Johnson's review of [Soame Jenyns], *A Free Inquiry into the Nature and Origin of Evil* in Samuel Johnson, *The Major Works*, ed. by Donald Green (Oxford: Oxford University Press, 1984), p. 536; and the last quotation is from Boswell's *Life of Johnson*, p. 618 in Womersley's edition.

passion to his vision; fertilizing his psychological imagination, it invests even his contempt for humanity and his outbursts of fury with pithy realism.'[5]

The benefits to future generations were beautifully articulated by the Swedish poet and painter Ernst Josephson: 'Tell me, why do we convey that torment to the world / Which we ought to have concealed from it? / After all, our world is a vale of tears, half-buried in sorrows. / The answer is that the howl from the poet, brought on by his wounded heart, / will sound like sad sweet music in the ears of posterity.'[6]

Let us conclude this account of pain and grief on a more cheerful note – with sweet music played in celebration of the happy outcome of medical treatment (see p. 173).

In the early eighteenth century, as we have seen, Marin Marais composed a piece for viola da gamba which illustrates an operation for the bladder stone and the patient's feelings during the procedure. A step-by-step account is found in the composer's score, from the fearful sight of the operating table by way of the binding of the patient's legs, the incision and withdrawal of the stone, and the gushing blood to the conclusion where the patient is put back to bed. The composer's relief is patent; when the gruesome effort to have his stone removed was over, he gave vent to his joy in three merry dances. In calling them 'Les Relevailles', Marais alluded to the old ceremony of churching, where a woman is received back into her congregation after giving birth – truly the happiest pain known to humanity.

---

5 Translated from Fredrik Böök, *Esaias Tegnér*, 2 vols (Stockholm: Bonniers, 1946), Vol. 2, p. 388. (Böök's statement specifically refers to Tegnér's creation of the hero of *Frithiofs saga.*)

6 Translated from Ernst Josephson, 'Svanesång' ('Swan Song'), in Josephson's *Svarta rosor och gula* (Stockholm: C. & E. Gernandts, 1901), p. 109.

Sources of illustrations

The source of each image in this book is stated below, the individual image being represented by its number in the volume. Except between illustrations 11–38, where the omission of one image and the addition of another affected the numbering, the numbers correspond to those in the Swedish version on which this translation is based, Philip Sandblom, *Skapande och sjukdom: Hur lidande påverkar litteratur, konst och music*, published in 2022 by Makadam Förlag (Gothenburg and Stockholm). That book was designed and its illustrative material edited by Johan Laserna, who graciously transferred his image files to Lund University Press and Manchester University Press for reproduction in the English version. We are deeply grateful to him.

One image is not present in the Swedish version, Ernst Josephson's painting which is now number 38, 'A summer day in the pine forest' of 1885. The painting was photographed by its owner, Philip Sandblom's grandson Stefan Gautschi.

Every reasonable effort has been made to obtain the approval of image owners of reproductions in this book, but if any have been missed Lund University Press will be happy to rectify the omission.

Alamy 47, 61–65; Alamy / photo: Peter Horree 10
Amherst College Archives & Special Collections 67
Aroseniusarkivet ('the Arosenius Archive') 89–92
Bridgeman Images / © Leonard de Selva 2; © Christie's Images 3; © Archives Charmet 26; © Bibliothèque Nationale Paris 27; © The British Library 40; © Succession Picasso / DACS, London 2024 73; ©Walter Henggeler / Photopress Archiv / Keystone 99
Fine Art America 8
Getty Foundation 60
Kunsthalle Basel / photo: Serge Hasenböhler 75
Litteraturbanken (Open Access website) 82
Madrid, Museo del Prado, P000763. Oil, 143.5x81.4cm. © Photographic Archive Museo Nacional del Prado 70
Museum der bildenden Künste, Leipzig 58
Musée du Louvre / photo: Stéphane Maréchalle 88
Musée d'Orsay, Paris 48
National Gallery of Art, Washington 11

Nationalmuseum, Stockholm 39, 57; photo: Hans Thorwid 5; photo: Anna Danielsson 69; photo: Erik Cornelius 87 (all images also at Wikimedia Commons)
RKD – Netherlands Institute for Art History 1
Scala Archives: Frontispiece, 59, 93
The Metropolitan Museum of Art, New York 12, 21, 36, 37 (all images in the public domain)
The Morgan Library and Museum 6
Web Gallery of Art 46
Wellcome Library 79 (image in the public domain)
Wikimedia Commons 5, 9, 14, 15, 24, 32, 39, 41, 42, 44, 45, 49, 50, 51, 57, 66, 68, 69, 72, 77, 80, 81, 87, 98
Zentrum Paul Klee 94, 95, 97

Reproductions of privately owned materials: 4, 7, 12, 16, 17, 18–20, 22–23, 25, 28, 29, 31, 33, 34, 35, 38, 43, 53, 54, 55, 56, 71, 76, 78, 83–85

Copyright permissions acquired through Bildupphovsrätt, a Swedish association of owners of pictorial copyright including 90,000 international copyright holders:

© 2022, Banco de México Diego Rivera & Frida Kahlo Museums Trust, México D.F / Bildupphovsrätt 2024 2–4
© Sam Francis Foundation, California / Bildupphovsrätt 2024 12
© Georges Braque / Bildupphovsrätt 2024 15–16
© Carl Fredrik Reuterswärd / Bildupphovsrätt 2024 18–20
© Maurice Utrillo / Bildupphovsrätt 2024 22–23
© Adagp / Comité Cocteau, Paris / Bildupphovsrätt 2024 26
© Henri Michaux / Bildupphovsrätt 2024 28
© Hilding Linnqvist / Bildupphovsrätt 2024 30
© Friedrich Schröder Sonnenstern / Bildupphovsrätt 2024 35
© Succession Picasso / Bildupphovsrätt 2024 52–54, 73; photo of 'La source' with the Sandbloms, Preface
© Raoul Dufy / Bildupphovsrätt 2024 55–56
© Francis Picabia / Bildupphovsrätt 2024 74
© Antoni Tàpies / Bildupphovsrätt 2024 86

Index

When names, titles, and concepts that occur in the running text also appear in footnotes, references to the latter have been omitted. Page numbers in italics refer to pages where illustrations occur.